D0495199

TELEPEN
6 20 015324 8

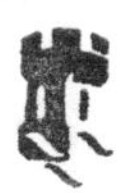

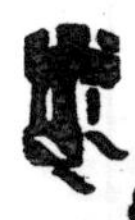

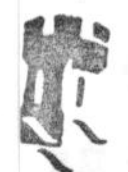

Butterworths International Medical Reviews

Obstetrics and Gynecology 1

Preterm Labor

Butterworths International Medical Reviews

Obstetrics and Gynecology 1

Future volumes to include

Fetal Monitoring

Diagnosis and Management of
Endocrine Causes of Infertility

Use of Drugs during Pregnancy:
Effects on Mother, Fetus and Newborn

Butterworths International Medical Reviews

Obstetrics and Gynecology 1

Preterm Labor

Edited by

M. G. Elder, MD, FRCS, FRCOG
Professor of Obstetrics and Gynaecology,
Institute of Obstetrics and Gynaecology,
Hammersmith Hospital,
Du Cane Road, London *and*

Charles H. Hendricks, MD
Professor and Emeritus Chairman,
Department of Obstetrics and Gynecology,
North Carolina Memorial Hospital,
Chapel Hill, North Carolina

Butterworths
London Boston
Sydney Wellington Durban Toronto

First published 1981

British Library Cataloguing in Publication Data
Obstetrics and gynecology. – (Butterworths international medical reviews ISSN 0144–9478).
1: Preterm labor
1. Gynecology 2. Obstetrics
1. Elder, M G 2. Hendricks, Charles H
618 RG101 80–41432

ISBN 0–407–02300–3

Photoset by Butterworths Litho Preparation Department
Printed and bound in England by Robert Hartnoll Ltd.

List of contributors

Mary Ellen Avery, AB, MD, SC D(HON.),
Thomas Morgan Rotch Professor of Pediatrics, Harvard Medical School, Physician-in-Chief, Children's Hospital Medical Center, Boston

Leiv S. Bakketeig, MD,
Professor of Social Medicine, Department of Community Medicine, University of Trondheim

Ian G. Chalmers, MB BS, M SC, DCH, MFCM, MRCOG,
Director of the National Perinatal Epidemiology Unit, Oxford

Ronald A. Chez, MD,
Chairman, Department of Obstetrics and Gynecology, Pennsylvania State University at Milton S. Hershey Medical Center, Hershey

Pamela A. Davies, MD, FRCP, DCH,
Reader in Paediatrics, Department of Paediatrics and Neonatal Medicine, Institute of Child Health, Hammersmith Hospital, London

Lilly M. S. Dubowitz, MD, DCH,
Research Fellow, Department of Paediatrics and Neonatal Medicine, Institute of Child Health, Hammersmith Hospital, London

Victor Dubowitz, BSC, PHD, MD, FRCP, DCH,
Professor of Paediatrics, Institute of Child Health, Hammersmith Hospital, London

M. G. Elder, MD, FRCS, FRCOG,
Professor of Obstetrics and Gynaecology, Institute of Obstetrics and Gynaecology, Hammersmith Hospital, London

Denys V. I. Fairweather, MD, FRCOG,
Professor of Obstetrics and Gynaecology, Faculty of Clinical Sciences, University College, London

Rudolph P. Galask, MD,
Professor of Obstetrics and Gynecology and Microbiology, University of Iowa Hospitals and Clinics, Iowa City

Louis Gluck, MD,
Professor of Pediatrics and Reproductive Medicine, University of California, San Diego

Charles H. Hendricks, MD,
Professor and Emeritus Chairman, North Carolina Memorial Hospital, Chapel Hill

Howard J. Hoffman, MA,
Mathematical Statistician, Epidemiology and Biometry Research Program, National Institute of Child Health and Human Development, National Institutes of Health, Bethesda

Rosamond A. K. Jones, MB BS, D OBST RCOG, MRCP,
Research Fellow, Department of Paediatrics and Neonatal Medicine, Institute of Child Health, Hammersmith Hospital, London

Ernest N. Kraybill, MD,
Associate Professor of Pediatrics, University of North Carolina, Chapel Hill

David T. Y. Liu, MPHIL (BIOENG.), MRCOG,
Lecturer, Department of Obstetrics and Gynaecology, Faculty of Clinical Sciences, University College, London

M. C. Macnaughton, MD, FRCOG, FRCP (GLAS.),
Muirhead Professor of Obstetrics and Gynaecology, University of Glasgow, Royal Maternity Hospital, Glasgow

M. D. Mitchell, MA, DPHIL,
MRC Senior Fellow, Nuffield Department of Obstetrics and Gynaecology, University of Oxford, John Radcliffe Hospital, Oxford

R. G. Newcombe, MA, PHD, FSS,
Lecturer in Medical Statistics, Welsh National School of Medicine, Cardiff

E. J. Quilligan, MD,
Professor and Director of Maternal and Fetal Medicine, University of California Irvine Medical Center, Orange

Jack M. Schneider, MD,
Director of The Perinatal Center, Sutter Memorial Hospital, Sacramento

A. C. Turnbull, MA, MD, FRCOG,
Nuffield Professor of Obstetrics and Gynaecology, University of Oxford, John Radcliffe Hospital, Oxford

Michael W. Varner, MD,
Fellow, Maternal–Fetal Medicine, Department of Obstetrics and Gynecology, University of Iowa Hospitals and Clinics, Iowa City

Nils Wiqvist, MD, PHD,
Professor and Chairman, Department of Obstetrics and Gynecology, University of Gothenburg

Contents

1

Extent and significance of the problem

Charles H. Hendricks

Of all the major problems in medical care, none has experienced such dramatic progress during the past decade as has the management of preterm birth and its sequelae. Only 20 years ago it was still somewhat unusual, although no longer rare, for an infant to survive if his birth weight was less than 1000 g or before 28 completed weeks gestation. Twenty years ago survivorship of infants born alive within the weight range 1001–1500 g was less than 50 percent on many services. Those low birth weight infants too often were destined to die of respiratory distress problems, feeding problems, sepsis or unrecognized stress from cold environmental temperature.

Table 1.1 Approximate chance of survival after atraumatic birth. North Carolina Memorial Hospital

Weight	*Percentage survival*
501–750	15
751–1000	50
1001–1500	90
1501–2000	96–97
2001–2500	97–98

Table 1.1 shows the approximate chances of survival for an infant born after atraumatic preterm birth at the North Carolina Memorial Hospital in 1980. The figures reflect *all* infants born preterm, including those with congenital malformations and those from pregnancies associated with premature rupture of the membranes and third trimester hemorrhage. The table indicates that we should have good expectation of survivorship among even the very low birth weight

infants. Today about 15 percent of infants weighing between 501–750 g are surviving and it appears that these results will become increasingly good within the next few years. As many as 50 percent of infants within the birth range 751–1000 g can be expected to survive. Among those born at birth weight 1001–1500 g, 90 percent of infants should survive and among those low birth weight infants weighing in excess of 1500 g more than 95 percent should survive.

Paradoxically the almost miraculous progress in this field has in turn bred a whole new set of problems as more and more infants survive after being born at lower and lower birth weights. Thus the long-range goal of obliterating preterm birth in human infants remains as elusive as ever because progressively more immature candidates for salvage are added to the preterm birth pool in the hope that smaller and smaller infants may be enabled to survive.

This publication is by no means a didactic 'cookbook' on how to treat various aspects of preterm birth. Rather it proposes to take a wide-gauge look at the nature of the problem as it exists today, considering both the pros and cons of various aspects of the subject. Two examples of major issues where the pros and cons are discussed in the book are (1) the question of whether or not one should intervene in spontaneously beginning preterm labor and (2) the question of whether or not one should administer corticosteroids to the mother prior to planned preterm delivery of the infant.

In general the book is designed to take an 'internationalized' look at various aspects of the subject, viewing the subject as a medical problem, a family problem, and a societal problem.

Preterm birth will be considered from the epidemiologic standpoint and also from the standpoint of predicting the likelihood of its occurrence. There will be examined afresh from new perspectives the age-old questions: *Why* should preterm birth occur? *What* is new about the problem in relationship to changing practices? *How* should preterm labor be best dealt with? *Where* should the delivery be conducted? *Who* should be primarily responsible for optimal care of the prematurely born infant? It is hoped that this book will serve in some measure to enhance the overall understanding of the reader since a good perspective forms the basis of successful and rational management of any difficult medical problem.

Finally one should hope that the book will reflect the conviction of the editors that the preterm aspect of perinatal practice today is satisfying, exciting and challenging. Rapid further progress in the field may be anticipated with confidence.

2
Endocrine aspects of preterm labour

A. C. Turnbull and M. D. Mitchell

The birth of a healthy viable infant depends heavily on the proper functioning of the mechanisms which initiate labour at term and then ensure a rapid progression to spontaneous delivery. These mechanisms are remarkably reliable in their timing and efficiency. This is necessary since any defect in the process which leads to undue prolongation of gestation, or even more seriously, to preterm delivery, predisposes to increased perinatal mortality and morbidity. Indeed, preterm delivery has been shown to account for 85 per cent of early neonatal deaths, when lethal congenital deformities are excluded[45]. In order to be able to anticipate and treat preterm labour, we need to achieve a greater understanding of its antecedent events and course. This review describes our present knowledge of the hormonal environment associated with preterm labour.

Studies in experimental animals have shown that increased production of cortisol by the fetal adrenals is a crucial step in the initiation of parturition[27, 51]. Results from human studies are less convincing although higher concentrations of cortisol have been found in umbilical plasma after delivery following spontaneous labour than delivery by elective caesarean section or following induced labour[5, 25, 37]. Measurements of cortisol levels in fetal scalp blood samples, however, have led to the suggestion that the elevated fetal cortisol concentrations found in labour are raised in response to the stress of labour, rather than preceding its onset[19]. It is impossible to obtain comparable data in relation to preterm labour. Although cord blood can be obtained after spontaneous preterm delivery, the induction of labour or elective caesarean section are only performed preterm in the face of serious pathology. However, Murphy[38, 39] has shown that umbilical plasma from preterm infants has a wide range of cortisol

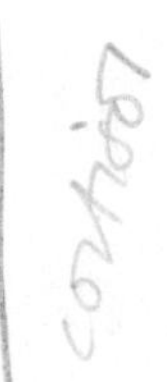

concentrations with lower levels in those who develop respiratory distress syndrome (RDS). Hence, preterm labour cannot be considered to occur always in conjunction with elevated fetal plasma cortisol concentrations.

In sheep, fetal hypophysectomy or adrenalectomy will prolong gestation[27,51]. Conversely, administration of cortisol or corticotropin (ACTH) to the fetus during late pregnancy will induce parturition. In human pregnancies complicated by anencephaly (but without hydramnios) there is an increase in the range of gestation at delivery[20], although only prolongation of gestation has been noted in some studies[9,29,32]. The extent of the prolongation of pregnancy complicated by anencephaly has been found to be inversely related to fetal adrenal weight at birth[1]. Data concerning gestational length in fetuses with adrenal hypoplasia without gross pituitary abnormality[16,41,44] or with congenital absence of the adrenals[43], have provided conflicting results. However, fetal adrenal hyperplasia has been described in babies born as a result of preterm labour of unexplained aetiology[1] which is consistent with the elevated urinary excretion of dehydroepiandrosterone sulphate (DHEAS) in prematurely delivered babies[24]. Administration of glucocorticoids does not induce preterm labour in women, although an effect has been observed in women past term[30,40].

Prenatal administration of betamethasone is used in an attempt to prevent RDS in infants destined to be born before term[26]. This treatment suppresses both maternal and fetal adrenal steroidogenesis[18,42] since betamethasone readily crosses the placenta[2]. Not only are cortisol levels depressed, but concentrations of DHEAS, which is a product of the fetal zone of the adrenal, are also reduced (*Figure 2.1*). Since DHEAS is the major precursor of oestrogens, as might be expected, levels of oestradiol-17β also decline.

Recent work[6,48] has suggested that there are maturational events occurring during late gestation in the fetal anterior pituitary, with a switch from the secretion of ACTH fragments similar to α-melanotropin (α-MSH) and corticotropin-like intermediate lobe peptide (CLIP) to 'real' ACTH. Furthermore, preliminary evidence has been provided that preterm delivery is associated with premature maturation of the fetal brain and hence, perhaps, a premature trophic drive to the adrenal. Although this may be consistent with the abnormally heavy fetal adrenals found after preterm delivery[1], it is not consistent with the high rates of urinary excretion of DHEAS in preterm infants[24] which suggests a relative lack of adrenal maturation.

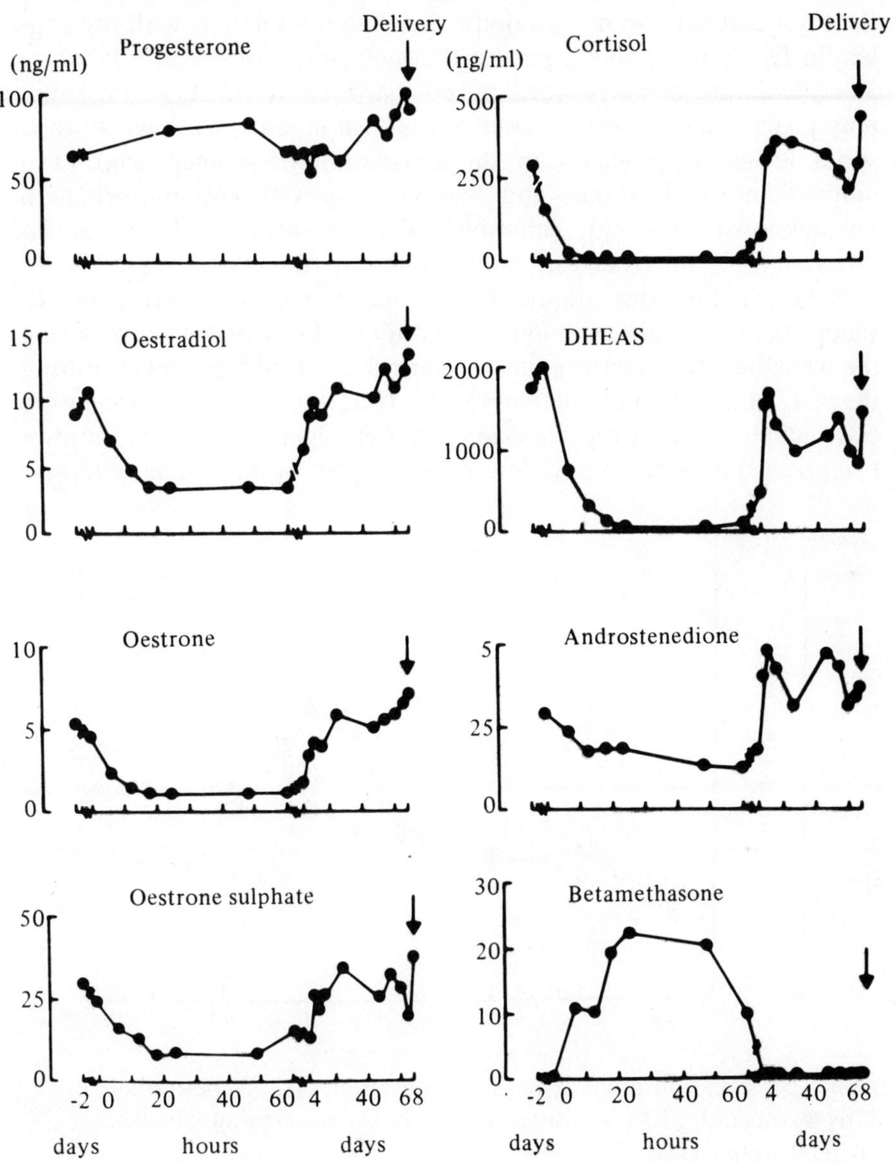

Figure 2.1 Concentrations of steroids in the plasma of a woman admitted to hospital in preterm labour of unexplained aetiology and treated (starting at time 0) with betamethasone (12 mg per 24 h for 48 h). (Unpublished observations)

It has been suggested that prolactin can provide a trophic stimulus to the fetal adrenal and may perhaps, through interactions with prostaglandin E_2 (PGE_2), play a part in the mechanism of preterm labour[7]. The possibility has also been raised that measurements of prolactin may provide a clue to the onset of preterm labour. We have studied serial levels of prolactin in the circulation of women who have delivered normally at term and those who have delivered preterm with an unknown aetiology (unpublished observations). There is no difference in the trends or levels between the two groups.

Next, we turn our attention to progesterone and oestrogens. In sheep there is an almost complete withdrawal of progesterone during the week before parturition and a sharp rise in oestrogen levels during the 24 hours before delivery[27,51]. Determination of circulating concentrations of progesterone and oestrogens in recent studies (*Figure 2.2*) on women have led to the suggestion that changes in their

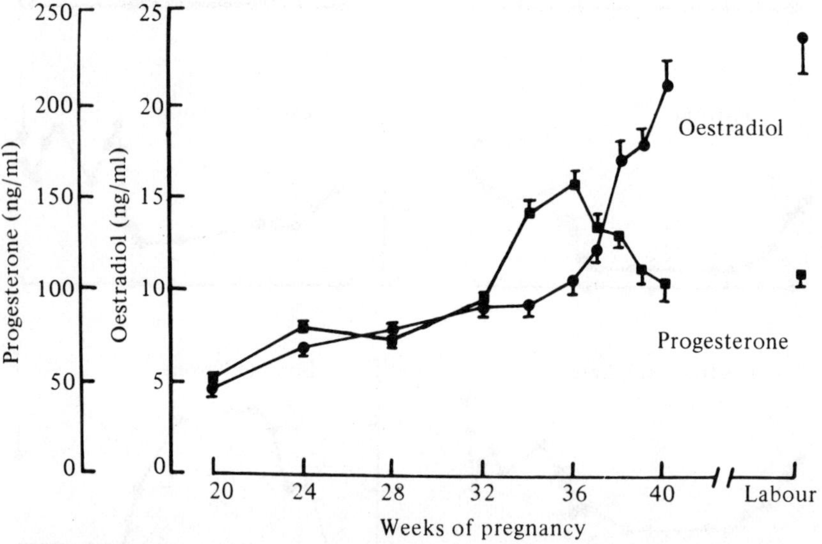

Figure 2.2 Concentrations of plasma progesterone (■) and oestradiol-17β (●) (mean ± SEM) measured serially in 33 normal primigravidae. (After Turnbull *et al.*[52])

concentrations during late gestation play a facilitatory rather than a stimulatory role in the onset of human labour[52,53]. Decreased plasma levels of progesterone before labour have only been demonstrated twice, in studies where the strictest criteria have been applied to patient selection[12,52]. Even so, progesterone withdrawal does not

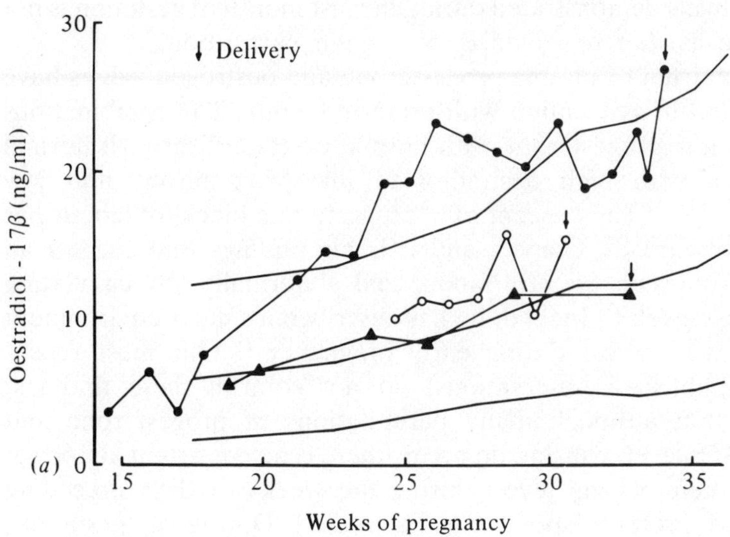

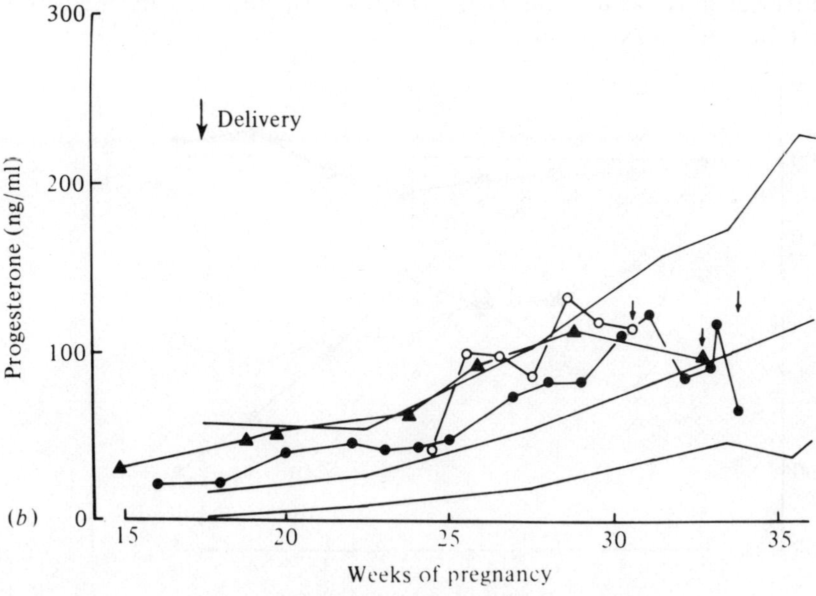

Figure 2.3 Serial plasma oestradiol-17β (*a*) and progesterone (*b*) concentrations before preterm delivery in three women. (Unpublished observations)

always occur and is never as complete as in sheep. Similarly, the rise in oestradiol levels demonstrated during the last month of gestation is not as dramatic as that observed during ovine parturition.

A full spectrum of plasma progesterone and oestrogen values have been reported in association with preterm labour. The combinations range from low progesterone with normal oestradiol through normal progesterone with high oestradiol to low progesterone and low oestradiol[10, 13, 49]. The concept of a 'progesterone block' of labour has been put forward by Csapo[11] and it is his findings that suggest an association between preterm labour and abnormally low circulating progesterone levels[13]. Indeed, he has described a similar environment in patients who abort during early pregnancy[13]. Our most recent results (unpublished observations) do not confirm these findings, suggesting that although many permutations of progesterone and oestradiol-17β levels can and do occur, there is no consistent abnormal change in their plasma levels during the weeks or days preceding 'unexplained' preterm labour (e.g. *Figure 2.3*). During late gestation, however, a unique progesterone binding protein has been shown to appear in the fetal membranes[46], and so a local progesterone withdrawal may occur near term which is not detected by measurements in peripheral plasma.

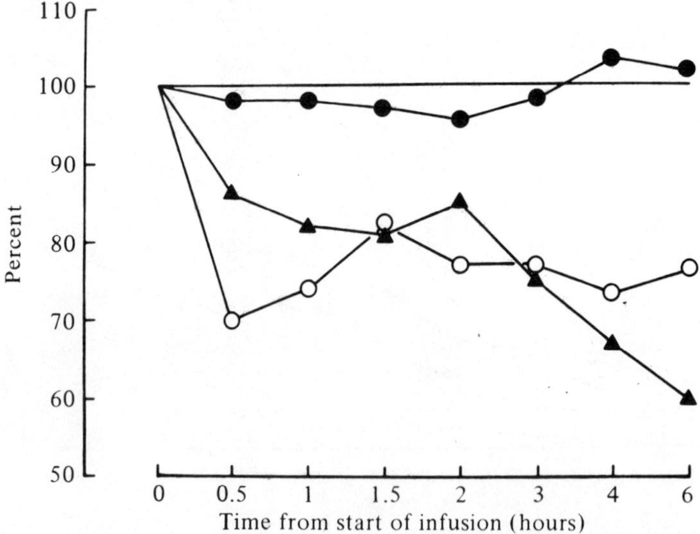

Figure 2.4 Mean ± SEM percentage change of progesterone (○) oestradiol-17β (▲) and human placental lactogen (●) during salbutamol infusion in six women admitted to hospital in preterm labour. (After Bibby *et al.*[3])

The administration of β-sympathomimetic drugs (e.g. salbutamol, ritodrine) is a common treatment for preterm labour. Interestingly the use of salbutamol in preterm labour is associated with a fall in the circulating concentrations of both progesterone and oestradiol, but not that of human placental lactogen[3] (*Figure 2.4*). The mechanism which results in these changes is uncertain, but it is unlikely that the resultant steroid hormone changes play a part in the inhibition of uterine activity produced.

Cervical cerclage is used prophylactically in cases of threatened abortion or preterm labour, although initially described for use in women with cervical incompetence[31,47]. This procedure causes a rapid increase in circulating levels of 13,14-dihydro-15-keto-prostaglandin F (PGFM), the major circulating metabolite of PGF, probably indicating uterine or cervical release[4] of $PGF_{2\alpha}$ (*Figure 2.5*). Since $PGF_{2\alpha}$ is a powerful myometrial stimulant, this may provide an explanation for

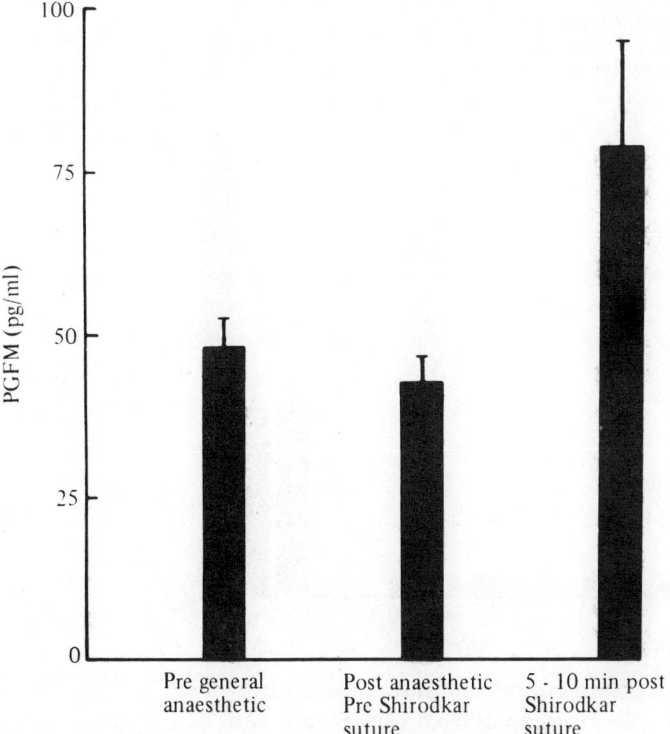

Figure 2.5 Peripheral plasma PGFM concentrations (mean ± SEM, n = 10) before and after cervical cerclage in women at 13–20 weeks gestation. (After Bibby *et al.*[4])

the enhanced uterine activity that has been noted in association with cervical cerclage. Whether the increased production of $PGF_{2\alpha}$ has any long term deleterious effects on the pregnancy is unknown. It should be noted that recent data[23] collected retrospectively point to a lack of effect of cervical cerclage in reducing the incidence of preterm labour. Prospective studies must, however, be performed before firmer conclusions may be drawn about the effectiveness of this manoeuvre.

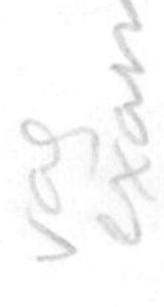

Our investigations of the effect of cervical cerclage on PGFM levels arose from observations that vaginal examination or amniotomy at term leads to a rapid (less than 5 min) increase in PGFM concentrations in both amniotic fluid and peripheral plasma[33, 34]. Amniotomy provided the stimulus for the greatest elevation of PGFM levels, which is not surprising since fetal membranes are a significant source of

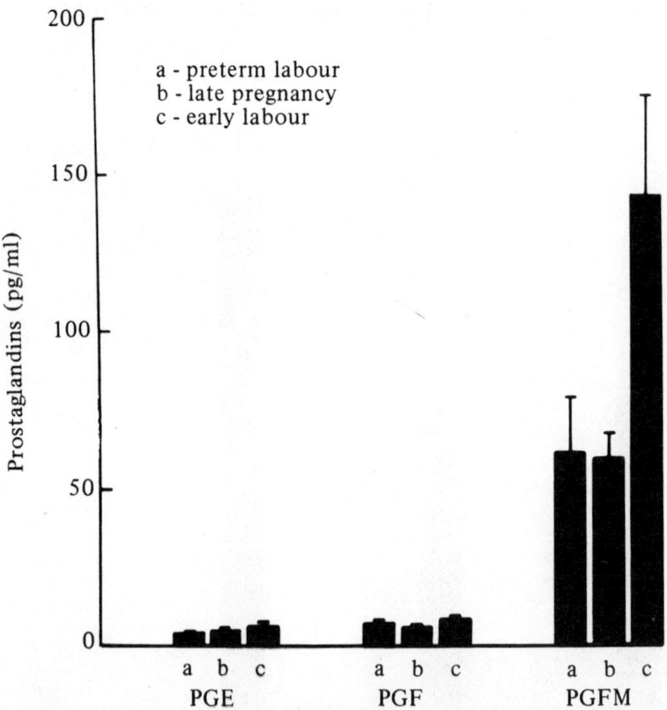

Figure 2.6 Concentrations of prostaglandins (mean ± SEM, n = 5–13) in plasma samples from women in preterm labour (less than 37 weeks of gestation), late pregnancy (more than 34 weeks of gestation) before the onset of labour, and in early term labour. (After Mitchell *et al.*[36])

prostaglandins[22,28,35]. Recently, we have obtained blood samples before and after vaginal examination from women in early preterm labour (cervix less than 4 cm dilated). The magnitude of the rise in PGFM levels exceeded that found in control patients of a similar gestational age and was even greater than that observed at term. It should be noted, however, that comparisons with the effects of vaginal examination during labour at term have not been available. Nevertheless, it is possible that an important part of the mechanism for preterm labour is a heightened uterine response to external stimuli such as vaginal examination or sexual intercourse. Such an hypothesis would be consistent with, and perhaps explain, the unusual finding that circulating levels of PGFM were not elevated during early preterm labour as they are during early term labour[36] (*Figure 2.6*). These findings have been confirmed by measurements both in plasma and amniotic fluid[21,50].

Oxytocin is generally considered to be released during labour, especially during the second stage, although only one group of workers has actually demonstrated such findings[14,15]. We are unable to find any increase in oxytocin levels during normal labour at term (*Figure 2.7*). This accords with previous reports[8,17,54]. It seems unlikely that increased oxytocin levels are involved in the mechanism of preterm labour, but alteration in the sensitivity of the myometrium perhaps via an increased receptor population cannot be excluded.

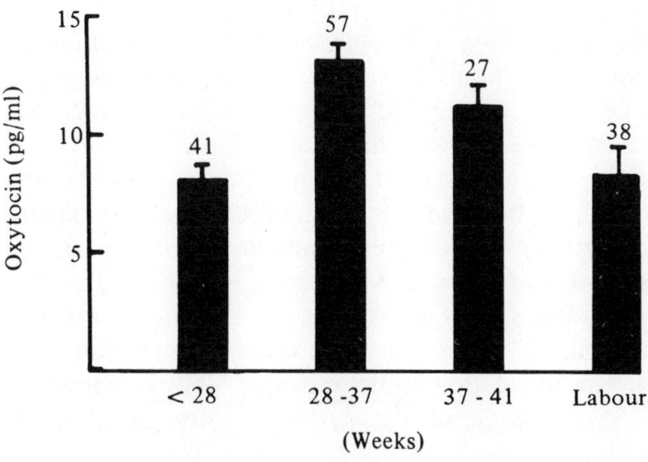

Figure 2.7 Concentrations of oxytocin (mean ± SEM, n = above bars) in peripheral plasma during pregnancy. (Unpublished observations)

Finally, we must stress that all our observations in preterm labour have been made in cases uncomplicated by obvious pathological processes causing too early birth and possibly also reducing fetal growth. Disorders such as antepartum haemorrhage, pre-eclampsia, intrauterine growth retardation, polyhydramnios, for example, all predispose to preterm birth, and their presence may well be associated with abnormal changes in plasma levels of steroid hormones, or prostaglandins, but our main concern is to discover the mechanisms which initiate labour prematurely in apparently normal pregnancy. Inclusion of cases of preterm delivery due to various pregnancy pathologies may have been responsible for the conflicting findings presented by different workers.

References

1 ANDERSON, A. B. M., LAWRENCE, K. M., DAVIES, K., CAMPBELL, H. and TURNBULL, A. C. Fetal adrenal weight and the cause of premature delivery in human pregnancy. *Journal of Obstetrics and Gynaecology of the British Commonwealth*, **78,** 481–488 (1971)

2 ANDERSON, A. B. M., SAYERS, L., JEREMY, J. Y., TURNBULL, A. C., OHRLANDER, S. and GENNSER, G. Placental transfer and metabolism of betamethasone in human pregnancy. *Obstetrics and Gynecology*, **49,** 471–474 (1977)

3 BIBBY, J. G., HIGGS, S. A., KENT, A. P., FLINT, A. P. F., MITCHELL, M. D., ANDERSON, A. B. M. and TURNBULL, A. C. Plasma steroid changes in preterm labour in association with salbutamol infusion. *British Journal of Obstetrics and Gynaecology*, **85,** 425–430 (1978)

4 BIBBY, J. G., BRUNT, J., MITCHELL, M. D., ANDERSON, A. B. M. and TURNBULL, A. C. The effect of cervical encerclage on plasma prostaglandin concentrations during early human pregnancy. *British Journal of Obstetrics and Gynaecology*, **86,** 19–22 (1979)

5 CAWSON, M. J., ANDERSON, A. B. M., TURNBULL, A. C. and LAMPE, L. Cortisol, cortisone and 11-deoxycortisol levels in human umbilical and maternal plasma in relation to the onset of labour. *Journal of Obstetrics and Gynaecology of the British Commonwealth*, **81,** 737–745 (1974)

6 CHARD, T., SILMAN, R. E. and REES, L. H. The fetal hypothalamus and pituitary in the initiation of labour. In *The Fetus and Birth*, edited by J. Knight and M. O'Connor, 359–370. Amsterdam, Elsevier (1977)

7 CHEZ, R. A. In *Pre-term Labour* (Proceedings of the fifth study group of the Royal College of Obstetricians and Gynaecologists), edited by A. B. M. Anderson, R. Beard, J.M. Brudenell, P. M. Dunn, 121. London, Royal College of Obstetricians and Gynaecologists (1977)

8 COBO, E. Uterine and milk-ejecting activities during human labor. *Journal of Applied Physiology*, **24,** 317–323 (1968)

9 COMERFORD, J. B. Pregnancy with anencephaly.*Lancet*, **1,** 679–680 (1965)

10 COUSINS, L. M., HOBEL, C. J., CHANG, R. J., OKADA, D. M. and MARSHALL, J. R. Serum progesterone and estradiol-17β levels in premature and term labor. *American Journal of Obstetrics and Gynecology*, **127,** 612–615 (1977)

11 CSAPO, A. I. Progesterone 'block'. *American Journal of Anatomy*, **98,** 273–291 (1956)

12 CSAPO, A. I., KNOBIL, E., VAN DER MOLEN, H. J. and WIEST, W. G. Peripheral plasma progesterone levels during human pregnancy and labor. *American Journal of Obstetrics and Gynecology*, **110**, 630–632 (1971)

13 CSAPO, A. I. The 'see-saw' theory of parturition. In *The Fetus and Birth*, Ciba Foundation Symposium No. 47 (new series) edited by J. Knight, M. O'Connor, 159–195. Amsterdam, Elsevier (1977)

14 DAWOOD, M. Y., RAGHAVAN, K. S. and POCIASK, C. Radioimmunoassay of oxytocin. *Journal of Endocrinology*, **76,** 261–270 (1978)

15 DAWOOD, M. Y., RAGHAVAN, K. S., POCIASK, C. and FUCHS, F. Oxytocin in human pregnancy and parturition. *Obstetrics and Gynecology*, **51**, 138–143 (1978)

16 FLEIGNER, J. R. H., SCHINDLER, I. and BROWN, J. B. Low urinary oestriol excretion during pregnancy associated with placental sulphatase deficiency or congenital adrenal hypoplasia. *Journal of Obstetrics and Gynaecology of the British Commonwealth*, **79,** 810–815 (1972)

17 GAZAREK, F., POHANKA, J., TALAS, M., FINGEROVA, H., JANOUSKOVA, M., KRIKAL, Z. and HAMAL, Z. Plasma oxytocin and oxytocinase levels in third trimester of pregnancy and at labour. *Endocrinologia Experimentalis*, **10,** 283–287 (1976)

18 GENNSER, G., OHRLANDER, S. and ENEROTH, P. Cortisol in amniotic fluid and cord blood in relation to prenatal betamethasone load and delivery. *American Journal of Obstetrics and Gynecology*, **124,** 43–50 (1976)

19 GENNSER, G., OHRLANDER, S. and ENEROTH, P. Fetal cortisol and the initiation of labour in the human. In *The Fetus and Birth*, edited by J. Knight and M. O'Connor, 401–420. Amsterdam, Elsevier (1977)

20 HONNEBIER, W. J. and SWAAB, D. F. The influence of anencephaly upon intra-uterine growth of fetus and placenta and upon gestation length. *Journal of Obstetrics and Gynaecology of the British Commonwealth*, **80,** 577–580 (1973)

21 JOHNSON, J. W. C., DUBIN, N. H., CALHOUN, S. GHODGAVANKAR, R. and BECK, J. Sequential prostaglandin metabolite values in pregnant patients delivering at term and pre-term. *Proceedings of Fourth International Prostaglandin Conference* (Washington), 55. (1979)

22 KEIRSE, M. J. N. C. and TURNBULL, A. C. The fetal membranes as a possible source of amniotic fluid prostaglandins. *British Journal of Obstetrics and Gynaecology*, **83,** 146–151 (1976)

23 KEIRSE, M. J. N. C., RUSH, R. W., ANDERSON, A. B. M. and TURNBULL, A. C. Risk of preterm delivery in patients with previous preterm delivery and/or abortion. *British Journal of Obstetrics and Gynaecology*, **85,** 81–85 (1978)

24 LAURITZEN, C. H. and LEHMANN, W. D. Levels of chorionic gonadotropin in the newborn infant and their relationship to adrenal dehydroepiandrosterone. *Journal of Endocrinology*, **39,** 173–182 (1967)

25 LEONG, M. K. H. and MURPHY, B. E. P. Cortisol levels in maternal venous and umbilical cord arterial and venous serum at vaginal delivery. *American Journal of Obstetrics and Gynecology*, **124,** 471–473 (1976)

26 LIGGINS, G. C. and HOWIE, R. N. A controlled trial of ante-partum glucocorticoid treatment for prevention of the respiratory distress syndrome in premature infants. *Paediatrics*, **50,** 515–525 (1972)

27 LIGGINS, G. C., FAIRCLOUGH, R. J., GRIEVES, S. A., KENDALL, J. Z. and KNOX, B. S. The mechanism of initiation of parturition in the ewe. *Recent Progress in Hormone Research*, **29**, 111–150 (1973)

28 MACDONALD, P. C., SCHULZ, F. M., DUENHOLTER, J. H., GANT, N. F., JIMENEZ, J. M., PRITCHARD, J. A., PORTER, J. C. and JOHNSTON, J. M. Initiation of human parturition: I, Mechanism of action of arachidonic acid. *Obstetrics and Gynecology*, **44,** 629–636 (1974)

29 MALPAS, P. Postmaturity and malformations of the fetus. *Journal of Obstetrics and Gynaecology of the British Commonwealth*, **40,** 1046–1053 (1933)

30 MATI, J. K. G., HORROBIN, D. F. and BRAMLEY, P. S. Induction of labour in sheep and in humans by single doses of corticosteroids. *British Medical Journal*, **2,** 149–151 (1973)

31 MCDONALD, J.A. Suture of the cervix for inevitable miscarriage. *Journal of Obstetrics and Gynaecology of the British Commonwealth*, **64,** 346–350 (1957)

32 MILIC, A. B. and ADAMSONS, K. The relationship between anencephaly and prolonged pregnancy. *Journal of Obstetrics and Gynaecology of the British Commonwealth*, **76,** 102–112 (1969)

33 MITCHELL, M. D., FLINT, A. P. F., BIBBY, J., BRUNT, J., ARNOLD, J. M., ANDERSON, A. B. M. and TURNBULL, A. C. Rapid increases in plasma prostaglandin concentrations after vaginal examination and amniotomy. *British Medical Journal*, **2,** 1183–1185 (1977)

34 MITCHELL, M. D., KEIRSE, M. J. N. C., ANDERSON, A. B. M. and TURNBULL, A. C. Evidence for a local control of prostaglandins within the pregnant human uterus. *British Journal of Obstetrics and Gynaecology*, **84,** 35–38 (1977)

35 MITCHELL, M. D., BIBBY, J., HICKS, B. R. and TURNBULL, A. C. Specific production of prostaglandin E by human amnion in vitro. *Prostaglandins*, **15**, 377–382 (1978)

36 MITCHELL, M. D., FLINT, A. P. F., BIBBY, J., BRUNT, J., ARNOLD, J. M., ANDERSON, A. B. M. and TURNBULL, A. C. Plasma concentrations of prostaglandins during late human pregnancy: influence of normal and preterm labour. *Journal of Clinical Endocrinology and Metabolism*, **46,** 947–951 (1978)

37 MURPHY, B. E. P. Does the human fetal adrenal play a role in parturition? *American Journal of Obstetrics and Gynecology*, **115,** 521–525 (1973)

38 MURPHY, B. E. P. Evidence of cortisol deficiency at birth in infants with the respiratory distress syndrome. *Journal of Clinical Endocrinology and Metabolism,*, **38,** 158 (1974)

39 MURPHY, B. E. P. Cortisol and cortisone levels in the cord blood at delivery of premature infants with and without the respiratory distress syndrome. *American Journal of Obstetrics and Gynecology*, **119,** 1112–1120 (1974)

40. NWOSU, U. C., WALLACH, E. E. and BOLOGNESE, R. J. Initiation of labour by intra-amniotic cortisol instillation in prolonged human pregnancy. *Obstetrics and Gynecology*, **47,** 137–142 (1976)

41 O'DONOHOE, N. V. and HOLLAND, P. D. J. Familial congenital adrenal hypoplasia. *Archives of Diseases of Childhood*, **43**, 717–723 (1968)

42 OHRLANDER, S., GENNSER, G., BATRA, S. and LEBECH, P. Effect of betamethasone administration on estrone, estradiol-17β and progesterone in maternal plasma and amniotic fluid. *Obstetrics and Gynecology*, **49**, 148–153 (1977)

43 PAKRAVAN, P., KENNY, F. M., DEPP, R. and ALLEN, A. C. Familial congenital absence of adrenal glands: evaluation of glucocorticoid, mineralocorticoid and oestrogen metabolism in the perinatal period. *Journal of Paediatrics*, **84,** 74–78 (1974)

44 ROBERTS, G. and CAWDERY, J. E. Congenital adrenal hypoplasia. *Journal of Obstetrics and Gynaecology of the British Commonwealth*, **77,** 654–656 (1970)

45 RUSH, R. W., KEIRSE, M. J. N. C., HOWAT, P., BAUM, J. D., ANDERSON, A. B. M. and TURNBULL, A. C. Contribution of preterm delivery to perinatal mortality. *British Medical Journal*, **2**, 965–968 (1976)

46 SCHWARZ, B. E., MILEWICH, L., JOHNSTON, J. M., PORTER, J. C. and MACDONALD, P. C. Initiation of human parturition. V. Progesterone binding substance in fetal membranes. *Obstetrics and Gynecology*, **48,** 685–689 (1976)

47 SHIRODKAR, V.N. A new method of operative treatment for habitual abortions in the second trimester of pregnancy. *Antiseptic*, **52**, 299–300 (1955)

48 SILMAN, R. E., CHARD, T., LOWRY, P. J., SMITH, I. and YOUNG, I. M. Human fetal pituitary peptides and parturition. *Nature* (London), 260, p. 716–718 (1976).

49 TAMBYRAJA, R. L., ANDERSON, A. B. M. and TURNBULL, A. C. Endocrine changes in premature labour. *British Medical Journal*, **4,** 67–71 (1974)

50 TAMBYRAJA, R. L., SALMON, J. A., KARIM, S. M. M. and RATNAM, S. S. F prostaglandin levels in amniotic fluid in premature labour. *Prostaglandins*, **13**, 339–348 (1977)

51 THORBURN, G. D., CHALLIS, J. R. G. and ROBINSON, J. S. Endocrine control of parturition. In *Biology of the Uterus*, edited by R. M. Wynn, 653–732. New York, Plenum Press (1977)

52 TURNBULL, A. C., PATTEN, P. T., FLINT, A. P. F., KEIRSE, M. J. N. C., JEREMY, J. Y. and ANDERSON, A. B. M. Significant fall in progesterone and rise in oestradiol levels in human peripheral plasma before the onset of labour. *Lancet*, **1**, 101–104 (1974)

53 TURNBULL, A. C., ANDERSON, A. B. M., FLINT, A. P. F., JEREMY, J. Y., KEIRSE, M. J. N. C. and MITCHELL, M. D. Human parturition. In *The Fetus and Birth*, Ciba Foundation Symposium No. 47 (new series), edited by J. Knight, M. O'Connor, 427–452. Amsterdam, Elsevier (1977)

54 VASICKA, A., KUMARESAN, P., HANS, G. S. and KUMARESAN, M. Plasma oxytocin in initiation of labor. *American Journal of Obstetrics and Gynecology*, **130,** 263–273 (1977)

3

Epidemiology of preterm birth: results from a longitudinal study of births in Norway

Leiv S. Bakketeig and Howard J. Hoffman

Introduction

Preterm labour resulting in preterm birth is one of the most important single causes of perinatal death[20, 23, 39] and neonatal morbidity as well as subsequent impairments[32]. Therefore, preterm labour is both an extremely important public health and clinical problem. For several decades epidemiologists have taken an interest in this field of research, but without much success in providing clues as to the aetiology.

Some women with preterm onset of labour avoid a preterm delivery either through spontaneous interruption of labour, or through successful medical intervention[37]. In focusing on the epidemiology of preterm birth, we are most likely studying a selected group of women from among those with preterm onset of labour. However, the onset of labour is poorly defined, and is easily confused with false labour[36]. As a result, preterm labour *per se* has scarcely ever been studied in any large scale epidemiological endeavour. Instead of the occurrence of preterm labour, epidemiologists have been concerned with the occurrence of preterm birth.

In spite of the large number of studies using preterm delivery as an outcome of interest, there is still a noticeable shortage of information about the epidemiology of these events. This situation is to some extent due to the lack of appropriate data being available in many epidemiological studies. There has also been a problem with changing definitions and terminology used in this field of research, which has made the interpretation of some of the earlier studies difficult[28]. The term 'prematurity,' which until recently has covered births delivered early, or with low birth weight, or both, has been responsible for confusion in some research studies. According to recent World Health Organization conventions and other international agreements[40, 47], the terminology of 'preterm' birth should be used for births of gestational age less than 37 completed weeks (or less than 259 days), as measured from the time between the first day of the last menstrual period and the delivery or expulsion of the fetus. The terminology of 'low birth weight' is recommended for births weighing *less* than 2500 g, instead of the previous definition which was equal to or less than 2500 g[47]. An earlier standard definition of preterm birth[9, 18] was based on less than 38 completed weeks of gestation (or less than 266 days). In an analogous fashion, post-term birth is still defined as any delivery which occurs two or more weeks after term.

For purposes of epidemiological studies, any of the above definitions, or perhaps other definitions, may be shown to be useful depending upon the rationale of the study. We have chosen an even more stringent criterion than the one currently recommended by the WHO. It has been acknowledged in previous studies and a WHO working group, that by making the cut-off point less than 36 completed weeks of gestation a better agreement with the less than 2500 g birth weight criterion is achieved[25, 46]. In addition, WHO has recommended that countries should provide statistics for preterm births in which births occurring at less than 36 weeks are available for analysis[28, 47]. Births between 36 and 38 weeks comprise those in which the majority weigh more than 2500 g and have much better prospects for survival. Based on these observations, we have defined preterm birth as being less than 36 completed weeks of gestation (or less than 252 days) for purposes of this study.

There is even less agreement as to what should constitute the lower limit of gestational age in defining preterm births. The source of data for this study is the notification system known as the Medical Registration of Births of Norway which covers all births, both live births and fetal deaths, with a gestational age of 16 or more weeks[5, 12]. In most other countries, or registration areas, the data routinely collected do not include preterm births with equally low gestational ages. Even obtaining reliable and comprehensive data on all gestations of 28 weeks or more is difficult in several developed countries. Thus, there are tremendous obstacles in attempting to compare the rate of occurrence and epidemiology of preterm birth from one country to another.

As a result of the limitations of the data available, most investigators have had to rely on rates of low birth weight deliveries, rather than the rate of preterm births, to reflect the incidence of prematurity[18, 24]. Unfortunately, the variation in the frequency of low birth weight deliveries may be due as much to the occurrence of small-for-dates births as it is to preterm births, and these two outcomes may have entirely different aetiologies. Likewise, the time trends in the frequency of preterm birth have been indirectly examined through the incidence of low-weight births[16,24]. In spite of some reduction of low-weight births through time there is little evidence to suggest that any substantial part of the considerable decline in perinatal mortality, which has been observed in recent years[1,3,13,16,24], is due to a reduction in the frequency of low-weight or preterm births.

In spite of the problems in conducting research studies on preterm birth, there have been several studies which have shown associations of various factors with the occurrence of preterm birth. For example, preterm birth has been associated with environmental factors such as place of residence[22,45], maternal occupation and work during pregnancy[22,44], social class indicators[7,15,21,22], and the amount of antenatal care received[22,41,43]. In addition, many characteristics of the mother and her pregnancy have also been found to be associated with preterm birth, such as race[14,15,16,25], maternal age and parity[15,22,25], multiple birth[26,29], maternal stature and weight[7,15,22,44], cigarette smoking[22,30], alcohol consumption[27,35], nutrition[24,42], certain diseases and other conditions during pregnancy and delivery[8,22,24,33], length of inter-pregnancy interval[19], and previous history of abortion, perinatal loss, or low birth weight infants[2,17,22,24,37].

Most of these earlier studies on the epidemiology of preterm birth have been based either on available vital statistics data, or on survey data, which are cross-sectional in nature. In this chapter, we shall examine the epidemiology of preterm birth using a longitudinal database. By identifying groups of mothers with different reproductive outcomes in successive deliveries (either preterm or not preterm births), it is possible to gain more understanding of the way in which various factors are associated with the occurrence of preterm births. For example, mothers with their first three births can be characterized as having either zero, one, two, or three preterm births. The mothers having one, as opposed to more than one, preterm birth may show entirely different associations with environmental and maternal risk factors. Also, mothers having a single preterm first birth may show different associations with risk factors as compared with mothers whose preterm birth occurs at a higher parity. Further, if a mother has had two preterm births, there may be differences depending upon whether these two preterm deliveries occurred in the first and second, first and third, or second and third deliveries. In addition, a normal birth to mothers with one or more previous preterm births may have an increased perinatal risk compared with births to mothers without any preterm deliveries. These and similar questions are addressed in the analysis of epidemiologic risk factors in this study. Using the longitudinal method based on successive births to the same women, some of the previously accepted associations between environmental or maternal factors and preterm birth are liable to change, or acquire new interpretations.

Material and methods

Births in Norway are registered through a notification system known as the Medical Registration of Births. This system which was introduced in 1967, covers all live births and fetal deaths of gestational age of 16 weeks or more. The registry includes information on birth weight, length of gestation, conditions of the newborn, mothers' health during pregnancy, as well as complications and interventions during labour and delivery.

During the 10-year period, 1967–1976, a total of 635 140 births were recorded in the registry. However, the analysis presented here is restricted to the 107 495 mothers who delivered their first and second singleton births, and the 30 979 mothers who delivered their first three or more single births during this 10-year period. Because unique identification numbers are assigned to all births and their parents, linkage of successive births to the same mother is easily accomplished[2, 5, 12]. Similarly, information regarding infant deaths as provided to the registry by the Central Bureau of Statistics of Norway has been linked to the birth information through the personal identification number[4, 12]. The Medical Registration of Births provides no information on social conditions apart from maternal age, parity, marital status and place of residence. In order to obtain some information on social variables such as parental education, an additional record linkage has been made between the birth registration data file and the 1970 Norwegian census data[13].

Gestational age has been calculated using the date of the first day of the last menstrual period and the date of birth or expulsion of the fetus. In this study, preterm birth is defined as any birth of gestational age less than 36 completed weeks (or less than 252 days). As mentioned above, births with gestational age of 36 weeks correspond more closely to births weighing 2500 g than do births of 37 weeks. Results for mothers with unknown length of gestation for one or more of their births are shown separately in most of the tables.

Non-spontaneous births have not been excluded from the analysis since the proportion of induced labours among births with gestational age less than 36 weeks is small. Also, there is uncertainty as to what is labelled 'induction' of labour as opposed to merely 'stimulation' of labour in this data set. When similar analyses were done based on spontaneous births only the findings were essentially unaffected. Thus, it was elected to show the results for all single preterm births without any exclusions from the data.

Results

The tendency to repeat gestational age

The risk of having a subsequent preterm birth after having already had one or two previous preterm births is shown in *Table 3.1* for all 27 677 mothers who had their first three singleton births during the study period. Out of the original total of 30 979 such mothers, 3302 mothers were excluded from the calculations since gestational age was not recorded for one or more of their three births.

From the table, we note that if the first birth is not preterm then only 4.4 per cent of second births are preterm. If, however, the first birth is preterm, then 17.2 per cent of second births are also delivered preterm. Comparing the latter rate with the previous, we find that mothers who have a preterm first birth have a relative risk for a subsequent preterm birth of 3.9. Also, based on this table, we can show that the risk of a

Table 3.1 The risk of preterm birth in subsequent births. Based on 27 677 mothers with their first three singleton births, Norway 1967–1976.

First birth	*Second birth*	*Number of mothers*	*Subsequent birth preterm*		
			Numbers	*%*	*Relative risk*
Not preterm		25 817	1128	4.4	1.0
Preterm		1860	320	17.2	3.9
Not preterm	Not preterm	24 689	637	2.6	0.6
Preterm	Not preterm	1540	88	5.7	1.3
Not preterm	Preterm	1128	125	11.1	2.5
Preterm	Preterm	320	91	28.4	6.5

subsequent preterm birth is further increased if the mother has had two previous preterm births (28.4 per cent of these mothers have a third preterm birth). On the other hand, for each birth which is not delivered preterm, the risk of a subsequent preterm birth decreases. Thus, if a mother has had two births, neither of which were preterm, the risk of a third birth being preterm is reduced to 2.6 per cent.

Parity

The accepted associations between parity and low birth weight and between parity and preterm birth are based on the analysis of data from cross-sectional studies. In a cross-sectional study, the proportion of preterm births is derived after combining all first births, all second births, all third births, and so forth. The relationship which emerges using the cross-sectional approach is 'U' shaped, and is shown for the data by the bold line in *Figure 3.1*.

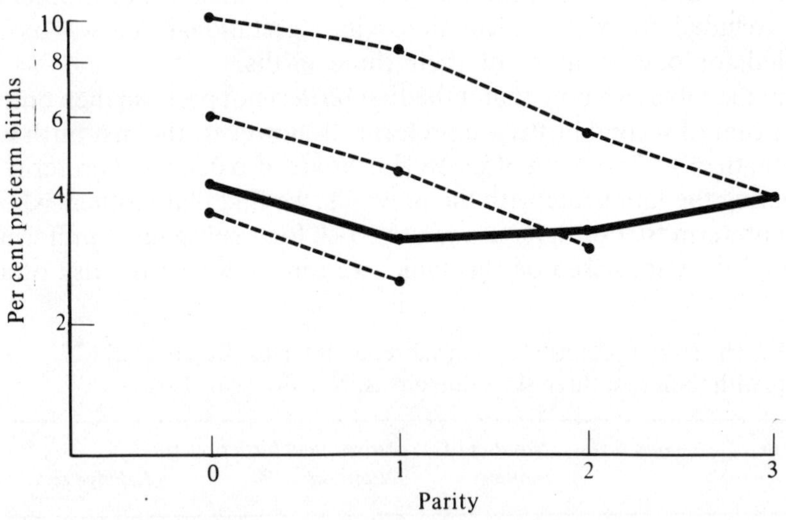

------ Based on cohorts of mothers by sibship size;

——— Based on cross sectional analysis.

Figure 3.1 Proportion (per cent) of preterm births by parity. Comparison of cross-sectional and longitudinal data analysis. Based on mothers with their first two, three or four singleton births, Norway, 1967–1976

If the relationship between parity and preterm birth is examined within groups of women based on their attained size of sibship, however, a very different pattern is found as shown by the stippled lines in this figure. These stippled lines are calculated based on women who delivered their first two births, their first three births, or their first four births within the study period. As shown in the figure, the proportion of preterm births decreases as parity increases, and the proportion is generally higher among mothers with larger sibships.

However, the 'U' shaped bold curve in *Figure 3.1* is based on exactly the same data set, except the data are pooled together for the cross-sectional analysis. Hence, in the cross-sectional analysis the frequency of preterm births is lower for second births compared with higher order births largely because the dominant contribution to second births comes from women having only two births who have lower overall rates of preterm birth. Since the frequency of preterm birth among third and fourth births necessarily must be based on women with larger sibships who have generally higher rates of preterm deliveries, a selection phenomenon occurs which accounts for the discrepancy between the cross-sectional and longitudinal results.

Although the longitudinal method of analysis discloses an artefact of cross-sectional studies, there are also methodological questions associated with the longitudinal results. One of the principal questions concerning the longitudinal method is based on the observation that mothers who have had a previous perinatal loss may tend to have larger sibships than they would have had otherwise. This tendency is known as 'self-selection for pregnancy'[4, 6, 11]. Also, if the interval for observation in a longitudinal study is too short then the results based on attained sibship size will not reflect results based on completed sibships.

Some understanding of these two potentially confounding influences can be obtained by comparing the results shown in *Figure 3.1* with those in *Figure 3.2.* The results of the longitudinal study by size of sibship are shown in *Figure 3.2a*, after the exclusion of all sibships in which one or more perinatal deaths occurred. Removing all sibships with perinatal deaths has reduced approximately by half all the rates of preterm birth. Nevertheless, the trend of fewer preterm births for higher parity within a given size of sibships still remains. Also, the relative difference in the overall rate of preterm deliveries for mothers of two, three or four births remains unchanged.

In *Figure 3.2b*, a further exclusion has been made in order to obtain results more indicative of complete sibships. Only mothers who delivered their first fetus in 1967 are used for this analysis. In addition,

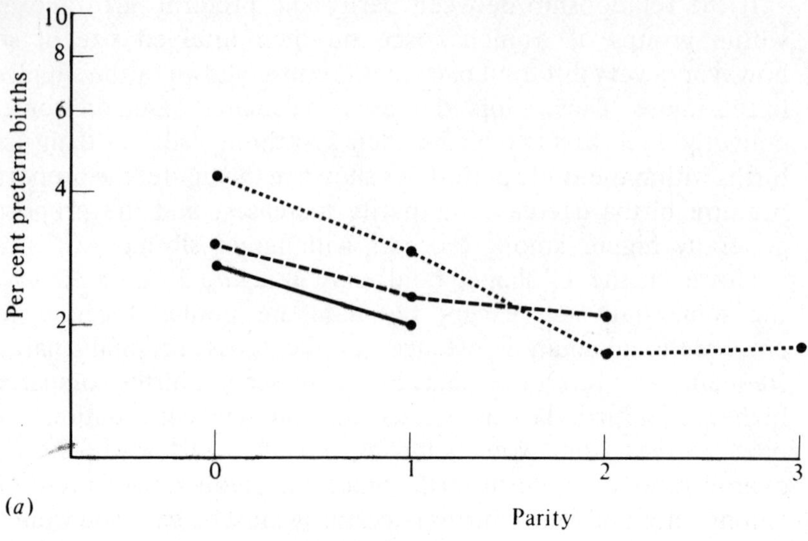

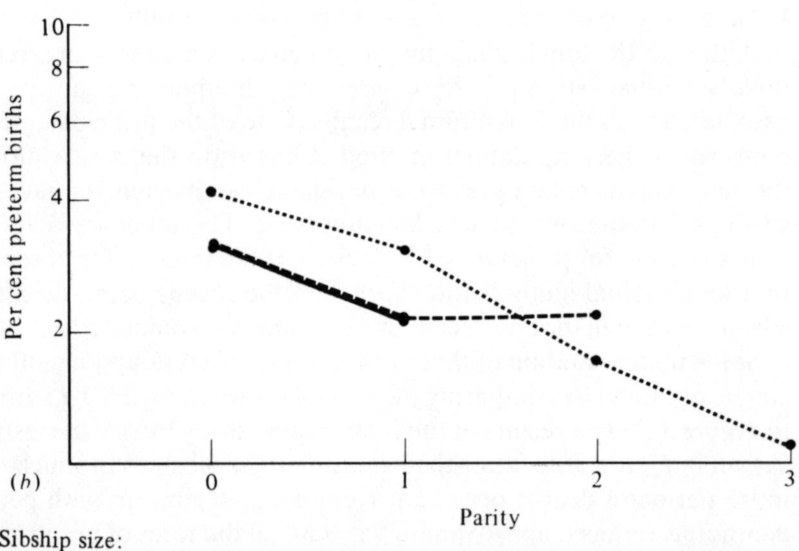

Figure 3.2 Preterm birth by parity and sibship size. (*a*) Single births 1967–1976. Excluding mothers with perinatal deaths. (*b*) Single births 1967–1976, first births in 1967. Excluding mothers with perinatal deaths

sibships of mothers having one or more perinatal deaths have also been excluded. Even with the exclusion of sibships where the first birth occurred after 1967, the preterm birth rates are basically the same as shown in *Figure 3.2a*. There is a difference in that *Figure 3.2b* shows that the preterm birth rates are nearly identical for the first two births of women having either two or three births. Also, the trend for mothers of four consecutive single births is more nearly linear.

It is clear from this figure, that the tendency to quickly replace a previous perinatal loss does not account for the longitudinal results. Even after exclusion of sibships containing perinatal losses, there is a marked decline in the rate of preterm births as parity increases within different sized sibships. Furthermore, the pattern is not much affected by the use of attained sibship size from the entire data set for the 10-year period.

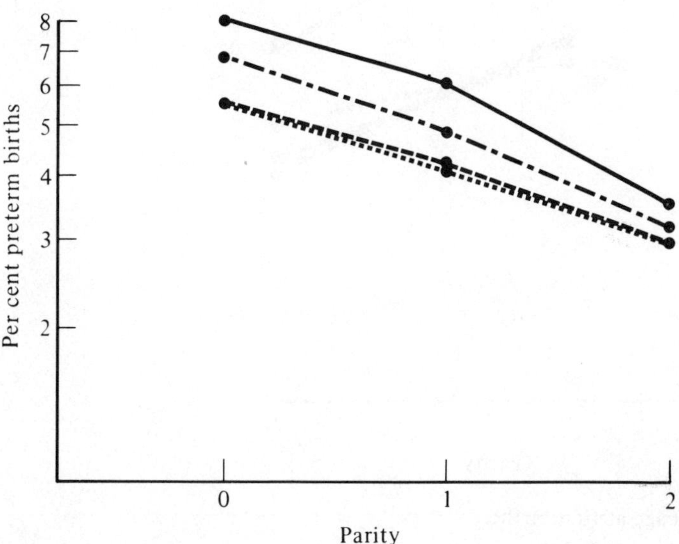

Maternal age at first birth:
——— < 20;
- - - - - 20 - 24;
·········· 25 - 29;
-·-·-·- 30+

Figure 3.3 Proportion (per cent) of preterm births by parity and maternal age at first birth. Based on mothers with their first three singleton births only, Norway, 1967–1976

Maternal age

Since parity and maternal age are closely interrelated, we have also examined the associations between these two variables jointly with the rate of preterm births in the longitudinal data set. In *Figure 3.3*, the proportion of preterm births among first, second and third births is shown for mothers with their first three singleton births during the

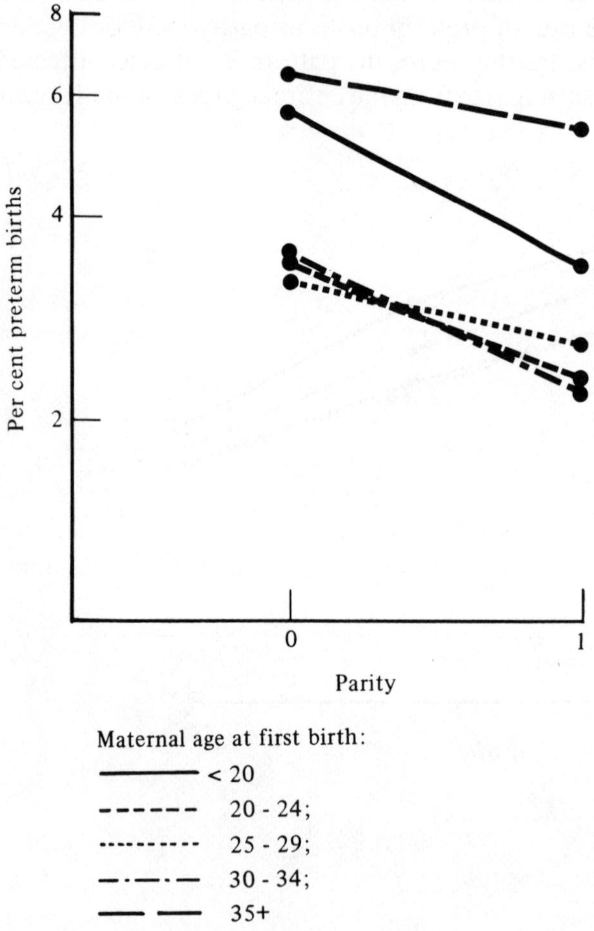

Figure 3.4 Proportion (per cent) of preterm births by parity and maternal age at first birth. Based on mothers with their first and second singleton births only, Norway, 1967–1976, and where all first births occurred in 1967.

10-year study period. The mothers are grouped according to the age at time of their first birth.

The proportion of preterm births is higher for the young mothers, and their rate of preterm births remains relatively higher also for their second and third births. Mothers who are between 20 and 29 years of age when they start childbearing have the lowest risk of preterm delivery. Even mothers aged 30 years or more have lower risks of preterm birth compared with mothers aged less than 20 years at the time of their first birth.

Similar relationships are shown in *Figure 3.4* which is based on mothers having only their first two singleton births during the study period, and whose first births all occurred in 1967. Thus, a cohort of mothers has been identified, most of whom will have a completed sibship size of two. In this figure, mothers aged 30 years or more have been split into two subgroups: those aged between 30 and 34 when they started childbearing, and those age 35 years or more.

When maternal age of 35 or more at first delivery is broken out separately, this group is shown to have the highest risk of preterm delivery. As before, the young mothers under the age of 20 also have a much higher risk of preterm birth. For the mothers aged 35 years or

Table 3.2 Proportion (per cent) of preterm births by parity and maternal age. Based on 30 979 mothers with their first three singleton births, Norway, 1967–1976.

Parity and age	*Total number of mothers*	*% Preterm births*
Para 0		
<20	5735	7.9
20–34	25 062	5.6
35+	182	7.1
Para 1		
<20	1246	8.4
20–34	29 317	4.5
35+	416	4.8
Para 2		
<20	72	13.9
20–34	29 663	3.0
35+	1244	2.7

more at their first delivery, the risk of preterm birth decreases only slightly between first and second births. For the younger mothers, however, there is a marked decrease in risk of preterm birth for their second delivery.

Another way of examining the joint effect of maternal age and parity on the risk of preterm birth is shown in *Table 3.2*. This table is based on all 30 979 mothers with their first three births in the 10-year study period. In this table, mothers are classified according to their age and parity at each birth, instead of their age at first birth only.

For primiparae the risk of preterm birth is higher for younger (less than 20 years) and older (35 years or more) mothers. For mothers having their second and third births, the risk of a preterm birth increases significantly for mothers aged less than 20 years. However, the risk of preterm birth declines for both the subgroups of mothers aged between 20 and 34 years and those aged 35 years or more as parity increases. For the young mothers, these results are different from that discussed above since there maternal age groups were defined based on first birth only.

Mothers who have had no preterm births have the lowest proportion of young mothers, less than 20 years of age, in each of the three parity groups, which are nulliparae and para one and two. Among mothers who had a preterm first birth, the proportion of young mothers was higher (23–27 per cent) than among mothers whose first births were not preterm (16–22 per cent). Among mothers having all three births preterm, 24.2 per cent were less than 20 years old when they had their first birth, 7.7 per cent were below 20 years of age at the time of their second birth, and 4.4 per cent were under the age of 20 at the time of all three of their births.

Marital status

The proportion of unmarried mothers by parity and sequence of outcomes (preterm or not) is shown in *Table 3.3*. Mothers with no preterm births in their first three deliveries were least likely to have been unmarried within each of the three parity groups: 11.4 per cent at the first birth, 2.8 per cent at the second birth, and 2.1 per cent at the third birth. As shown above for young maternal age, the proportion of unmarried mothers is higher for mothers whose first birth is preterm regardless of subsequent outcomes.

There is a marked association between the proportion of unmarried mothers and the occurrence of a preterm birth at higher parities as well.

Table 3.3 Illegitimacy by occurrence of preterm births. Based on 30 979 mothers with their first three singleton births, Norway, 1967–1976.

Sequence of births			P = preterm N = not preterm	*Proportion (%) of unmarried mothers in each parity group. (Bold italics indicate preterm births).*		
First birth	*Second birth*	*Third birth*	*Total number of mothers*	*Para 0*	*Para 1*	*Para 2*
No preterm births:						
N	N	N	24 052	11.4	2.8	2.1
One preterm birth:						
P	N	N	1452	***18.2***	4.9	2.3
N	P	N	1003	16.7	***5.1***	2.9
N	N	P	637	12.1	4.6	***4.6***
Two preterm births:						
P	P	N	229	***21.0***	***7.0***	3.9
P	N	P	88	***20.5***	4.5	***8.0***
N	P	P	125	15.2	***8.0***	***5.6***
Three preterm births:						
P	P	P	91	***23.1***	***3.3***	***1.1***
Unknown			3302	18.7	5.1	4.1
Total			30 979	12.8	3.3	2.5

The one exception to these findings occurred for women who had three consecutive preterm births. Although 23.1 per cent of these mothers were unmarried at the time of their first delivery, only 3.3 per cent were unmarried at their second delivery and an overall minimum of 1.1 per cent were unmarried at their third delivery.

Education

The relationship between maternal educational level and the number of preterm births is shown in *Table 3.4*. Among mothers with no preterm births there are relatively fewer with low educational achievement: 7.5 per cent of these mothers had completed only 7 years of education compared with 10.2 per cent for all the rest of the mothers combined. On the other hand, 8.3 per cent of the mothers with no preterm births had more than 12 years of education, compared with 5.9, 6.8 and 5.5 per cent of mothers with one, two, or three preterm births, respectively.

Table 3.4 Mothers' education (completed years) by number of preterm births. Based on 30 979 mothers with their first three singleton births, Norway, 1967–1976.

Number of preterm births	*Total number of mothers*	*Years of education (%)*				
		7	*9*	*12*	*>12*	*Unknown*
0	24 052	7.5	66.6	9.1	8.3	8.5
1	3092	8.9	69.1	8.6	5.9	7.6
2	442	12.0	60.4	9.0	6.8	11.8
3	91	7.7	73.6	4.4	5.5	8.8
Unknown	3302	10.9	67.0	6.8	6.8	8.6
Total	30 979	8.1	66.8	8.8	7.9	8.4

Father's education has also been examined using data on couples married at the time of their second birth. Thus, for mothers with no preterm births, 13.4 per cent of the fathers had more than 12 years of education. The corresponding percentage of fathers with more than 12 years of education were 10.9, 9.2 and 11.4 per cent for mothers with one, two, or three preterm births, respectively. Conversely, the percentage of fathers with only 7 years of education was 12.4 for mothers with no preterm births, compared with 13.8, 13.8 and 17.0 per cent for mothers with one, two, and three preterm births, respectively. These findings are consistent, then, using either father's or mother's educational level, but do not demonstrate any sizable relative risk. It is possible that the importance of parental education has been masked by the fact that only the 1970 Norwegian census information was available for study. If similar information had been available in 1976, at the end of the study period, then a more realistic assessment of parental education could have been obtained.

Complications of pregnancy and delivery

In the data set, toxaemia during pregnancy is reported only slightly more frequently among mothers with preterm births than in mothers without preterm births. The relative risk is only 1.2. However, as shown in *Table 3.5*, there is a tendency for an increased frequency of toxaemia among mothers whose first birth was preterm but whose subsequents births were not preterm. The frequency of toxaemia for these mothers was nearly twice as high as for other primiparae, and is also higher in subsequent births of these mothers.

Some caution is necessary in interpreting this table since toxaemia is not a well-defined diagnostic entity. Also, in the reporting system on which this study is based, there is some reason to believe that toxaemia has been under-reported[31]. Nevertheless, these data demonstrate that the frequency of toxaemia is nearly 50 per cent higher in third births

Table 3.5 Toxaemia by occurrence of preterm births. Based on 30 979 mothers with their first three singleton births, Norway, 1967–1976.

Sequence of births			P = preterm N = not preterm	*Proportion (%) with toxaemia (Bold italics indicate preterm births)*		
First birth	*Second birth*	*Third birth*	*Total number of mothers*	*Para 0*	*Para 1*	*Para 2*
No preterm births:						
N	N	N	24 052	6.5	3.9	5.6
One preterm birth:						
P	N	N	1452	***10.1***	7.2	7.9
N	P	N	1003	4.6	***2.8***	5.6
N	N	P	637	7.9	3.5	***5.7***
Two preterm births:						
P	P	N	229	***5.2***	***3.9***	4.4
P	N	P	88	***6.8***	5.7	***8.0***
N	P	P	125	7.2	***3.2***	***5.6***
Three preterm births:						
P	P	P	91	***6.6***	***2.2***	***5.5***
Unknown			3302	8.1	3.9	5.8
Total			30 979	6.8	4.0	5.7

than in to second births in this cohort, regardless of the occurrence of preterm birth. First births were at slightly higher increased risk of toxaemia compared with second births.

In *Table 3.6* the results are shown for another medical complication during pregnancy, bleeding or threatened abortion, which is more directly related to the occurrence of preterm birth. Among women

Table3.6 Bleeding during pregnancy by occurrence of preterm births. Based on 30 979 mothers with their first three singleton births, Norway, 1967–1976.

Sequence of births			P = preterm N = not preterm	*Proportion (%) with bleeding during pregnancy (Bold italics indicate preterm births)*		
First birth	*Second birth*	*Third birth*	*Total number of mothers*	*Para 0*	*Para 1*	*Para 2*
No preterm births:						
N	N	N	24 052	1.5	1.9	2.4
One preterm birth:						
P	N	N	1452	***13.1***	3.1	3.0
N	P	N	1003	2.3	***22.1***	5.3
N	N	P	637	2.7	3.5	***22.8***
Two preterm births:						
P	P	N	229	***17.9***	***17.9***	5.2
P	N	P	88	***14.8***	8.0	***11.4***
N	P	P	125	8.0	***28.0***	***0.8***
Three preterm births:						
P	P	P	91	***16.5***	***11.0***	***24.2***
Unknown			3302	2.1	3.4	4.3
Total			30 979	2.4	3.1	3.3

whose first birth was preterm, bleeding during pregnancy is relatively less frequent for those women whose subsequent two births were not preterm (the same subgroup of mothers who were at highest risk for toxaemia). Unlike toxaemia, bleeding during pregnancy is least likely to occur at first birth, and is also much less likely to occur for women all of whose births were not preterm. Indeed, the association between preterm birth and bleeding during pregnancy is strong: 18.1 per cent of preterm births also had reported bleeding during pregnancy while only

2.1 per cent of the births had reported bleeding during pregnancy. The relative risk for preterm birth among women with bleeding during pregnancy is 7.4

The frequency of either placenta praevia or abruptio placentae in relation to the occurrence of preterm birth is reported in *Table 3.7.* The pattern of results is quite similar to that shown in *Table 3.6* for bleeding during pregnancy. However, the association between the occurrence of preterm birth and either placenta praevia or abruptio placentae is even stronger: 14.6 per cent of preterm births compared with 0.9 per cent of births which were not preterm, in this case the relative risk is 10.5. Thus, the appearance of either of these two pathological conditions of the placenta is very closely related to the occurrence of preterm birth. The degree of overlap between placenta praevia or abruptio placentae and bleeding during pregnancy as reported in the Medical Birth Registry is

Table 3.7 Proportion with placenta praevia or abruptio placentae by parity and by occurrence of preterm births. Based on 30 979 mothers with their first three singleton births, Norway, 1967–1976.

Sequence of births			P = preterm N = not preterm	*Proportion (%) with placenta praevia or abruptio placentae. (Bold italics indicate preterm births)*		
First birth	*Second birth*	*Third birth*	*Total number of mothers*	*Para 0*	*Para 1*	*Para 2*
No preterm births:						
N	N	N	24 052	0.7	0.9	1.0
One preterm birth:						
P	N	N	1452	***13.0***	1.2	1.8
N	P	N	1003	0.9	***15.3***	1.8
N	N	P	637	0.8	2.4	***17.0***
Two preterm births:						
P	P	N	229	***15.7***	***13.1***	0.4
P	N	P	88	***15.9***	0	***14.8***
N	P	P	125	1.6	***18.4***	***16.0***
Three preterm births:						
P	P	P	91	***16.5***	***11.0***	***12.1***
Unknown			3 302	1.7	2.0	2.3
Total			30 979	1.6	1.7	4.7

Table 3.8 Position anomaly by parity and by occurrence of preterm births. Based on 30 979 mothers with their first three singleton births, Norway, 1967–1976

Sequence of births			P = preterm N = not preterm	*Position anomaly (%) as complication of birth (Bold italics indicate preterm births.)*		
First birth	*Second birth*	*Third birth*	*Total number of mothers*	*Para 0*	*Para 1*	*Para 2*
No preterm births:						
N	N	N	24 052	2.3	2.4	2.5
One preterm birth:						
P	N	N	1452	***5.8***	3.9	3.2
N	P	N	1003	3.1	***9.6***	3.4
N	N	P	637	2.7	1.7	***10.2***
Two preterm births:						
P	P	N	229	***7.0***	***13.5***	5.2
P	N	P	88	***10.2***	8.0	***8.0***
N	P	P	125	7.2	***14.4***	***12.8***
Three preterm births:						
P	P	P	91	***7.7***	***11.0***	***12.1***
Unknown			3302	2.9	3.0	3.0
Total			30 979	2.7	2.9	2.9

only about 20 per cent. Altogether, then, these complications of pregnancy and delivery occur in about 30 per cent of all preterm births.

Position anomalies, mostly breech presentation, were reported to occur in nearly three per cent of the births as shown in *Table 3.8*. If a preterm birth occurred, however, these complications were considerably more frequent. The relative risk of position anomalies for preterm births is 3.3 times that reported for births which were not preterm, which is in accordance with other reports[10]. From the table, it appears that among mothers who had one or two preterm births position anomalies occurred more frequently even for their births which were not preterm.

Apart from bleeding during pregnancy (threatened abortion), placenta praevia or abruptio placentae, and breech presentation, no other reported diseases or complications during pregnancy or delivery were closely associated with the occurrence of preterm birth. It should be emphasized, however, that the available data in this registry do not permit a detailed analysis of conditions such as premature rupture of the membranes, 'incompetent' cervix, or uterine malformations.

Conditions of the new born

Congenital malformations were generally more common in preterm than in term birth, if only one preterm birth occurred in a sibship. The results reported in *Table 3.9* also suggest that there is no increased rate of malformation among not preterm births of the mothers who had a single preterm birth. For mothers with more than one preterm birth, there is no apparent increase in the rate of congenital malformation compared with mothers who had no preterm births.

Table 3.9 Congenital malformations by parity and by occurrence of preterm births. Based on 30 979 mothers with their first three singleton births, Norway, 1967–1976.

Sequence of births		P = preterm N = not preterm		*Congenital malformations per 1000 births. (Bold italics indicate preterm births.)*		
First birth	*Second birth*	*Third birth*	*Total number of mothers*	*Para 0*	*Para 1*	*Para 2*
No preterm births:						
N	N	N	24 052	31.1	26.8	27.9
One preterm birth:						
P	N	N	1452	***81.3***	24.8	31.0
N	P	N	1003	26.9	***72.8***	31.9
N	N	P	637	29.8	40.8	***45.5***
Two preterm births:						
P	P	N	229	***17.5***	***26.2***	30.6
P	N	P	88	***34.1***	56.8	***22.7***
N	P	P	125	48.0	***64.0***	***16.0***
Three preterm births:						
P	P	P	91	***54.9***	***0***	***22.0***
Unknown			3302	27.0	22.1	29.1
Total			30 979	32.9	28.1	28.6

A more detailed breakdown by specific malformation categories is shown in *Table 3.10*. There is a tendency for multiple malformations to be associated with the occurrence of preterm birth. However, the increased rate of central nervous system malformations is primarily

Table 3.10 Congenital malformations by number of preterm births. Based on 30 979 mothers with their first three singleton births, Norway, 1967–1976.

Number of preterm births	*Total number of mothers*	*Total number of births*	*Congenital malformations per 1000 births*				
			CNS	*Cardio-vascular*	*Down's syndrome*	*Multiple*	*All other*
0	24 052	72 156	2.4	2.4	0.9	0.6	22.3
1	3092	9276	8.6	2.7	1.2	3.6	27.6
2	442	1326	3.8	2.3	0	3.0	23.4
3	91	273	3.7	0	0	0	22.0
Unknown	3302	9906	3.0	2.3	0.7	1.1	18.9
Total	30 979	92 937	3.0	2.4	0.9	1.0	22.5

responsible for the higher risk of malformation of preterm births in sibships with only one preterm delivery.

The frequency of occurrence of low birth weight in conjunction with preterm birth is shown in *Table 3.11*. At each parity the per cent of births less than 1500 g is given in the left-hand column, and the percentage of births with weight greater than 1500 g but less than 2500 g is shown in the adjacent column to the right. Overall, 72 per cent of the preterm births were low birth weight (less than 2500 g). If these low birth weight outcomes are split into births less than 1500 g and those above, then we find that 35 per cent of the preterm births were very low birth weight (less than 1500 g) and 37 per cent were above this cut-off.

This table also contains information about the differences in the low birth weight distributions according to the number of preterm births and parity. The preterm births of mothers with two or three preterm deliveries were more often low weight compared with the preterm births of mothers of only one preterm birth (78 per cent compared with 69 per cent). In addition, among the not preterm births the percentage of low weight deliveries was 9.7, 4.3 and 1.9 for mothers of two, one or

Table 3.11 Birth weight by parity and by occurrence of preterm births. Based on 30 979 mothers with their first three singleton births, Norway, 1967–1976

Sequence of births			P = Preterm N = Not preterm	*Proportion (%) with birth weight less than 1500 g and birth weight 1500–2499 g (Bold italics indicate preterm births).*					
			Total number	*Para 0*		*Para 1*		*Para 2*	
First birth	*Second birth*	*Third birth*	*of mothers*	*<1500*	*1500–2499*	*<1500*	*1500–2499*	*<1500*	*1500–2499*
No preterm births:									
N	N	N	24 052	0.2	2.9	0.1	1.3	0	1.2
One preterm birth:									
P	N	N	1452	***39.3***	***34.0***	0.1	3.4	0	2.2
N	P	N	1003	0.1	5.8	***37.4***	***31.7***	0.1	3.9
N	N	P	637	2.0	6.1	0.3	4.4	***24.0***	***35.8***
Two preterm births:									
P	P	N	229	***47.2***	***34.9***	***35.8***	***41.5***	0	5.7
P	N	P	88	***35.2***	***45.5***	1.1	11.4	***26.1***	***37.5***
N	P	P	125	0.8	14.4	***49.6***	***29.6***	***40.8***	***33.6***
Three preterm births:									
P	P	P	91	***50.5***	***37.4***	***46.2***	***41.8***	***26.4***	***40.7***
Unknown			3302	3.1	6.5	2.1	4.8	1.4	3.8
Total			30 979	3.0	5.4	2.1	3.4	1.0	2.7

no preterm births, respectively. Hence, the birth weight distributions are different even for births which were not preterm deliveries.

Perinatal mortality rates in relation to the occurrence of preterm births are shown in *Table 3.12*. For mothers with no preterm births the perinatal mortality rate decreased from 30.6 to 15.8 and to 6.3 per 1000 births for first, second, and third births, respectively. Perinatal mortality is defined here as the number of fetal deaths of 16 weeks or more gestational age plus the number of live births who die within the first week of life per 1000 births (including the fetal deaths in the denominator). There is also a tendency for the perinatal mortality of preterm births to decrease with increasing parity, which is particularly evident for the third birth. The tendency of self-selection for pregnancy

Table 3.12 Perinatal mortality by parity and by occurrence of preterm births. Based on 30 979 mothers with their first three singleton births, Norway, 1967–1976.

Sequence of births			P = preterm N = not preterm	*Perinatal deaths per 1000 (Bold italics indicate preterm births)*		
First birth	*Second birth*	*Third birth*	*Total number of mothers*	*Para 0*	*Para 1*	*Para 2*
No preterm births:						
N	N	N	24 052	30.6	15.8	6.3
One preterm birth:						
P	N	N	1452	***533.7***	12.4	11.7
N	P	N	1003	25.9	***539.4***	10.0
N	N	P	637	28.3	34.5	***298.3***
Two preterm births:						
P	P	N	229	***545.9***	***436.7***	13.1
P	N	P	88	***443.2***	45.4	***352.3***
N	P	P	125	24.0	***552.0***	***400.0***
Three preterm births:						
P	P	P	91	***582.4***	***615.4***	***296.7***
Unknown			3302	63.3	40.3	23.6
Total			30 979	64.1	42.7	18.0

obviously affects this pattern as mentioned previously. *Table 3.12* further indicates that the mortality of second and third births which are not preterm is higher in sibships containing preterm births.

Discussion

The purpose of this study has been to examine the characteristics of groups of mothers with different reproductive experience in terms of having preterm deliveries or not. In doing so, we have used a longitudinal analysis of the outcome of successive births to mothers with their first three singleton births during the 10 year study period.

Non-spontaneous births were included in the analysis presented here. However, separate analyses of the data were done on the study mothers excluding non-spontaneous births. There were 19 665 mothers with known gestational ages for each of their first three consecutive births after excluding mothers with one or more non-spontaneous deliveries. In general, the associations found on the restricted data set were very similar to those reported above, and if anything, the associations were usually stronger and the relative risks were slightly higher. Since the distinction between 'induced' or 'spontaneous' birth as ascertained in data such as these is often misleading, we have preferred to report analyses based on the entire data set.

The sizable number of mothers, 3302, who were listed as 'unknown' for preterm birth outcomes in the tables deserves some additional comments. Since a mother is listed as 'unknown' if any of her three births had missing gestational age information, we have examined further the pattern of missing gestational age data for these mothers. For mothers with 'unknown' gestational age births, we found that in 93.2 per cent of them only one of their three births had unknown gestational age. Also, there were no mothers in which all three of their births were unknown for gestational age. In this study we have not attempted to impute 'preterm' birth from the ancillary information on birth weight and crown–heel length which is often recorded in the Medical Birth Registry even though gestational age may be unknown. It may well be worthwhile to attempt to estimate the occurrence of preterm birth when gestational age is unknown using the combined information on birth weight and crown–heel length, but this effort will require a separate study. After inspection of the patterns of known and unknown gestational age data for these mothers, we are fairly confident that our conclusions based on the known data will not be much affected by the unknown preterm births. For instance, the unknown births will not contribute more than 15 per cent additional births to any of the eight subgroups of mothers having successive preterm or not preterm births.

In a review of the literature on the epidemiology of 'prematurity', Terris and Gold[44] in 1969 concluded that too often associations found with presumed aetiologic factors have been due to lack of comparability of the study and control groups. They especially stressed the importance of controlling for such factors as maternal age, parity, marital status, social class and race. In this analysis we have shown that the associations between preterm birth and factors such as parity and maternal age are indeed hard to disentangle. This complicates the analysis of epidemiological risk factors since parity and age are themselves related to other factors which may be significant in the aetiology of preterm birth.

It is clear that some observations derived from cross-sectional analyses have been influenced by the method of study, and consequently, the interpretation of findings from these studies may have to be revised. Thus, until recently [4,38] it has been considered unquestionable that mothers of higher parity carry an increased risk of perinatal mortality, and also, an increased risk of preterm birth. However, based on the present analysis there is no evidence that the risk of a preterm birth increases for individual women with increasing parity.

The association between maternal age and preterm birth is also influenced by the method of analysis. In either a longitudinal or cross-sectional analysis, young maternal age (less than 20 years) is closely related to an increased risk of preterm birth. Likewise, mothers aged 35 or more years carry an increased risk of a preterm first birth. However, using the longitudinal analysis presented in this report, high maternal age is not clearly associated with an increased risk of a preterm second or later birth, with the possible exception of those mothers who start childbearing after age 35.

Also, the longitudinal approach allows for a rather detailed examination of medical risk factors in successive pregnancies to the same mothers. For example, the present study shows that vaginal bleeding during pregnancy is closely associated with a preterm birth, especially where a preterm birth occurs subsequent to a normal (not preterm) first birth. The study also confirms the close association between preterm birth and either abruptio placentae or placenta praevia, but without indicating a marked tendency to occur more frequently in multiparous women[34,36,37]. The results indicate no clear association between toxaemia and preterm birth, except possibly where toxaemia occurs in the first pregnancy. No additional associations between preterm birth and other maternal conditions (prior to or during pregnancy) were found in this study. Again, it is stressed that limitations of the data collected may have prevented detection of some actual associations with variables which were not ascertained.

The present study has shown a strong and cumulative risk for repeating preterm birth. Thus, a mother who has a preterm first birth is four times as likely to have a preterm second birth. And, if a mother's second birth is also preterm, then she has between a six and seven fold increased risk of a preterm subsequent birth. This tendency to repeat a preterm birth has been shown in previous reports to be part of a very general tendency to repeat both gestational age and birth weight in successive pregnancies[2,5].

Table 3.13 provides a summary comparing several of the risk factors for preterm birth based on the tables presented earlier. Among the maternal factors shown, the multiparous mothers who were less than 20 years old have the highest relative risk, 5.2. The only other maternal condition associated with at least a two fold increased risk is illegitimacy among multiparous women. Women with all three of these risk factors, young age, multipara, and unmarried, have an even higher relative risk, but comprise less than one per cent of the mothers at risk for preterm birth. On the other hand the multiparous, older mothers (more than 35 years) have a considerably reduced risk of preterm delivery.

Table 3.13 Summary of risk factors for preterm birth. Based on 27 677 mothers with their first three singleton births, Norway, 1967–1976.

	Percent with condition	*Relative risk*	*Predictive value (%)**
Maternal factors:			
Primipara, < 20 years	17.6	1.5	9
Primipara, ⩾ 35 years	0.6	1.1	8
Primipara, unmarried	12.1	1.7	10
Multipara, < 20 years	1.8	5.2	11
Multipara, ⩾ 35 years	2.7	0.4	2
Multipara, unmarried	2.7	2.0	8
Education: 12 years or less	92.0	1.4	5
Factors relating to preceding birth†:			
Preterm	6.7	3.9	17
Low birth weight	8.3	3.5	15
Bleeding during pregnancy	2.4	2.6	13
Placenta praevia/abruptio	1.6	2.8	14
Toxaemia	6.6	0.7	4
Position anomaly	2.6	1.7	9
Congenital malformation	3.4	0.8	5
Complications of current pregnancy/delivery:			
Bleeding during pregnancy	2.9	7.4	32
Placenta praevia/abruptio	1.6	10.5	46
Toxaemia	5.5	1.2	6
Position anomaly	2.8	3.3	16
Congenital malformation	3.0	2.0	10

*Predictive value is defined as the proportion of preterm births when the factor is present.
† Preceding birth is restricted to first birth only, and the risks for subsequent preterm birth are computed based on the second delivery.

The highest relative risks in this table are associated with placenta praevia or abruptio, and bleeding during pregnancy. In fact, 46 and 32 per cent, respectively, of women with either of these two conditions deliver a preterm birth. Also, a previous pregnancy characterized by either of these two conditions is predictive of a subsequent preterm birth. Congenital malformation in a previous birth does not, however, indicate an increased risk of a subsequent preterm birth. Neither is a toxaemia of pregnancy in a previous birth associated with a subsequent preterm birth. However, there is an association between a position anomaly in a prior birth and the delivery of a preterm subsequent birth.

Many of the possible aetiological factors associated with preterm birth mentioned in the introduction have not been dealt with in the present study. This is due to the lack of available information on these factors within the study data set. Also, interactions between risk factors need to be examined in more detail but will require additional studies.

There are still large gaps in the understanding of the aetiology of preterm birth. This lack of knowledge is illustrated by the rather poor behaviour of the present risk prediction schemes which will be discussed elsewhere in this volume.

Conclusion

Practically all studies focusing on the epidemiology of preterm birth have been based on study populations defined cross-sectionally. As shown in the present study, this approach has been partially misleading. By using a longitudinal study design based on successive pregnancies to the same mothers, some of the associations between maternal factors, perinatal events, and preterm birth appear to be different, some have been strengthened, but others seem to be much weaker or even disappear.

In the study of perinatal events, it is desirable to take advantage of the heterogeneity of reproductive careers which exists within the population of childbearing women. Data collected longitudinally on successive pregnancies to the same mother facilitates comparison between groups of women with contrasting reproductive outcomes. The results from such studies are more directly related to understanding different outcomes as they relate to the reproductive careers of individual women.

Since longitudinal data sets similar to the one used in the present study have recently become available in other populations, it is hoped that the studies using these longitudinal data will add appreciably to the understanding of the epidemiology of preterm birth, and perinatal epidemiology in general.

Acknowledgements

We wish to thank Professor Tor Bjerkedal and his staff at the Medical Birth Registry of Norway for having made these data available for study. We are grateful to Mr Leif Gullberg and Mr Per Balstad for their skilful computer processing of the data required in our analyses. Also, we thank Mrs Berit Eggen and Mrs Brit Fladvad for their assistance in typing the manuscript and in preparing the tables.

This study has been supported by research contract No. 1 HD-82826 from the National Institute of Child Health and Human Development, National Institutes of Health, Bethesda, Maryland, USA. Also, we wish to acknowledge the valuable support received from the Norwegian Research Council for Science and the Humanities.

References

1 ASHFORD, J. R., FRYER, J. G. and BRIMBLECOMBE, F.S W. Secular trends in late fetal deaths, neonatal mortality and birth weight in England and Wales. *British Journal of Preventive and Social Medicine*, **23,** 154–162 (1969)

2 BAKKETEIG, L. S. The risk of repeated preterm or low birth weight delivery. In *The Epidemiology of Prematurity*, edited by D. M. Reed and F. J. Stanley. Baltimore, Urban and Schwarzenberg, 231–241 (1977)

3 BAKKETEIG, L. S., HOFFMAN, H. J. and STERNTHAL, P. M. Obstetric service and perinatal mortality in Norway. *Acta Obstetrica et Gynecologica Scandinavica*, Supplement **77,** 19pp. (1978)

4 BAKKETEIG, L. S. and HOFFMAN, H. J. Perinatal mortality by birth order within cohorts based on sibship size. *British Medical Journal*, **2,** 693–696 (1979)

5 BAKKETEIG, L. S., HOFFMAN, H. J. and HARLEY, E. E. The tendency to repeat gestational age and birth weight in successive births. *American Journal of Obstetrics and Gynecology*, **135,** 1086–1103 (1979)

6 BAKKETEIG, L. S. and HOFFMAN, H. J. Pregnancy order and reproductive loss. *British Medical Journal*, **1,** 716 (1980)

7 BAIRD, D. The epidemiology of low birth weight: changes in incidence in Aberdeen, 1948–72. *Journal of Biosocial Science*, **6,** 323–341 (1974)

8 BATTAGLIA, F. C. and SIMMONS, M. A. The low-birth-weight infant. In *Human Growth*, edited by F. Falkner and J. M. Tanner. London, Balliere Tindal (1978)

9 BATTAGLIA, F. C. and LUBCHENCO, L. O. A practical classification of newborn infants by weight and gestational age. *Journal of Pediatrics*, **71,** 159–163 (1967)

10 BERENDES, H. W., WEISS, W., DEUTSCHBERGER, J. and JACKSON, E. Factors associated with breech delivery. *American Journal of Public Health*, **55,** 708–719 (1965)

11 BILLEWICZ, W. Z. Some implications of self-selection for pregnancy. *British Journal of Preventive and Social Medicine*, **27,** 49–52 (1973)

12 BJERKEDAL, T. and BAKKETEIG, L. S. *Medical Registration of Births in Norway during the 5-Year Period 1967–71*. Institute of Hygiene and Social Medicine, University of Bergen, Norway, 71 (1975)

13 BJERKEDAL, T.and LUND, T. E. *Yrke og fodsel (Occupation and birth)*, Hygienisk Institutt, Universitetet i Oslo, Norway (1978) (in Norwegian only)

14 BOLDMAN, R. and REED, D. M. Worldwide variations in low birth weight. In *The Epidemiology of Prematurity*, edited by D. M. Reed and F. J. Stanley. 39–52. Baltimore, Urban and Schwarzenberg (1977)

15 CHAMBERLAIN, R., CHAMBERLAIN, G., HOWLETT, B. and CLAIREAUX, A. *British Births, 1970. The First Week of Life*. London, Heinemann (1975)

16 CHASE, H. C. and BYRNES, M. E. Trends in 'prematurity': United States, 1950–1967. *American Journal of Public Health*, **60,** 1967–1983 (1970)

17 DALING, J. R. and EMANUEL, I. Induced abortion and subsequent outcome of pregnancy. *Lancet*, **2,** 170–172 (1975)

18 DUBOWITZ, V. The infant of inappropriate size. In *Size at Birth* (Ciba Foundation Symposium 27, new series), 47–64. Amsterdam, Elsevier (1974)

19 ERICKSON, J. D. and BJERKEDAL, T. Interpregnancy interval: Association with birth weight, stillbirth, and neonatal death. *Journal of Epidemiology and Community Health*, **32**, 124–130 (1978)

20 ERHARDT, C. L., JOSHI, G. B., NELSON, F. G., KROLL, B. H. and WEINER, L. Influence of weight and gestation on perinatal and neonatal mortality by ethnic group. *American Journal of Public Health*, **54,** 1841–1855 (1964)

21 FEDRICK-GOLDING, J. Predisposing factors of risk. In *Perinatal Medicine*, edited by O. Thalhammer, K. Baumgarten and A. Pollak. Stuttgart, Thieme (1979)

22 FEDRICK, J. and ANDERSON, A. B. M. Factors associated with spon-

taneous pre-term birth. *British Journal of Obstetrics and Gynaecology*, **83,** 342–350 (1976)

23 GRUENWALD, P. Growth and maturation of the fetus and its relationship to perinatal mortality. In *Perinatal Problems–The Second Report of the 1958 British Perinatal Mortality Survey*, edited by N. R. Butler and E. D. Alberman, 141–162. Edinburgh, Livingstone (1969)

24 HEMMINKI, E. and STARFIELD, B. Prevention of low birth weight and pre-term birth. *Milbank Memorial Fund Quarterly Bulletin*, **56,** 339–361 (1978)

25 HOFFMAN, H. J., LUNDIN, F. E. JR., BAKKETEIG, L. S. and HARLEY, E. E. Classification of births by weight and gestational age for future studies of prematurity. In *The Epidemiology of Prematurity*, edited by D. M. Reed and F. J. Stanley, 297–333. Baltimore, Urban and Schwarzenberg (1977)

26 HOFFMAN, H. J., BAKKETEIG, L. S. and STARK, C.R. Twins and perinatal mortality: A comparison between single and twin births in Minnesota and in Norway, 1967–1973. In *Twin Research, Part B–Biology and Epidemiology*, edited by W. E. Nance, G. Allen and P. Parisi, 133–142. New York, Alan R. Liss (1978)

27 KAMINSKI, M., RUMEAU-ROUQUETTE, C, and SCHWARTZ, D. Alcohol consumption in pregnant women and the outcome of pregnancy. *Alcoholism Clinical and Experimental Research*, **2,** 155–163 (1978)

28 KEIRSE, M. J. N. C. Epidemiology of preterm labour. In *Human Parturition*, (Boerhaave Series, Vol. 15), edited by M. J. N. C. Keirse, A. B. M. Anderson, J. Bennebroek Gravenhorst, 219–234. The Hague, Martinus Nijhoff (1979)

29 MCKEOWN, T and RECORD, R. G. Observations on foetal growth in multiple pregnancy in man. *Journal of Endocrinology*, **8,** 386–401 (1958)

30 MEYER, M. B., JONAS, B. S. and TONASCIA, J. A. Perinatal events associated with maternal smoking during pregnancy. *American Journal of Epidemiology*, **103**, 464–476 (1976)

31 NATIONAL CENTRAL BUREAU OF STATISTICS. Medical Birth Registration in 1975 and 1976. *Statistics of the National Board of Health and Welfare*. Stockholm (1980)

32 NELIGAN, G. A., KOLVIN, I., SCOTT, D. MCL. and GARSIDE, R. F. *Born too Soon or Born too Small*. London, Heinemann (1976)

33 NISWANDER, K. R. Obstetric factors related to prematurity. In *The Epidemiology of Prematurity*, edited by D. M. Reed and F. J. Stanley, 249–264. Baltimore, Urban and Schwarzenberg (1977)

34 NISWANDER, K R. and GORDON, M. *The Women and their Pregnancies*. DHEW (NIH) Publication No. 73–379, Washington DC (1972)

35 OULETTE, E. Adverse effects on offspring of ethanol alcohol abuse during pregnancy. *New England Journal of Medicine*, **297**, 528–530 (1978)

36 PRITCHARD, J. A. and MACDONALD, P. C., In *Williams Obstetrics*, 15th Edn., New York, Appleton-Century-Crofts (1976)

37 RITCHIE, K. and MCCLURE, G. Prematurity. *Lancet*, **2**, 1227–1229 (1979)

38 ROMAN, E., DOYLE, P., BERAL, V., ALBERMAN, E. and PHAROAH, P. Fetal loss, gravidity and pregnancy order. *Early Human Development*, **212**, 131–138 (1978)

39 RUSH, R. W., KEIRSE, M. J. N. C., HOWAT, P., BAUM, J. D., ANDERSON, A. B. M. and TURNBULL, A. C. Contributions of preterm delivery to perinatal mortality. *British Medical Journal*, **2**, 965–968 (1976)

40 SECOND EUROPEAN CONGRESS OF PERINATAL MEDICINE. Working Party to discuss nomenclature. Based on gestational age and birth weight. *Archives of Disease in Childhood*, **45**, 730 (1970)

41 STANLEY, F. J. Medical care of the fetus and the risk of prematurity. In *The Epidemiology of Prematurity*, edited by D. M. Reed and F. J. Stanley, 269–278. Baltimore, Urban and Schwarzenberg (1977)

42 SUSSER, M. and STEIN, Z. Prenatal nutrition and subsequent development. In *The Epidemiology of Prematurity*, edited by D. M. Reed and F. J. Stanley, 177–188. Baltimore, Urban and Schwarzenberg (1977)

43 TERRIS, M. and GLASSER, M. A life table analysis of the relation of prenatal care to prematurity. *American Journal of Public Health*, **64**, 869–875 (1974)

44 TERRIS, M. and GOLD, E. M. An epidemiologic study of prematurity. I. Relation to smoking, heart volume, employment and physique. *American Journal of Obstetrics and Gynecology*, **103**, 358–370 (1969)

45 TERRIS, M. and GOLD, E. M. An epidemiologic study of prematurity. II. Relation to prenatal care, birth interval, residential history and outcome of previous pregnancies. *American Journal of Obstetrics and Gynecology*, **103**, 371–379 (1969)

46 WORLD HEALTH ORGANIZATION. *Report on Methodology Related to Perinatal Events*. WHO Document ICD/74.4, 32. Geneva (1974)

47 WORLD HEALTH ORGANIZATION. Recommended definitions, terminology and formulae for statistical tables related to the perinatal period and use of a new certificate for cause of perinatal death. *Acta Obstetrica et Gynecologica Scandinavica*, **56**, 247–253 (1977)

4

Assessing the risk of preterm labour

R. G. Newcombe and I. Chalmers

Introduction

A considerable number of factors have been identified which are both ascertainable in early pregnancy and associated with spontaneous preterm labour. The concept of using such factors to allocate individual pregnant women to certain 'risk categories' is immediately appealing. Theoretically, there should be advantages in such an approach. It should facilitate rationally-based variations in the nature and intensity of the antenatal care offered to the individuals so assessed. Consequently it should make possible the earlier identification of departures from normality which may be amenable to beneficial intervention.

Several formalized risk assessment systems, which permit simultaneous weighing of a number of such factors, each of relatively weak adverse effect, have been published. Such systems aim to identify women at high risk of preterm labour or other adverse outcomes of pregnancy, but the question arises as to whether such formalized risk assessment is worthwhile. Can it lead to improved management and outcome of pregnancy, and if so, would the experienced clinician using his own unformalized expertise achieve equally good results?

Widely accepted criteria exist for evaluating both formalized and unformalized risk assessment. Such screening procedures should be safe and acceptable to the individuals assessed. If possible, they should be cheap, and this must be judged in relation to the relatively low incidence of adverse outcome in pregnancy. They should be reliable as judged by acceptably low proportions of 'false positives' and 'false negatives'; and this is a necessary but not sufficient condition for the most important criterion of all: that use of the test can lead to a net balance of benefit in the population screened.

Predictive factors

The roles of the individual factors predictive of outcome of pregnancy have been reviewed comprehensively elsewhere[31]. The sets of factors predictive of different adverse outcomes of pregnancy, e.g. preterm delivery, intrauterine growth retardation, stillbirth, neonatal death, overlap considerably but are not identical. The associations of general factors (such as maternal height and weight, marital status, social class, cigarette smoking, race, and area of residence) with birth weight, duration of gestation and perinatal death are well established, e.g.[8, 9]. The increased incidence of both preterm labour and fetal growth retardation among deliveries to small women may be explained by constraint on intrauterine growth[49]. Smoking has relatively little effect on the duration of gestation, but rather seems to inhibit the rate and quality of fetal growth[9]. The remaining factors are probably indicative rather than causal, but this does not necessarily contraindicate their inclusion in a risk assessment system.

Maternal age and parity

Information on the mother's age, parity and inter-pregnancy interval is readily ascertained. Nevertheless it is very difficult to establish precisely how these factors are implicated in the aetiology of adverse outcome, or the rather different issue of how they are best used in risk assessment. Childbearing is largely a matter of selection on the part of the parents, especially now, as termination and highly effective contraception are available. The decision by a woman with a given number of past pregnancies to bear a child, and the timing of her decision in relation to her age and the interval since her last pregnancy, are largely voluntary and she will normally cease reproduction when the desired family size is attained. Two hypotheses have been postulated involving systematic differences between groups with women of different eventual family size: reproductive compensation[37], the attempt to replace a lost baby, which often occurs very soon after the loss, and excess fertility among women prone to regularly lose their babies[24]. These phenomena would suggest the use of longitudinal methods of analysis in which successive pregnancies of the same woman are studied. However, such analysis is unfortunately associated with other artefacts.[54]. Similarly, the association of maternal age with outcome of pregnancy is complicated by selection artefacts in that the best outcome of pregnancy in a given population is regularly associated with the modal age at childbearing, whether this is in the early twenties, late twenties or early thirties[36]. In addition to problems associated with the variables maternal age and parity taken individually, there are further problems in separating age and parity effects from cohort and secular trends[38].

Inter-pregnancy interval

Related problems apply to inter-pregnancy interval, and it is particularly difficult to assess the risk of preterm labour when the preceding pregnancy was very recent. Here statistics based on the interval between births are grossly biased: cases in which the last menstrual period (LMP) preceding the index pregnancy occurs 16 weeks after a previous delivery will be included in a group defined by an inter-birth interval of under one year only if delivery occurs at 36 weeks gestation or earlier. Thus it is inevitable that short gestations will be over-represented. The interval between the two LMPs is a more appropriate measure but even this is difficult to interpret. There may be no return of menstruation between the pregnancies or the menstrual cycle may not have been fully re-established. Uncertainty of menstrual dates prejudices the interpretation of this factor and indeed all data on preterm delivery. In summary, it *may* prove possible to make intelligent use of information on age, parity and inter-pregnancy interval; but these variables must be used with great caution and assessed primarily in the light of individual past reproductive histories.

Reproductive history

By contrast, reproductive history is a very informative risk predictor, particularly as the factors giving rise to risk in the current pregnancy may well have done so previously. The extreme example occurs in the study of Freeman and Graves[17] in which four out of seven women whose first three babies were of low birth weight delivered a fourth low birth weight baby. However, the recurrence risk is generally very much lower than this.

Maternal illness

Many risk assessment systems include medical factors such as diabetes, cardiac and renal disease, epilepsy, tuberculosis, malignant disease and

Rhesus isoimmunization alongside the less specific factors already discussed. However, as the presence of such factors will be a specific determinant of the management of the pregnancy, it is preferable not to include them in scoring systems[39] and restrict risk assessment to women free of these conditions. Similarly, it is appropriate to make risk assessment conditional upon the absence of multiple pregnancy and major fetal malformation. As with maternal disease, early identification is often possible, different questions of management arise, and statistical evaluation of a risk assessment system on a mixture of singleton and multiple pregnancies is impaired by the violation of a one-to-one correspondence of maternal and fetal information. Likewise, conditions of established mendelian heritability are to be regarded as a different matter.

All the factors so far discussed can be ascertained in early pregnancy. As pregnancy proceeds, risk assessment can only improve, either as alarming signs and test results lead to an increase in risk level or their non-occurrence leads to a shading down of the level of risk.

Risk assessment systems

The following authors and their co-workers have produced formalized risk assessment systems which relate not only to preterm delivery, but to a wide range of adverse outcomes of pregnancy.

(1)*British Perinatal Mortality Survey Team[16, 18]
(2)*Goodwin[19]
(3)*Nesbitt[30, 4]
(4) Papiernik-Berkhauer[33, 34, 26, 27]
(5) Rantakallio[35]
(6) Štembera[44, 45]
(7) Saling[42], [32]
(8) Bompiani[7, 21]
(9) Donahue[13]
(10)*Hobel[23]
(11) Mercier[29]
(12)*Rumeau-Rouquette[39–41], [25, 20]
(13) Thalhammer[47, 48]
(14) Wilson[52]
(15) Davies[12]
(16)*Haeri[22]
(17)*Fedrick[15, 1]
(18)*Williams[51]

*Validated risk assessment system (*see* p. 52).

Although such risk assessment systems have been proposed for both educational[19] and resource allocation[2] purposes, interest in them has mainly been prompted by a desire to provide a rational basis for identifying individuals for differential prophylactic or therapeutic intervention. However, even if a perfectly effective intervention to delay delivery were available, it could not be assumed that the benefits to the fetus would necessarily outweigh the hazards to the mother and the fetus. Assuming that there are some members of the parturient population for whom a specific intervention is indicated, the risk assessment system should aim to identify such women[10].

The structure of the risk assessment system would have to be rather more complicated to give appropriate weight to factors regarded as absolute contraindications to the intervention. The hazards of specific interventions, such as cervical cerclage and tocolytic drugs, are well established and are discussed at length in Chapter 7. When predictive power is imperfect, there are necessarily 'false positives' and 'false negatives'. Those who have been inappropriately allocated to a high-risk category may be subjected needlessly to the hazards of intervention, whilst there is the danger that a low-risk score may instil an unwarranted sense of security[11,46].

Predictive power

A risk assessment system, however derived, is useful only to the degree that it permits prospective identification of high-risk groups and discriminates between levels of risk[53]. The incidence of preterm delivery within a group assessed to be at high risk is of importance in the practical application of a risk assessment system; but is not solely a characteristic of the system itself, being also heavily dependent on the overall incidence of preterm delivery in the obstetric population.

Since the threshold separating the high- and low-risk groups is arbitrary, an appropriate measure of predictive power is P – the estimated probability that if two pregnancies are chosen at random, one delivering preterm and the other delivering at term, the former will have received the more unfavourable score[5,6]. The method generalizes the sensitivity and specificity and is equivalent to the statistics of Wilcoxon[50] and Mann and Whitney[28] cast in a form which is free of sample size. Being non-parametric it permits comparison of systems derived by elaborate, often multivariate, analyses of specific source databases with systems in which the score components have been assigned arbitrarily. A value of 1.0 denotes perfect discrimination whilst, in the absence of predictive power, P takes the value 0.5.

The authors of a risk assessment system often seek to indicate the performance of the system by referring it back to the set of deliveries from which it was derived; this may be termed back-validation. The assessment of predictive power thus obtained is over-optimistic, and there are two main reasons for this. First, the coefficients used in the risk assessment score have been chosen specifically in such a way as to maximize discrimination, and if the source database is finite, they will reflect its sampling vagaries as well as the underlying effects. Secondly, the interpretation of predictive factors, and even of an outcome such as preterm labour, may vary between clinicians, even when an apparently definite risk assessment system is used, with the result that those using it will find it a less precise instrument in their hands than in those of its originator. Accordingly it is appropriate to supplement back-validation results with independent validation, either prospectively or retrospectively using other data already collected.

All of the risk assessment systems listed on p. 50 have been assessed in terms of the statistic *P*. Suitable systems (asterisked) have been validated independently using two target databases: the control week singletons of the Brtish Perinatal Mortality Survey of 1958[8,9] and the Cardiff Births Survey[3]. Obstetric history is such an informative factor that it is appropriate to present validation data separately for primiparae and multiparae; predictive power is necessarily better for multiparae.

Table 4.1, which refers not only to the prediction of preterm delivery but a range of possible outcomes, shows the best predictive performance in the literature by a given stage of pregnancy. The independent retrospective validation referred to above indicated rather poorer predictive power. Predictive power improves as gestation advances; tautologically it cannot deteriorate, but the order of magnitude of the improvement is impressive. Values of *P* that might be regarded as an adequate basis for intervention are not found until it is too late to try to postpone the onset of labour; at this stage prognostication rather than prediction would be a more apt description of function.

If attention is restricted to prediction at, say 28 weeks gestation, the best performance available is that of the Fedrick predictor[15] applied to multiparae. This predictor involves multiplication of relative risk factors for the following variables: maternal age, weight, smoking habits, social class; whether a threatened abortion has taken place in the index pregnancy; and abortion, perinatal death, antepartum haemorrhage and birth weights in previous pregnancies. The score was derived from and applied to the British Perinatal Mortality Survey data of 1958.

Table 4.1 Best prediction performance in the literature at a given stage of pregnancy.

Stage	*Author*	*Restricted to*	*Outcome predicted*	*Validated on*	*P*
Early pregnancy	Rumeau-Rouquette, Kaminski and Goujard[39]	Multigravidae	Stillbirth	Source	0.75
6th month	Thalhammer *et al.*[48]	All	Low birth weight	Independent	0.80
28 weeks	Fedrick[15]	Multiparae	Spontaneous preterm labour	Source	0.81
Prenatal	Lambotte[27]	All	Preterm	Arbitrary	0.87
Prenatal including gestational age	Goodwin, Dunne and Thomas[19]	All	Neonatal death	Arbitrary	0.95
Intrapartum	Mercier and Desjardins[29]	All	Perinatal death	Arbitrary	0.96

A sensitivity and specificity of 0.78 and 0.76 respectively were obtained using the arbitary dichotomy point suggested by the author; the predictive power was assessed as $P = 0.81$ using the full information from the frequency distribution of the scores. The outcome to be predicted was defined as spontaneous preterm labour leading to the delivery of an infant weighing under 2500 g. This occurs in only 1.6 per cent of the multiparae studied, and only 5.1 per cent of the high-risk group in fact go into spontaneous preterm labour. Accordingly, the hazards of applying an intervention in 20 cases must be weighed against the possible advantages accruing to one.

Improvements in two directions may be contemplated. First, when prediction of an outcome as specific as preterm labour is envisaged, it is appropriate to quantify directly relevant variables such as those relating to the condition of the cervix. In such a study[14] three risk groups were identified. In the lowest risk group cervical cerclage was found to be unnecessary; in the middle group the intervention was judged to have been beneficial whilst in the highest risk group it was insufficient to prevent spontaneous abortion or very early labour.

Secondly, it is possible to narrow down the outcome to be predicted in order to choose preventive measures more appropriately. With this in mind, tabulations from the Cardiff Births Survey were obtained with a view to discriminating between those spontaneous preterm labours in which contractions started with membranes intact and those in which membranes ruptured spontaneously prior to the onset of contractions. On this very restricted sample no predictive power could be found. Moreover a predictor designed for one of these two modes of onset, even were it to have a higher P, would relate to an outcome of lower incidence, and thus the predictive power of a high-risk score would be lower. This could not be regarded as an improvement.

Randomized controlled trials

How is the clinical worth of a risk assessment system to be tested? The prospective uncontrolled study is particularly liable to be uninformative. It does not provide information on the effectiveness of the treatment used since the identified low-risk cases do not provide an adequate control group against which to assess the effectiveness of the treatment applied to the high-risk group. Equally it does not yield adequate information on predictive power. For, unless the treatment applied to those at high risk is of no benefit, in which situation even ideal discrimination would lead to no practical benefit, such treatment of the high-risk cases improves their prognosis and narrows the gap in outcome between high-risk and low-risk groups, whence P is underestimated.

The prospective randomized controlled trial is the only adequate test of the clinical worth of a risk assessment system. This should be linked to a specific treatment for identified high-risk cases; if the aim is to apply non-specific extra care, maintenance of such differential standards is very difficult, the regimes actually used tending to converge rapidly towards each other[40].

From most points of view, the model randomized controlled trial for evaluating the usefulness of an item of information in the perinatal field is the trial of Spellacy *et al.*[43] who investigated the value of knowing the level of human placental lactogen in a group of high-risk pregnant women. Cases were entered into the trial prior to obtaining the item of information, half were treated on the basis of this information, the remainder in ignorance of it. This was quite readily done in the original context, where the piece of information was a laboratory test result and it was possible to 'ignore' this entirely by not looking at it until the analysis stage. However, when the item of information is the synthesis of information already routinely collected and on which management would otherwise be based in an unformalized way, the contrast between experimental and control groups will be attenuated, especially when the clinician is fully conversant with the form of the risk assessment system.

It is *a priori* most unlikely that a risk assessment system of sound mathematical derivation from a definite source database would give a P that failed to exceed 0.5 appreciably; but the clinical judgement of an experienced obstetrician might well give rise to a P commensurately greater than 0.5 and it is by no means a foregone conclusion that the formalised risk assessment system would show superior performance prospectively, especially in view of its limited transferability. For reasons given above it is the P derived from the control group that would more closely reflect the natural history quantified by the risk assessment system. Indeed, the shortfall of P derived from the experimental group when compared with P derived from the controls might be used as a measure of the effectiveness of the treatment in diluting the predictive relationship, though a rather large sample size would be required in order to show that such a shortfall was not merely a result of sampling fluctuation.

Finally, the ideal must be to identify a group of cases likely to experience net benefit from a particular proposed intervention. Derivation of the scoring system will be complicated by the fact that the intervention might be contemplated at various stages of the pregnancy.

Once a suitable system has been found, a randomised controlled trial is required to compare use of the intervention as prompted by the system against use of the intervention as prompted by clinical judgement. The choice of outcome variables is difficult, especially when potential benefits for the fetus are to be weighed against possible hazards to the mother.

Conclusion

If an effective method of preventing spontaneous preterm labour existed, *and* there were no hazards associated with it, there would be less cause to feel concerned about the imperfect predictive power of risk assessment systems. The use of existing risk assessment systems to select women for treatment with the interventions currently available to obstetricians cannot yet be regarded as of established benefit. The hazards of applying an intervention unnecessarily to numerous 'false positives' must be balanced against the possible advantages accruing to each 'true positive' among those treated.

References

1 ADELSTEIN, P. and FEDRICK, J. Antenatal identification of women at increased risk of being delivered of a low birth weight infant at term. *British Journal of Obstetrics and Gynaecology*, **85,** 8–11 (1978)

2 ALBERMAN, E. D. and GOLDSTEIN, H. The 'at risk' register: a statistical evaluation. *British Journal of Preventive and Social Medicine*, **24,** 129–135 (1970)

3 ANDREWS, J., DAVIES, K., CHALMERS, I. and CAMPBELL, H. The Cardiff Birth Survey: development, perinatal mortality, birth weight and length of gestation. In *Genetic and Population Studies in Wales*, edited by Harper, P. S., Sunderland, E. University of Wales Press (In press)

4 AUBRY, R. H. and PENNINGTON, J. C. Identification and evaluation of high risk pregnancy. *Clinical Obstetrics and Gynecology*, **16,** 3–27 (1973)

5 BERKSON, J. Cost-utility as a measure of the efficiency of a test. *Journal of the American Statistical Association*, **42,** 246–255 (1947)

6 BIRNBAUM, Z. W. On a use of the Mann-Whitney statistic. *Proceedings of the 3rd Berkeley symposium on Mathematical Statistics and Probability*, **1,** 13–17 (1956)

7 BOMPIANI, A., ROMANINI, C., OLIVA, G. C., PALLA, G. P. and LIVERANI, A. Selezione di alcuni indici di 'alto rischio perinatale' e valutazione della loro attendibilità. *Annali di Ostetricia, Ginecologia, Medicina Perinatale*, **93,** 624–639 (1973)

8 BUTLER, N. R. and BONHAM, D. G. *Perinatal Mortality*. Edinburgh, Livingstone (1963)

9 BUTLER, N. R. and ALBERMAN, E. D. *Perinatal Problems*. Edinburgh, Livingstone (1969)

10 CHALMERS, I. and RICHARDS, M. Intervention and causal inference in obstetric practice. In *Benefits and Hazards of the New Obstetrics*, edited by T. Chard, M.P.M. Richards. Clinics in Developmental Medicine, London, Spastics Publications/Heinemann (1977)

11 CURZEN, P. and MOUNTROSE, U. M. The general practitioner's role in the management of labour. *British Medical Journal*, **2,** 1433–1434 (1976)

12 DAVIES, A. M. and HARLAP, S. Antenatal prediction of perinatal and neonatal mortality risk. World Health Organisation, MCH/WP/HR74, 1. (1974)

13 DONAHUE, C. L. and WAN, T. T. H. Measuring obstetric risks of prematurity. *American Journal of Obstetrics and Gynecology*, **116,** 911–915 (1973)

14 DUMONT, M. and POIZAT, C. L. Etude d'un coefficient de la béance cervico-isthmique. *Journal de Gynécologie, d'Obstetrique et de Biologie de la Reproduction.***3,** 981–995 (1974)

15 FEDRICK, J. Antenatal identification of women at high risk of spontaneous preterm birth. *British Journal of Obstetrics and Gynaecology*, **83,** 351–354 (1976)

16 FELDSTEIN, M. S. and BUTLER, N. R. Analysis of factors affecting perinatal mortality. *British Journal of Preventive and Social Medicine*, **19,** 128–134 (1965)

17 FREEMAN, M. G. and GRAVES, W. L. Risk of premature delivery among indigent Negro women based on past reproductive performance. *Obstetrics and Gynecology*, **34,** 648–654 (1969)

18 GOLDSTEIN, H. Predictors of birthweight and mortality risk. In *Perinatal Problems*, edited by N. R. Butler, E. D. Alberman, 42, 56. Edinburgh, Livingtone (1969)

19 GOODWIN, J. W., DUNNE, J. T. and THOMAS, B. W. Antepartum identification of the fetus at risk. *Canadian Medical Association Journal*, **101,** 458–464 (1969)

20 GOUJARD, J., HENNEQUIN, J. F., KAMINSKI, M., MARENDAS, R. and RUMEAU-ROUQUETTE, C., Prévision de la prématurité et du poids de naissance en début de grossesse. *Journal de Gynécologie, Obstetrique et Biologie de la Reproduction*, **3,** 45–59 (1974)

21 GRELLA, P. and FEDE, T. La gravidanza ed il parto a rischio. *Minerva Ginecologica*, **27,** 837–842 (1975)

22 HAERI, A. D., SOUTH, J. and NALDRETT, J. A scoring system for identifying pregnant patients with a high risk of perinatal mortality. *Journal of Obstetrics and Gynaecology of the British Commonwealth*, **81,** 535–538 (1974)

23 HOBEL, C. J., HYVARINEN, M. A., OKADA, D. M. and OH, W. Prenatal and intrapartum high-risk screening. *American Journal of Obstetrics and Gynecology*, **117,** 1–9 (1973)

24 JAMES, W. H. Stillbirth and birth order. *Annals of Human Genetics* (London), **32**, 151–162 (1968)

25 KAMINSKI, M., GOUJARD, J. and RUMEAU-ROUQUETTE, C. Prediction of low birth weight and prematurity by a multiple regression analysis with maternal characteristics known since the beginning of pregnancy. *International Journal of Epidemiology*, **2,** 195–204 (1973)

26 KAMINSKI, M. and PAPIERNIK, E. Multifactorial study of risk of prematurity at 32 weeks. II. *Journal of Perinatal Medicine*, **2,** 37–44 (1974)

27 LAMBOTTE, R. Epidemiology of preterm labour. In *Pre-term Labour* (Proceedings of the 5th Study Group of the Royal College of Obstetricians and Gynaecologists), edited by A. B. M. Anderson, R. Beard, J. M. Brudenell, P. M. Dunn, 40–41. London, Royal College of Obstetricians and Gynaecologists (1977)

28 MANN, H. B. and WHITNEY, D. R. On a test of whether one of two random variables is stochastically larger than the other. *Annals of Mathematical Statistics*, **18,** 50–60 (1947)

29 MERCIER, G. and DESJARDINS, P. D. Evaluation numérique de risque pendant la grossesse. *L'Union Médicale du Canada*, **102,** 102–106 (1973)

30 NESBITT, R. E. L. and AUBRY, R. H. High risk obstetrics II. *American Journal of Obstetrics and Gynecology*, **103,** 972–985 (1969)

31 NEWCOMBE, R. G. A critical review of risk prediction with special reference to the perinatal period. *Ph.D. Thesis*, University of Wales (1979)

32 OLIVA RODRIQUEZ, J. A., FARNOT CARDOSO, U., POMMIER GOMEZ, M. and VALDES VIVO, P. Evalucion de un sistema de puntucion del riesgo durante la atencion prenatal. *Ginecologia y Obstetricia de Mexico*, **39,** (232) 85–89 (1976)

33 PAPIERNIK-BERKHAUER, E. Coefficient de risque d'accouchement prématuré. *Presse Médicale*, **77,** 793–794 (1969)

34 PAPIERNIK, E. and KAMINSKI, M. Multifactorial study of risk of prematurity at 32 weeks. I. *Journal of Perinatal Medicine*, **2,** 30–36 (1974)

35 RANTAKALLIO, P. Groups at risk in low birth weight infants and perinatal mortality. *Acta Paediatrica Scandinavica*, supplement **193,** (1969)

36 RESSEGUIE, L. J. Changes in stillbirth ratios resulting from changing fashions in age at childbearing. *Social Biology*, **20,** 173–184 (1973)

37 RESSEGUIE, L. J. Influence of age, birth order and reproductive compensation on stillbirth ratio. *Journal of Biosocial Science*, **5,** 443–452 (1973)

38 RESSEGUIE, L. J., Comparison of longitudinal and cross-sectional analysis. *American Journal of Epidemiology*, **103,** 551–559 (1976)

39 RUMEAU-ROUQUETTE, C., KAMINSKI, M. and GOUJARD, J. Prediction of perinatal mortality in early pregnancy. *Journal of Perinatal Medicine*, **2,** 196–207 (1974)

40 RUMEAU-ROUQUETTE, C., BRÉART, G., DENIEL, M., HENNEQUIN, J. F. and DU MAZAUBRUN, C. La notion de risque en perinatologie. Revue d'Epidémiologie et de Santé Publique, **24,** 253–276 (1976)

41 RUMEAU-ROUQUETTE, C., GOUJARD, J., KAMINSKI, M., BRÉART, G., DU MAZAUBRUN, C., DENIEL, M. and HENNEQUIN, J. F. Risk indicators and environment – investigations in France. In *Proceedings of the 8th World Congress of Gynaecology and Obstetrics, Mexico City, 1976*, edited by L. Castelazo-Ayala, C. MacGregor, 81–85. Amsterdam, Excerpta Medica (1977)

42 SALING, E. Prämaturitäts–und Dysmaturitäts–Präventions–Programm. In *Perinatale Medizin* (4th German Congress for Perinatal Medicine, Berlin, 1971), edited by E. Saling, and J. W. Dudenhausen. Stuttgart, Thieme (1972)

43 SPELLACY, W. N., BUHI, W. C. and BIRK, S. A. The effectiveness of human placental lactogen measurements as an adjunct in decreasing perinatal deaths. *American Journal of Obstetrics and Gynecology*, **121,** 835–844 (1975)

44 ŠTEMBERA, Z. and ZNAMENÁČEK, K. Screening and differentiation of the high-risk pregnancy. *Praktický Lékař,* **50,** 874–876 (1970)

45 ŠTEMBERA, Z. K., ZEZULÁKOVÁ, J., DITTRICHOVA, J. and ZNAMENÁCEK, K. Identification and quantification of high risk factors affecting fetus and newborn. *4th European Congress of Perinatal Medicine*, (Prague, 1974), edited by Z. K. Štembera, K. Poláček, V. Šabata, 400–406. Stuttgart, Thieme (1975)

46 SUREAU, C. Le concept du haut risque dans la surveillance prénatale. *Revue Internationale de Pediatrie*, **72,** 39–44 (1977)

47 THALHAMMER, O. Verhütung von Frühgeburtlichkeit und přanataler Dystophie. I. Zeitschrift für Geburtshilfe und Perinatologie, **177,** 169–177 (1973)

48 THALHAMMER, O., CORADELLO, H., POLLAK, A., SCHEIBENREITER, S. and SIMBRUNER, G. Prospective and retrospective examination of an easily applicable score to predict the probability of premature birth defined by weight. *Journal of Perinatal Medicine*, **4,** 38–44 (1976)

49 WALTON, A. and HAMMOND, J. The maternal effects on growth and conformation in Shire horse–Shetland pony crosses. *Proceedings of the Royal Society* (London), Series B, **125,** 311–335 (1938)

50 WILCOXON, F. Individual comparisons by ranking methods. *Biometrics Bulletin*, **1,** 80–83 (1945)

51 WILLIAMS, J. A perinatal scoring system, currently undergoing prospective evaluation. (In preparation)

52 WILSON, E. W. and SILL, H. K. Identification of the high risk pregnancy by a scoring system. *New Zealand Medical Journal*, **78,** 437–440 (1973)

53 WORLD HEALTH ORGANISATION. Risk approach for maternal and child health care. Offset publication 39, (1938)

54 YUDKIN, P. Pregnancy order and reproductive loss. *British Medical Journal*, **1,** 715–716 (1980)

5
Pathologic causes of preterm labor

E. J. Quilligan

Prematurity remains one of the major causes of neonatal morbidity and mortality. The University of Southern California study showed that infants born weighing less than 1500 g account for 65 percent of the neonatal mortality[41]. The devastation of prematurity is not limited to death. The incidence of neurological damage in these small infants is significant, varying between 30–50 percent[10,28].

We while we know that certain conditions in the mother or fetus are associated with an increased incidence of prematurity, to assign cause is presumptious, since we don't even know precisely the cause of *term* labor. For the purposes of discussion in this chapter, I shall treat the associations with maternal and fetal conditions separately, realizing of course, that they may be interrelationships.

Maternal factors

General reproductive performance

The general reproductive capability of an individual seems to be reflected by her past performance. Niswander[38] has shown a striking relationship between the incidence of children born weighing less than 2500 g in the present pregnancy and the outcome of a previous pregnancy in terms of infant survival. If the mother had sustained a previous neonatal loss she had a 21.8 percent chance, if white, and 30.5 percent chance, if black, of having a baby weighing less than 2500 g in the present pregnancy. Kaltrieder and Johnson[20] have shown that women with three previous preterm births and no term deliveries have a

59.7 percent incidence of another preterm birth while for women with four previous term births and no preterm births, the incidence of a preterm birth in the next pregnancy is 9.8 percent. This striking difference has been confirmed by the studies of Hobel[16] who demonstrated, using a multiple regression analysis technique, that a history of a preterm birth was the single best indication of the possibility of a preterm birth in the present pregnancy. Kierse *et al.*[21] have shown that preterm birth in the present pregnancy is associated with a history of abortion as well as a history of prematurity. In their study of 8404 patients, the incidence of prematurity was 12.2 percent in those women who had experienced two or more spontaneous abortions prior to the present pregnancy and 2.3 percent in gravida threes without a prior history of spontaneous abortion. The same group found that with a history of two prior preterm deliveries the incidence of preterm delivery was 62.5 percent; however the number of cases was small (five of eight cases).

These women with poor reproductive histories are at least partially a product of their environment. Many studies have demonstrated a higher incidence of prematurity in the lower socio-economic groups[5, 12, 14]. The factors responsible for this difference are hard to dissect. Nutrition would appear to be an obvious choice. The studies in Guatemala[25] have shown an increase in birth weight of infants whose mothers received caloric supplementation; however, whether there was a decrease in the incidence of preterm infants was not determined.

Sir Dugald Baird[2] in his classic studies of perinatal mortality in England, Wales and Scotland demonstrated a significant difference in perinatal mortality depending on the height of the mother, the shorter mother (less than 1.5 m) having a higher perinatal mortality. The lower social classes had a preponderance of the women of short stature; however the association between maternal height and perinatal mortality held regardless of social class. He felt that the evidence implicated the diet from birth to maturity as being of prime importance in the final stature and general health of the mother. If one can assume an increased number of preterm infants as one factor in the increased mortality these studies would also seem to implicate nutritional deficiencies in the etiology of prematurity. Nevertheless, it is very difficult to find studies making the direct link, the reason being the difficulty in precisely determining the gestation. This difficulty applies particularly to the nutritionally deprived, who usually seek prenatal care late in their pregnancy and are frequently uncertain of the date of their last menstrual period.

Therapeutic abortion

The significant increase in therapeutic abortions during the last decade may account for an increasing incidence of preterm births. The initial reports from Hungary[23] would seem to indicate there was an increased risk of premature delivery following induced abortion. Studies in Britain[51] confirmed this finding. On the other hand a study in the Netherlands[46] showed no significant difference in the incidence of delivery before 32 weeks in three groups of primiparae: the rate for those with one previous therapeutic abortion was 3.6 percent; for those with one spontaneous abortion, 3.0 percent; and for those with no abortion, 2.1 percent.

In a large World Health Organization collaborative study[50], three city clusters were examined. Debrecen, Lodz and Warsaw were in one cluster, Copenhagen, Newcastle and Helsinki in a second, and Ljubljana and Stockholm in yet a third. The study showed an increase in prematurity when the abortion was done by vacuum extraction in one city but this was not confirmed in the others. In Debrecen, Lodz and Warsaw, there was a significant difference in preterm delivery in the group whose only previous pregnancy had been an abortion by D & C compared with those who had had a live birth. This was not the case in the other city clusters. It is interesting that the original reports of an increase in preterm births came from those cities of Eastern Europe which continued to have a high incidence of preterm birth. This is perhaps due to excessive cervical dilatation at the time of abortion in some centers. Overall, the WHO report did not seem to demonstrate an increased risk of preterm birth in pregnancies following an abortion.

Cervical conization

Conization of the uterine cervix was reported in 1938 by Miller and Todd[34] to be associated with a higher rate of prematurity. The recent review by Weber and Obel[47] of 17 articles on the subject noted prematurity rates ranging from 0 to 33 percent. Most of the series were relatively small and none took into account other factors such a previous pregnancies. Weber and Obel thought the literature failed to support the assertion that cervical conization was associated with an increased rate of preterm delivery.

Jones, Sweetnam and Hibbard[18] examined the reproductive performance of 76 women who had 91 pregnancies following cervical conization. They matched each study patient with four controls for the following:

(1) singleton birth;
(2) maternal age;
(3) parity;
(4) social class;
(5) date of delivery.

Patients who had previous conization had a significantly higher incidence of preterm deliveries than did the controls. It is interesting to note that the incidence of preterm deliveries in the first pregnancy after conization was 11 percent (six out of 55) while in the second pregnancy it was 40 percent (four out of 10 pregnancies). It is unfortunate that the numbers are too small to draw definitive conclusions and that the study did not seem to be controlled for previous preterm births.

In Lee's[26] study a comparison of pregnancy outcome was made in those patients who had an adequate versus an inadequate conization. 'Adequate' was defined as a conization that was not torn, not different in any part and was 2 cm in diameter and 2 cm in length up the cervical canal including the squamo-columnar junction. The incidence of preterm labor was three of 26 in the adequate cone group and five of 16 in the inadequate group.

Congenital malformations

Congenital malformations of the uterus such as septate uterus and uterus didelphys are known to be associated with a significant increase in the incidence of preterm deliveries[5], the incidence being as high as 30 percent. Bennett and Berry[4] examined by ultrasound the uteri of women who delivered prior to the 37th week. Eight women (16.3 percent) were found to have a congenital fundal abnormality; whereas no fundal abnormalities were demonstrated in 100 control patients who delivered at term. Since the incidence of this anomaly is less than 0.5 percent in a general parous population, it behooves the prudent physician to examine all women delivering prematurely, either manually, by ultrasound, hysterosalpingography or by hysteroscopy to detect any problem. This is particularly important since surgical correction may be of real benefit[17] in salvaging subsequent pregnancies.

Maternal smoking

The most marked difference noted in the fetus of a mother who smokes during her pregnancy is a reduction in fetal weight. *Figure 5.1* from MacMahon, Alpert and Salper[30] shows a marked shift to the left in the distribution of birth weights of infants of mothers who smoke. There is

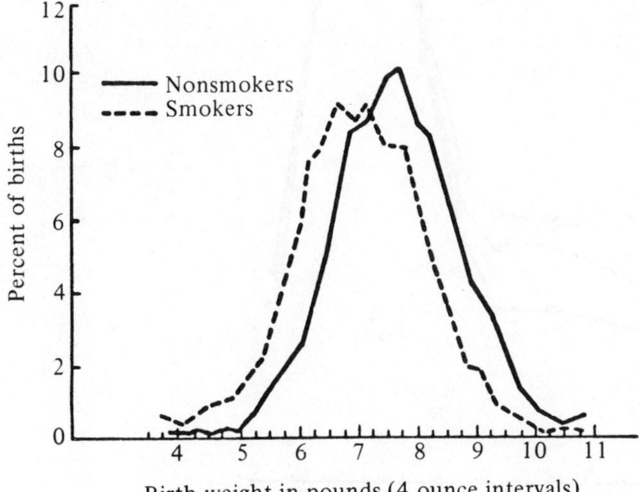

Figure 5.1 Distribution of birth weight by maternal smoking status. Smokers were those who consumed 20 or more cigarettes per day during pregnancy. (From MacMahon, Alpert and Salper[30], courtesy of the Editor and publishers, *American Journal of Epidemiology*)

also a decrease in gestational length associated with smoking, which is somewhat dependent on the number of cigarettes smoked per day (*Figure 5.2*)[33]. The effect of cigarette smoking on the fetus seems to involve at least two constituents of the cigarette smoke, carbon monoxide and nicotine. Carbon monoxide binds with hemoglobin to reduce available oxygen sites; thus the more carbon monoxide the less oxygen available to the fetus. Cole, Hawkins and Roberts[7] found the mean maternal carboxyhemoglobin to be 1.2 percent in nonsmokers and 4.1 percent in smokers. Nicotine is a vasoconstrictor and also causes release of epinephrine. Lehtovista and Forss[27] studied the effects on intervillous blood flow following smoking and noted an immediate decrease which did not return to normal for 15 minutes. It is easy to see

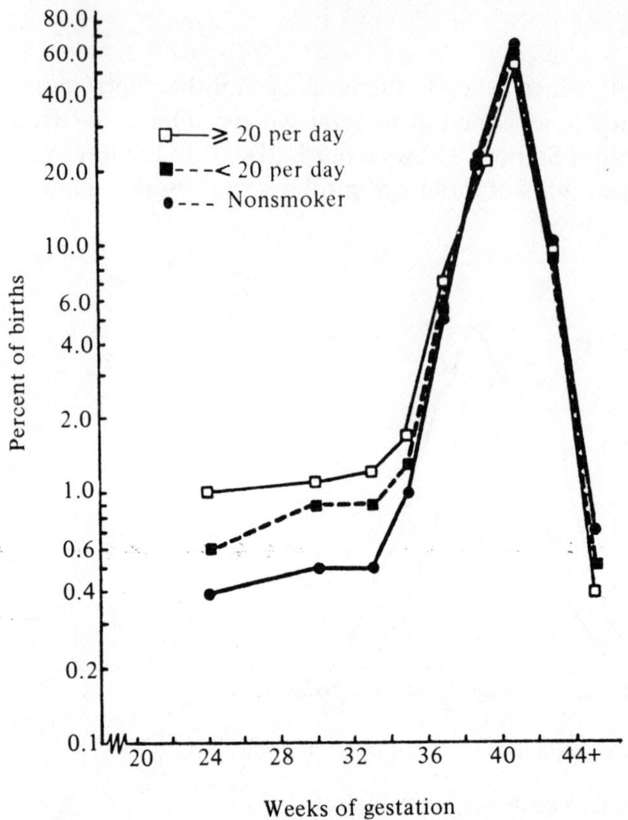

Figure 5.2 Distribution of gestation lengths by maternal smoking level, Ontario Perinatal Mortality Study. (From Meyer[33], courtesy of Urban and Schwarzenberg)

how these two effects, increase in carbon monoxide and reduced uterine blood flow, could result in decreased fetal weight. Why the labor also begins prematurely has not yet been explained.

Iatrogenic conditions

Bennett and Berry[4] noted that 27 percent of their preterm births resulted from deliberate obstetric interventions. The majority of these were for valid obstetric indications, but a few inadvertently preterm births in every series are brought about by elective induction or elective repeat cesarean section. Flaksman, Vollman and Benfield[11] reported that 5.4 percent of their preterm deliveries were iatrogenic. In no case was amniotic fluid L/S ratio analysis, or ultrasonic measurements of fetal size performed prior to delivery. There was one death in this group of 32 infants, and three infants were handicapped. With the techniques available today there should be no elective repeat cesarean section performed unless the pregnancy has been dated by ultrasound prior to 20 weeks gestation or there is a mature L/S ratio (greater than 2.0) in the amniotic fluid. The same criteria should apply to elective induction of labor although there must be very few modern indications for this procedure.

Medical problems

Diabetes and hypertension are not necessarily associated with *spontaneous* preterm delivery, but certain medical conditions do tend to shorten pregnancy. Niswander[13, 39, 40] has shown a higher incidence of low birth weight infants in asthmatics, patients with hyperthyroidism, glomerulonephritis, genitourinary tract infection with a temperature of 38.0°C (100.4°F) or higher, alcoholism, drug habituation and heart disease.

Acute pyelonephritis and appendicitis in pregnancy are associated with an increased incidence of preterm labors. In both instances one of the theories of the etiology of the labor is uterine irritation from the adjacent inflamed organ. Two other factors have been implicated in labor associated with a febrile illness – temperature elevation and the release of bacterial endotoxins. Kullander[54] demonstrated that lipopolysaccharides injected into pregnant rabbits caused significant temperature elevation. Subsequently, these animals had a preterm delivery rate (50 percent) similar to a second group given oxytocin to induce labor, and a significantly higher preterm delivery rate than the saline controls. One could postulate a direct action of the lipopolysaccharide on the myometrium; however, the fact that the majority of the births occurred during the second hour after injection of lipopolysaccharide and all the births occurred during the first hour after the oxytocin injection speaks against a direct action. On the other hand, Wiedermann, Stone and Pataki[49] have demonstrated a direct stimulatory effect on the myometrium *in vitro* of the endotoxin from *Escherichia coli*.

Pregnant women previously treated for pituitary adenomas had a preterm delivery rate of 37 percent[31]. Jurgensen and Taubert[19] reported cervical incompetence and prematurity in six of 10 women treated with bromocriptine while Singer, Cooke and Tachman[45] found no increase in prematurity in 43 patients treated with bromocriptine.

Cervical incompetence

Cervical incompetence is primarily associated with second trimester abortion but may also be a cause of preterm delivery. The classic history is a painless rapid labor in a woman who has had either a spontaneous or therapeutic abortion or term pregnancy. This is probably one of the most over-diagnosed conditions in obstetrics and it is almost a diagnosis made in retrospect; that is, if there is a history of a painless, rapid, second trimester abortion or preterm labor, and a suture is placed around the cervix during the next pregnancy with a successful conclusion at term, the woman is said to have an incompetent cervix. The exact cervical pathology is usually unknown, although in some cases there appears to be a defect in the fibers of the internal os of the cervix.

Fetal problems

Multiple pregnancy

Patients with multiple pregnancy are known to have a shorter period of gestation than those carrying a single fetus. McKeown and Record[29] found the average duration of pregnancy to be 280.5 days for singleton pregnancies, 261.6 days for twins, 246.8 days for triplets and 236.8 days for quadruplets. This decrease in gestational length has been postulated to be due to overdistension of the uterus with contractions ensuing when the muscle fibers reach a critical length.

Polyhydramnios

Polyhydramnios also produces uterine overdistension, and its incidence varies between 0.4 percent and 1.6 percent[43]. Kirbinen and Jouppila[22] found an incidence of polyhydramnios of 0.4 percent in 14 248 deliveries occurring at the Department of Obstetrics and Gynecology, University of Oulu. Preterm delivery occurred in 37.8 percent of the singleton pregnancies and in 35.7 percent of the multiple pregnancies. Fetal anomalies were noted in 30.0 percent of those pregnancies. Many authors have found a high incidence of diabetes and erythroblastosis associated with polyhydramnios[3,22,43,35]. The high fetal mortality of 42–69 percent is attributable to the increase in congenital malformations and prematurity.

Position anomalies

Patients with breech presentation have a prematurity rate of about 20 percent. During the early third trimester about 20 percent of babies are in a breech presentation; thus if labor commences during this period there will be a significantly increased incidence of breech delivery.

Placental factors

Some authors state that women with placenta previa have an incidence of preterm birth roughly five times that of gravidae with normally implanted placentas[40]. The exact frequency of preterm birth will depend to some extent on the management program elected once the diagnosis is made.

Premature separation of a normally implanted placenta is also associated with a high preterm delivery rate, roughly four times normal[40]. The reason for the premature separation is unknown. Mengert *et al.*[32] found that compression of the vena cava could cause abruption of the placenta, but this is not felt by Pritchard[42] to be a major factor. Folic acid deficiency[15] was also implicated in abruptio placenta; however Whalley *et al.*[48] found normal folate levels in patients with abruptio placenta. Trauma to the maternal abdomen is responsible for premature separation of the placenta in less than one percent of cases[42]. Both placenta previa and premature separation of the normally implanted placenta have a tendency to recur in subsequent pregnancies, and so both are continuing contributors to prematurity.

Premature rupture of membranes

Premature rupture of the membranes is variously defined. A useful working definition is the failure of labor to ensue within one hour following rupture of the membranes. Burchell[6] found a 23 percent incidence of premature rupture, using this definition. The reason the membranes rupture prematurely is not well understood. Danforth, McElin and States[8] did not find any weakness in the membranes when tested for bursting strength. Artal *et al.*[1] had similar findings, but they did demonstrate that the prematurely ruptured membranes were thinner at the rupture site than membranes which had ruptured spontaneously during labor. They also found that the modules of elasticity in the periplacental area of the membrane was lower in the membrane which ruptured prematurely.

Infection

Infection of the fetus or amniotic fluid is associated with an increased frequency of preterm delivery. The following infective agents are associated with preterm delivery.

(1) Viruses.
Cytomegalovirus
Herpes simplex
Rubella
Smallpox
Hepatitis

(2) Bacteria.
Treponema pallidum
Mycobacterium tuberculosis
Listeria monocytogenes
Vibrio fetus
Salmonella typhosa

(3) Protozoa
Toxoplasma gondii

(From Remington and Klein[44].)

Naeye[36] found 17 percent of the fetal and neonatal deaths in the Collaborative Perinatal Project to be associated with amniotic fluid infections in the presence of intact membranes. The majority of these deaths were due to prematurity. He[37] has shown that the major associated factor is low socio-economic status.

There are many other factors associated with the premature onset of parturition. Until we know more about the basic mechanisms of term labor, we must consider all these associations to be potential causes and try to eliminate or treat them.

References

1 ARTAL, R., SOKOL, R. J., NEUMAN, M., BURSTEIN, A. H. and STOJKOV, J. The mechanical properties of prematurely and non-prematurely ruptured membranes: Methods and preliminary results. *American Journal of Obstetrics and Gynecology*, **125,** 655–659 (1976)

2 BAIRD, D. The evolution of modern obstetrics. *Lancet*, **2,** 557–564 (1960)

3 BARRY, A. P. Hydramnios. A survey of 100 cases. *Irish Journal of Medical Science*, **6,** 257–264 (1953)

4 BENNETT, M. J. and BERRY, J. V. J. Preterm labor and congenital malformation of the uterus. *Ultrasound in Medicine and Biology*, **5,** 83–85 (1979)

5 BLAIR, R. G. Pregnancy associated with congenital malformations of the reproductive tract. *Journal of Obstetrics and Gynaecology of the British Empire*, **67,** 36–42 (1960)

6 BURCHELL, R. Premature spontaneous rupture of the membranes. *American Journal of Obstetrics and Gynecology*, **88**, 251–255 (1964)

7 COLE, P. V., HAWKINS, L. H. and ROBERTS, D. Smoking during pregnancy and its effect on the fetus. *Journal of Obstetrics and Gynaecology of the British Commonwealth*, **79,** 782–787 (1972)

8 DANFORTH, D., MCELIN, T. and STATES, H. Bursting tension of fetal membranes. *American Journal of Obstetrics and Gynecology*, **65,** 480–490 (1953)

9 FEDRICK, J. and ANDERSON, A. B. M. Factors associated with spontaneous preterm birth. *British Journal of Obstetrics and Gynaecology*, **83,** 342–350 (1976)

10 FITZHARDINGE, P. M. Follow-up studies on the low birth weight infant. *Clinics in Perinatology*, **3,** 503–516 (1976)

11 FLAKSMAN, R. J., VOLLMAN, J. H. and BENFIELD, D. G. Iatrogenic prematurity due to elective termination of the uncomplicated pregnancy. A major perinatal health care problem. *American Journal of Obstetrics and Gynecology*, **132,** 885–888 (1978)

12 GARDINER, S. In discussion of Hendricks' paper. (reference 14) *American Journal of Obstetrics and Gynecology*, **97,** 619–620 (1967)

13 GORDON, M., NISWANDER, K., BERENDES, H. and KANTOR, A. Fetal morbidity following potentially anoxigenic conditions. VII. Bronchial asthma. *American Journal of Obstetrics and Gynecology*, **106,** 421–429 (1970)

14 HENDRICKS, C. H. Delivery patterns and reproductive efficiency among groups of different socioeconomic status and ethnic origins. *American Journal of Obstetrics and Gynecology*, **97,** 608–624 (1967)

15 HIBBARD, B. and JEFFCOATE, T. Abruptio placenta. *Obstetrics and Gynecology*, **27,** 155–167 (1966)

16 HOBEL, C. J. The ABC's of Perinatal Medicine. In *Major Mental Handicap: Methods and Cost of Prevention*. Ciba Foundation Symposium 59 (new series), 53. Amsterdam, Elsevier (1978)

17 JONES, H. W., DELFS, E. and JONES, G. E. S. Reproductive difficulties in double uterus. The place of plastic reconstruction. *American Journal of Obstetrics and Gynecology*, **72,** 865–883 (1956)

18 JONES, J. M., SWEETNAM, P. and HIBBARD, B. M. The outcome of pregnancy after cone biopsy of the cervix: a case control study. *British Journal of Obstetrics and Gynaecology*, **86,** 913–916 (1979)

19 JURGENSEN, O. and TAUBERT, H-D. Cervical incompetence and premature delivery after bromocriptine therapy for infertility. *Lancet*, **2,** 203–204 (1977)

20 KALTRIEDER, B. and JOHNSON, J. Patients at high risk for low birth weight delivery. *American Journal of Obstetrics and Gynecology*, **124,** 251–256 (1967)

21 KIERSE, M. J. N. C., RUSH, R. W., ANDERSON, A. B. M. and TURNBULL, A. C. Risk of preterm delivery with previous preterm delivery and/or abortion. *British Journal of Obstetrics and Gynaecology*, **85,** 81–85 (1978)

22 KIRBINEN, P. and JOUPPILA, P. Polyhydramnion. A clinical study. *Annales Chirurgiae et Gynaecologiae Fenniae*, **67,** 117–122 (1978)

23 KOTOSEK, A. In *4th European Congress of Perinatal Medicine*, (Prague, 1974) edited by Z. K. Štembera, K. Polàček, V. Šabata, Stuttgart, Thieme (1975)

24 KULLANDER, S. Fever and parturition. An experimental study in rabbits. *Acta Obstetrica Gynaecologica Scandinavica*, (Supplement) **66,** 77–85 (1977)

25 LECHTIG, A., DELGADO, H., LASKY, R., YARBROUGH, C., KLEIN, R. E., HABICHT, J. P. and BEHAR, M. Maternal nutrition and fetal growth in developing countries. *American Journal of Diseases in Children*, **129,** 553–556 (1975)

26 LEE, N. H. The effect of cone biopsy on subsequent pregnancy outcome. *Gynecologic Oncology*, **6,** 1–6 (1978)

27 LEHTOVISTA, P. and FORSS, M. The acute effect of smoking and the intervillous blood flow of the placenta. *British Journal of Obstetrics and Gynaecology*, **85,** 729–731 (1978)

28 LUBCHENCO, L. D., DELEVORIA-PAPADOPOULOS, M. and SEARES, D. Long-term follow-up studies of prematurely born infants. II. Influence of birth weight and gestational age on sequellae. *Journal of Pediatrics*, **80,** 509–512 (1972)

29 MCKEOWN, T. and RECORD, R. Observations on fetal growth in multiple pregnancies in man. *Journal of Endocrinology*, **8**, 386–401 (1952)

30 MACMAHON, B., ALPERT, M. and SALPER, E. J. Infant weight and parental smoking habits. *American Journal of Epidemiology*, **83,** 247–261 (1965)

31 MAGYAR, D. M. and MARSHALL, J. R. Pituitary tumors and pregnancy. *American Journal of Obstetrics and Gynecology*, **132,** 739–751 (1978)

32 MENGERT, W., GOODROU, J., CAMPBELL, R. and HAYNES, D. Observations on the pathogenesis of premature separation of the normally implanted placenta. *American Journal of Obstetrics and Gynecology*, **66,** 1104–1112 (1953)

33 MEYER, M. B. Effect of maternal smoking at altitude on birth weight and gestation. In *The Epidemiology of Prematurity*, edited by D. M. Reed, F. J. Stanley, 81–104 Baltimore, Urban and Schwarzenberg (1977)

34 MILLER, N. G. and TODD, O. E. Conization of the cervix. *Surgery, Gynecology and Obstetrics*, **67,** 265–268 (1938)

35 MURRAY, S. R. Hydramnios. A study of 846 cases. *American Journal of Obstetrics and Gynecology*, **88,** 65–67 (1964)

36 NAEYE, R. L. Causes of perinatal mortality in the US. Collaborative Perinatal Project. *Journal of the American Medical Association*, **237,** 228–229 (1977)

37 NAEYE, R. L. Coitus and associated amniotic fluid infections. *New England Journal of Medicine*, **301,** 1198–1200 (1979)

38 NISWANDER, K. and GORDON, M. *The Women and their Pregnancies*. Philadelphia, DHEW Publication, NIH No. 73–379 (1972)

39 NISWANDER, K. and BERENDES, H. Effect of maternal cardiac disease on the infant. *Clinical Obstetrics and Gynecology*, **11,** 1026–1040 (1968)

40 NISWANDER, K. C. Obstetric factors related to prematurity. In *The Epidemiology of Prematurity*, edited by D. M. Reed, F. J. Stanley. 249. Baltimore, Urban and Schwarzenberg (1977)

41 PAUL, R. H., KOH, K. S. and MONFARED, A. H. Obstetric factors influencing outcome in infants weighing from 1001–1500 g. *American Journal of Obstetrics and Gynecology*, **133,** 503–507 (1979)

42 PRITCHARD, J. Genesis of severe placenta abruption. *American Journal of Obstetrics and Gynecology*, **108,** 22–27 (1970)

43 QUEENAN, J. T. and GADOW, E. C. Polyhydramnios chronic versus acute. *American Journal of Obstetrics and Gynecology*, **108,** 349–355 (1970)

44 REMINGTON, J. T. and KLEIN, J. O. *Infectious Disease of the Fetus and Newborn Infant*, 6. Philadelphia, W. B. Saunders (1976)

45 SINGER, A., COOKE, I. D. and TACHMAN, E. Cervical incompetence and premature delivery after bromocriptine therapy for infertility. *Lancet*, **2,** 503 (1977)

46 VANDER SLIKKE, J. W. and TREFFERS, P. E. Influence of induced abortion on gestational duration in subsequent pregnancies. *British Medical Journal*, **1,** 270–272 (1978)

47 WEBER, T. and OBEL, E. Pregnancy complications following conization of the uterine cervix. *Acta Obstetrica et Gynecologica Scandinavica*, **58,** 259–263 (1979)

48 WHALLEY, P. G., SCOTT, D. E., and PRITCHARD, J. A. Maternal folate deficiency and pregnancy wastage. *American Journal of Obstetrics and Gynecology*, **105,** 670–678 (1969)

49 WIEDERMANN, J., STONE, M. L. and PATAKI, R. Urinary tract infections and uterine activity. I. Effect of *Escherichia coli* endotoxins on uterine motility in vitro. *American Journal of Obstetrics and Gynecology*, **84,** 290–296 (1962)

50 WORLD HEALTH ORGANIZATION TASK FORCE. Gestation, birth weight and spontaneous abortion in pregnancy after induced abortion. *Lancet*, **1,** 142–145 (1979)

51 WRIGHT, C. S. W., CAMPBELL, S. and BRAGLEY, S. Second-trimester abortion after vaginal termination of pregnancy. *Lancet*, **1,** 1278–1279 (1972)

52 ZABRISKIE, J. R. Pregnancy and the malformed uterus. Report of 92 cases. *Western Surgery*, **70,** 293–296 (1962)

6

Preterm premature rupture of the membranes

Michael W. Varner and Rudolph P. Galask

The subject of preterm premature rupture of the membranes (PPRM) has generated a myriad of diagnostic and therapeutic regimens. The majority of these protocols have concentrated on the duration of rupture as related to the dichotomous threats of prematurity from early delivery and infection resulting from prolonged observation. With the continued improvements in the fields of maternal health and neonatology, past recommendations require re-evaluation. In order to accomplish this, a critical review of the literature was undertaken. In addition, all instances of PPRM occurring at the University of Iowa Hospitals from July 1, 1977 through December 31, 1979 were analyzed.

While not proposing absolute or final solutions to this problem we believe that a review of the current theories of etiology and management of PPRM is vitally important to the practicing obstetrician.

Etiology

The etiology of PPRM, while probably secondary to multiple factors, continues to remain an enigma. The incidence varies between 0.7 percent[22] and 2.1 percent[5] of all pregnancies and contributes signficantly to perinatal mortality. Possible etiologic factors include cervical and vaginal infections or colonization by certain bacteria, nutritional deficiencies, abnormal membrane physiology, incompetent cervix or other uterine anomalies, and uterine overdistention due to either polyhydramnios and/or multiple gestation. PPRM is more often associated with a similar episode with or without premature labor in a previous pregnancy.

The opinion of many clinicians is that ascending infection is not a problem with intact membranes, and that the risk is directly proportional to the duration of rupture[61]. However, it is increasingly evident that the amniotic membrane is more than simple mechanical barrier against infection. Many studies have reported amniotic fluid colonization and/or infection in labor with intact membranes[16, 35, 54, 57, 64]. The incidence of amniotic fluid colonization has been estimated to be as high as 10 percent of term pregnancies in labor[42]. Once reaching the amniotic fluid, bacteria may either be aspirated by the fetus, causing pneumonia; enter the auditory canal, causing otitis or meningitis; or the newborn may be clinically uninfected. The occurrence of amnionitis and perinatal sepsis with intact membranes is most commonly described in premature infants from patients in the lower socio-economic group.

Intra-amniotic infection with *intact* membranes has been postulated as an explanation for the early onset of neonatal group B β-hemolytic streptococcal infection, since the occurrence of fatal sepsis in the newborn may be observed too soon after membrane rupture to postulate acquisition of the organisms through cervical passage alone. Therefore, identification of a gravida whose vagina is colonized with group B streptococci and with PPRM is considered by some to be an appropriate indication for antepartum antibiotic treatment[22, 63], even though the frequency of neonatal sepsis is low as compared to the incidence of vaginal colonization. The absence of maternal antibody to type III group B streptococci in the presence of maternal cervical colonization may indicate fetal susceptability as described by Baker and Casper[9]. Since the eradication of genital tract colonization is difficult, the use of antibiotics to treat vaginal colonization before term should not be routine until the problem is fully understood.

Several authors[3, 27, 34, 47] have reported a relationship between maternal *Neisseria gonorrhoeae* infection and PPRM. The potential for neonatal disease with the organism is well established and has been recently reviewed[39]. Ward *et al.*[67] have convincingly outlined the mechanism of gonococcal invasion of tubal epithelium. Although as yet undocumented, a similar mechanism of cellular invasion and subsequent cellular lysis may underlie the increased frequency of PPRM seen with maternal gonococcal colonization or infection.

Bobitt and Ledger[18] studied amniotic fluid at the time of rupture and noted a high incidence of positive cultures. They reported an association between large numbers of bacteria (greater than 1000 per milliliter of amniotic fluid) and either low birth weight infants or subsequent infection, and suggested that an occult intra-amniotic fluid infection may precede premature rupture of the membranes. While the relationship between the presence of leukocytes in amniotic fluid sediment and subsequent infections has been reported[44], other authors feel that this is not diagnostic of infection[18, 26]. The literature appears to indicate that the absence of white cells correlates well with the absence of infection but the presence of white cells is not always associated with infection.

Bacteria which are able to cause disease in either the mother or the neonate have been shown to comprise part of the indigenous flora of the vagina and cervix of the pregnant patient. These women are often asymptomatic even when subsequent infection of the newborn occurs. Although it has been shown that a progressive decrease in the prevalence of certain Gram negative facultative and anaerobic bacteria occurs as term approaches, the increased incidence of infections among premature newborns is commonly associated with these organisms, suggesting that several mechanisms are involved in causing the disease[31].

Endotoxins from Gram negative bacteria enhancing uterine irritability have been described and histologic examinations of animal decidua have revealed significant necrosis following exposure to endotoxin[72]. Recent studies have shown that decidua and chorioamniotic membranes are responsible for the synthesis of prostaglandins involved in uterine activation, especially $PGF_{2\alpha}$, and these tissues may function as a reservoir for esterified arachidonic acid. Potential destruction of decidua by endotoxin, either from local or systemic infection, could release quantities of prostaglandin precursors that in turn would be converted by prostaglandin synthase to prostaglandins, causing premature labor. Whether Gram negative endotoxin has a direct effect on membrane potentials, stabilities, and subsequent rupture, has not been examined.

Nutritional deficiencies as a cause of PPRM are suggested by the work of Artal *et al.*[5] who have demonstrated significantly lowered serum copper levels in both fetuses and in mothers presenting with premature rupture of membranes at term. Although copper levels from the chorioamniotic membranes were similar in both premature rupture and control groups, they suggested that a limited availability of copper could alter the growth and maturation of the connective tissue components of the chorioamniotic membranes. The lower copper levels may reflect the lower progesterone and estradiol levels seen in patients with premature rupture[25]. An increased frequency of PPRM in patients with severe ascorbic acid deficiency has been reported by Wideman, Baird and Balding[69].

In pregnancies requiring cervical cerclage for incompetent cervix, PPRM has been reported to be the most frequent complication of the procedure[1].

The mechanical properties of the chorioamniotic membranes have been studied. No relationship between the strength of membranes and PPRM has been demonstrated[56]. Membranes from patients with and without premature rupture have been shown to withstand greater pressures than those present during labor. Trauma to the uterus is not thought to be an important factor, but may explain certain isolated cases.

Artal *et al.*[6] studied membranes of term pregnancies with and without premature rupture and showed that the prematurely ruptured membranes were thinner and less elastic near the site of rupture than near the site of placental implantation in the same patients. Parry-Jones and Priya[55] also demonstrated a significant decrease in elasticity of those membranes that ruptured before the onset of labor, irrespective of the duration of pregnancy. More recently, Lavery and Miller[45] suggested that premature rupture may be related to changes in membrane thickness associated with acute and chronic mechanical stress.

A report by Milingos *et al*[51] demonstrated a significant relationship between premature rupture of membranes and lower daily barometric pressures, although no distinction was made between term and preterm rupture.

Complications

Concern with intrauterine infection was first raised with Ballantyne's[10] description of sepsis *in utero*, reported in 1902. However, as late as the 1950's attention was directed towards documenting maternal morbidity and mortality with relatively infrequent advocacy of active intervention for fetal indications. In the 1960's maternal infection was still considered important but there was increasing recognition that prematurity rather than infection was the primary cause of perinatal morbidity and mortality, especially in cases of PPRM[52]. During the past decade neonatal survival has been enhanced by significant technical advances which have improved the prediction of fetal lung maturity and have allowed successful treatment of both the infant with immature lungs and the infant with sepsis.

Today the complications remain maternal and fetal infection and fetal immaturity, most commonly the respiratory distress syndrome (RDS). Accordingly, the decision of whether to intervene or delay following PPRM rests not only on the clinical and diagnostic information obtained for each patient but on the overall morbidity and mortality rates within each care facility as well. It is apparent that marked differences occur between various population groups, areas of the country and even between hospitals in the same city. Therefore, the recommendations from a metropolitan center with a predominantly indigent population may not be the same for a rural, middle-class population.

Diagnosis

The diagnosis of PPRM is based on a history of an uncontrollable, watery, vaginal discharge. Although the membranes may rupture with a sudden and obvious gush of fluid, PPRM may pose a diagnostic problem if the watery leakage is slight and intermittent. The discharge must be distinguished from a leukorrheal discharge, loss of urine, or the liquefaction of cervical mucus that often precedes the onset of labor. The physician should look for vaginal vault pooling of amniotic fluid by sterile speculum examination as well as the conversion of nitrazine paper from yellow to purple[15]. False-positive nitrazine reactions can occur in the presence of urine, blood, cervical mucus, examination glove powder, or examination lubricant, so care in the interpretation is necessary. Ferning will be observed when air-dried amniotic fluid from the vaginal pool is examined microscopically, while vaginal discharge does not produce ferning[40]. Vaginal fluid may also be stained with 0.1 percent Nile blue sulfate, allowed to react for five minutes, and examined for orange-stained fetal squamous cells. Atlay and Sutherst[7] have also recommended confirmation by transabdominal intra-amniotic instillation of 5 ml Evans blue dye. If the membranes are ruptured, the dye will appear in the vagina within 30–40 minutes. This technique should be reserved only for the rare situation that requires absolute diagnosis.

Management

When the diagnosis of PPRM has been established the obstetrician must decide the most appropriate management of the patient and her fetus. The accessability of a neonatal intensive care unit having a reasonable perinatal survival rate in the community will permit adequate care locally. However, if facilities are not available or have an unacceptably low perinatal survival rate then transport of the undelivered patient to a regional referral center is warranted. This is further discussed in Chapter 15.

Management should be based upon both maternal and fetal considerations, recognizing several generalizations from the literature:

(1) PPRM is more frequent in women of lower socio-economic status[53];
(2) infectious complications are more common in women of lower socio-economic status[65];
(3) the incidence of infectious morbidity rises with increasing duration of PPRM and is inversely related to gestational age;
(4) complications of prematurity, especially those involving inadequate lung maturation, are inversely related to gestational age;
(5) the earlier PPRM occurs in pregnancy, the higher is the incidence of cord prolapse, reflecting a relationship between fetal size and malpresentation[17].

The establishment of PPRM protocols by many obstetric services reflects their experience with the generalizations stated. Although rigidly applied by some services, they vary widely between institutions. The predominant consideration is balancing the risk of infection if the pregnancy is allowed to continue against the risk of prematurity associated with early intervention. All of these protocols clearly depend on the clinical experience of a specific institution and emphasize the importance of reviewing the experience of the institution(s) with which the practitioner is associated.

Most clinicians agree that when the diagnosis of PPRM is established and the gestation is greater than 36 weeks, induction of labor is appropriate unless other obstetric contra-indications are present.

When PPRM occurs in the absence of labor at less than 36 weeks gestation, or when the duration of gestation is uncertain, a wide range of recommendations are reported. Since spontaneous labor occurs less frequently prior to 36 weeks than at term, the obstetrician is compelled to make a decision based on the risks of prematurity from early induction versus the risk of infection by allowing the pregnancy to continue.

Investigators studying urban and/or indigent patient populations[68] have advocated immediate delivery in all cases of premature rupture of membranes because of the danger of maternal morbidity and mortality.

The underlying tenet of this recommendation is the reported relationship between increased duration of premature rupture and the development of chorioamnionitis. Chorioamnionitis has been reported to occur as frequently as 46 percent[41] in this patient population. Burchell[20] reported that the perinatal mortality rate doubled for every 24 hours following premature rupture, and cited a progressively increasing risk of maternal mortality as the duration of PPRM increased.

Several investigators[19, 20, 30] have recommended prophylactic antibiotics in cases of premature rupture of the membranes. However, double-blind studies have failed to show an advantage to either fetus or neonate from antepartum antibiotic therapy even though maternal puerperal morbidity was variably decreased[36, 46]. Other potential complications of prophylactic antibiotics include the possibility of inducing antibiotic resistant bacteria, interference with neonatal culture results, masking of subsequent perinatal infections, and causing drug reactions. Some authors have recommended the use of antibiotics at the onset of labor if the latent period is greater than 24 hours, but this has not been shown to significantly decrease perinatal morbidity or mortality[32].

The majority of studies recommending aggressive management were conducted prior to 1970 on urban, lower socio-economic populations before many of the advances in neonatology occurred. Recently a report from a similar patient population failed to demonstrate the severity of many of these previously reported complications[60].

The aggressive management of PPRM carries a rather high incidence of perinatal problems associated with immaturity, primarily those related to lung maturation.

Although several retrospective studies[8, 37] failed to document a protective effect, recent data suggests that maturation of the fetal lung occurs more rapidly with PPRM. Richardson *et al.*[58] have shown an earlier than otherwise anticipated increase in the L/S ratio in such patients and a decreased incidence of RDS with PPRM has been noted by others[13, 14, 66, 70, 71]. Most authors report the decrease in incidence of RDS only after a latent period of 16–48 hours. Bauer, Stern and Colle[12] have demonstrated that cord blood corticosteroid levels were increased in pregnancies complicated by PPRM. Smith, Worthington and Maloney[62] have shown similar increases of corticosteroids in amniotic fluid in cases of PPRM. The latter observation supports the speculation that the benefit accruing to the fetus is due to 'stress' between the event and delivery.

Most authors agree that fetal pulmonary studies should be employed whenever safely feasible to aid individual patient management, particularly in those patients in whom the duration of gestation or fetal pulmonary maturity is unknown. This should include ultrasound-directed amniocentesis, since vaginally collected amniotic fluid may yield a falsely elevated L/S ratio due to maternal blood contamination. The determination of amniotic fluid phosphatidylglycerol may circumvent this problem[33] in the future and it appears that PPRM may accelerate phosphatidylglycerol production[21]. In some patients, the easily performed foam stability, or shake, test is an alternative technique that may be employed in the absence of blood or meconium contamination to estimate fetal lung maturity[23]. Although its value is still unknown[4], interest has also been expressed in the spectrophotometric absorbance at 650 nm of amniotic fluid as an assessment of fetal pulmonary maturity[24, 59]. Recently, expectant management with PPRM has been advocated to allow fetal lung maturation[14, 29, 38, 49], and fetal growth appears to progress at a normal rate[2].

However, if maternal genital herpes infection is present, then expectant mangement is contra-indicated. The coexistence of PPRM, a viable fetus, and an active Herpes simplex virus infection of the cervix, vagina, or vulva is an indication for abdominal delivery within four hours of rupture. Although only 50 percent of intrapartum exposures to the virus result in clinical neonatal disease, the mortality rate of 65 percent and the frequency of devastating neurologic sequelae in survivors make this an unacceptable risk.

The policy of expectant management has been followed at the University of Iowa. Management includes a single sterile speculum examination at the time of admission for documentation of PPRM and collection of fluid for maturity studies and cultures. Bimanual examinations are not performed until obstetrically indicated. Cervical cultures are performed at the time of confirmation of PPRM for the identification of group A or B β-hemolytic streptococci or *Neisseria gonorrhoeae* to identify a population at increased risk of infection. The patient is hospitalized while amniotic fluid is leaking and daily white blood cell counts are obtained. The maternal temperature and pulse, as well as the fetal heart rate, are checked every four to six hours. Prophylactic antibiotics are not employed.

An ultrasound examination is performed when indicated to confirm the duration of gestation. Amniocentesis is performed when feasible at the time of ultrasound examination to obtain amniotic fluid for maturity studies and culture. Amniotic fluid obtained by amniocentesis is the only valid sample for culture to identify occult intrauterine infection. In addition, the amniotic fluid collected can be examined microscopically for leukocytes and bacteria, although the significance of these findings is controversial at present. The phosphate to zinc ratio[43], which has been reported to correlate with the antibacterial effect of amniotic fluid, is also performed. The lack of antibacterial activity in the future may prove to be useful in predicting an increased likelihood of ascending infection. However, further evaluation of this technique is necessary before it can be recommended for general use.

In order to substantiate the clinical impression that few complications were encountered with the aforementioned conservative management protocol, a review of all cases of PPRM treated at the University of Iowa Hospitals between July 1, 1977, and December 31, 1979, was undertaken. During this period 91 patients were admitted with documented PPRM and gave birth to 100 infants between 28 and 36 weeks gestation. There were no stillbirths and no cases were excluded. The gestational age was based on information obtained from the last menstrual period, early examinations, ultrasound studies, and gestational age assessment by the method of Ballard[11].

Table 6.1 Comparison of perinatal survival and gestational age in the presence of PPRM.

Weeks gestation	*All newborns (%)*	*PPRM total (%) (n = 100)*	*PPRM > 48 h (%) (n = 65)*
28–29	46.5	100	100
30–31	76.7	82	90
32–33	96.1	100	100
34–35	97.1	100	100
36	99.5	100	100
Total	89.6	97	98.4

During this 30 month interval there were three neonatal deaths in the study group, all associated with severe RDS and subsequent intracranial hemorrhage, for a perinatal mortality rate of three percent. *Table 6.1* shows the percent survival of all newborns[28] from pregnancies complicated by PPRM. Because of the relatively small numbers involved, statistical significance is not achieved. However, it is apparent from the data that conservative management of PPRM has not increased the perinatal mortality rate on this service.

Table 6.2 Comparison of various studies of the effect of duration of PPRM on the incidence of amnionitis

Duration (hours)	*Thibeault and Emmanouildes*[66]		*Miller, Pupkin and Crenshaw*[52]		*Schrieder and Benedetti*[60]		*University of Iowa*	
	Incidence	*%*	*Incidence*	*%*	*Incidence*	*%*	*Incidence*	*%*
< 24	4/100	4	3/79	4	5/17	29	0/11	0
24–48	4/18	22	4/41	10	Not reported		2/20	10
> 48	12/35	33	5/31	16	Not reported		4/60	6.7
> 1 week	Not reported		Not reported		6/23	26	1/15†	6.6
Total	20/153	13.1	12/151	7.7	24/90*	26.7	6/91	6.6

*Report also includes 50 patients with PPRM from 24 hours to 1 week with incidence of amnionitis of 26 percent (13/50)
†Included in the total of the preceding 4/60 in the line above

Table 6.3 Effect of duration of PPRM on the incidence of culture proven neonatal sepsis

Duration (hours)	*Miller, Pupkin and Crenshaw*[52]		*Thibeault and Emmanouildes*[66]		*University of Iowa*	
	Incidence	*%*	*Incidence*	*%*	*Incidence*	*%*
< 24	2/79	2.5	2/100	2	0/13	0
24–48	2/41	4.8	3/53*	5.6	1/22	4.5
> 48	2/31	6.4	Not reported		4/65	6.1
Total	6/151	3.8	5/153	3.3	5/100	5

*Includes all PPRM > 24 hours.

The data presented in *Tables 6.2* and *6.3* show the infectious complications that occurred. The incidence of amnionitis, 6.6 percent, was not greater than that reported in several other recent studies[52, 60, 66], and may be a reflection of the generally good nutritional status of the patient population.

Five of the 100 infants had sepsis confirmed by culture. The organisms isolated included either group B β-hemolytic streptococci, *Enterobacter cloacea, Staphylococcus epidermidis*, chlamydia, or a mixed culture of peptostreptococcus and peptococcus organisms from each of the five infants respectively.

Table 6.4 Effect of duration of PPRM on incidence of RDS

Duration (hours)	*Thibeault and Emmanouildes*[66]		*Richardson* et al.[58]		*Miller, Pupkin, Crenshaw*[52]		*University of Iowa*	
	Incidence	*%*	*Incidence*	*%*	*Incidence*	*%*	*Incidence*	*%*
< 24	60/100	60	27/42	64	7/79	8.8	7/13	53.8
24–48	6/18	33	4/10	40	7/41	17.1	5/22	22.7
48–72	1/10	10	1/3	33	4/31*	12.9	5/23	21.7
> 72	0/25	0	2/9	22	Not reported		9/42	21.4
Total	67/153	43.8	34/64	53	18/151	11.9	26/100	26

*Includes all PPRM > 48 hours

Table 6.4 demonstrates a decreasing risk of RDS after 24 hours of membrane rupture. Comparison of those neonates delivered following membrane rupture of either less than or greater than 48 hours is seen in *Figure 6.1*. The data show that those infants with over 48 hours duration of membrane rupture have a lower incidence of RDS than those who deliver earlier.

The results support the impression that a conservative plan of management of PPRM is appropriate for the patient population of our institution.

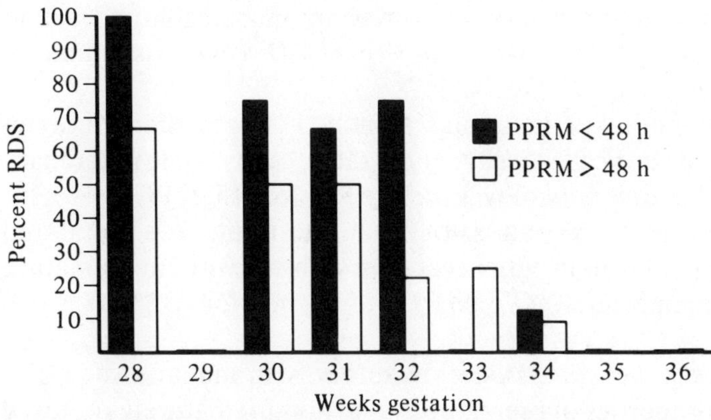

Figure 6.1 Effect of duration of PPRM at various gestational ages on the incidence of RDS

An alternative plan to the conservative management of the preterm pregnancy complicated by premature rupture of membranes is timed delivery following the administration of steroids. Although controversial, experimental data exists to suggest that antepartum glucocorticoid administration may accelerate fetal lung maturity without an increased infectious morbidity[48, 50]. The advantages and drawbacks of glucocorticoid administration discussed in more detail in Chapters 10 and 11.

Conclusion

Preterm premature rupture of the membranes occurs in 0.7–2.1 percent of pregnancies. The two major concerns are infection, which increases with duration of PPRM, and complications of neonatal prematurity, especially RDS, which decreases with duration of PPRM. The point at which expectant management must be replaced by intervention varies with each specific patient, the patient population, and the respective care facility. It is essential that the practitioner be familiar with these factors so that serious errors in management can be minimized.

References

1 AARNOUDSE, J. G. and HUISJES, H. J. Complications of cerclage. *Acta Obstetrica et Gynecologica Scandinavica*, **58,** 225–257 (1979)

2 ALBRECHT, R. C., CEFALO, R. C., LEWIS, P. E. and SMITH, J. P. Fetal growth after premature rupture of membranes. *American Journal of Obstetrics and Gynecology*, **127,** 869–870 (1977)

3 AMSTEY, M. S. and STEADMAN, K. T. Asymptomatic gonorrhea and pregnancy. *Journal of the American Venereal Disease Association*, **3,** 14–16 (1976)

4 ARIAS, F., ANDRINOPAULOS, G. and PINEDA, J. Correlation between amniotic fluid optical density, L/S ratio, and fetal pulmonary maturity. *Obstetrics and Gynecology*, **51,** 152–155 (1978)

5 ARTAL, R., BURGESON, R., FERNANDEZ, F. J. and HOBEL, C. J. Fetal and maternal copper levels in patients at term with and without premature rupture of membranes. *Obstetrics and Gynecology*, **53,** 608–610 (1979)

6 ARTAL, R., SOKOL, R. J., NEUMAN, M., BURSTEIN, A. H. and STOKJOV, J. The mechanical properties of prematurely and non-prematurely ruptured membranes. *American Journal of Obstetrics and Gynecology*, **125,** 655–659 (1976)

7 ATLAY, R. D. and SUTHERST, J. R. Premature rupture of the fetal membranes confirmed by intra-amniotic injection of dye (Evans blue T–1824). *American Journal of Obstetrics and Gynecology*, **108,** 993–994 (1970)

8 BADA, H. S., ALOJIPAN, L. C. and ANDREWS, B. F. Premature rupture of membranes and its effect on the newborn. *Pediatric Clinics of North America*, **24,** 491–500 (1977)

9 BAKER, C. J. and KASPER, D. L. Correlation of maternal antibody deficiency with susceptability to neonatal group B streptococcal infection. *New England Journal of Medicine*, **294,** 753 (1976)

10 BALLANTYNE, J. W. *Manual of Antenatal Pathology and Hygiene: The Foetus.* 221. Edinburgh, Wm. Green and Son, (1902)

11 BALLARD, J. L., KAZMAIER, K. and DRIVER, M. A simplified assessment of gestational age. *Pediatric Research*, **11,** 374 (1977)

12 BAUER, C. R., STERN, L. and COLLE, E. Prolonged rupture of membranes associated with a decreased incidence of respiratory distress syndrome. *Pediatrics*, **53,** 7–12 (1974)

13 BERKOWITZ, R. L., BONTA, B. W. and WARSHAW, J. E. The relationship between premature rupture of the membranes and the respiratory distress syndrome. *American Journal of Obstetrics and Gynecology*, **124,** 712–718 (1976)

14 BERKOWITZ, R. L., KANTOR, R. D., BECK, G. J. and WARSHAW, J. E. The relationship between premature rupture of the membranes and the respiratory distress syndrome. *American Journal of Obstetrics and Gynecology*, **131,** 503–508 (1978)

15 BERLIND, M. W. Test for ruptured bag of waters. *American Journal of Obstetrics and Gynecology*, **24,** 918 (1932)

16 BENIRSCHKE, K. Routes and types of infection in the fetus and newborn. *American Journal of Diseases of Children*, **99,** 714–721 (1960)

17 BISKIND, J. J. and BISKIND, L. A. Premature rupture of the membranes. *American Journal of Obstetrics and Gynecology*, **73,** 750–753 (1957)

18 BOBITT, J. R. and LEDGER, W. R. Unrecognized amnionitis and prematurity: a preliminary report. *Journal of Reproductive Medicine*, **19,** 8–12 (1977)

19 BREESE, M. W. Spontaneous premature rupture of the membranes. *American Journal of Obstetrics and Gynecology*, **81,** 1086–1093 (1961)

20 BURCHELL, R. C. Premature spontaneous rupture of the membranes. *American Journal of Obstetrics and Gynecology*, **88,** 251–255 (1964)

21 BUSTOS, R., KULOVICH, M. V., GLUCK, L., GABBE, S. G., EVERTSON, L., VARGAS, C. and LOWENT, E. Significance of phosphatidylglycerol in amniotic fluid of complicated pregnancies. *American Journal of Obstetrics and Gynecology*, **133,** 899–903 (1979)

22 CHRISTENSEN, K. K., CHRISTENSEN, P., INGEMARSSON, J., MARDH, P., NORDENFELT, E., RIPA, T., SOLUM, T. and SVENNINGSEN, N. A study of complications in preterm deliveries after prolonged premature rupture of the membranes. *Obstetrics and Gynecology*, **48,** 570–677 (1976)

23 CLEMENTS, J. A., PLATZKER, A. C., TIERNEY, D. F., HOBEL, C. J., CREASY, R. K., MARGOLIS, A. J., THIBEAULT, D. W., TODEY, W. H. and OH, W. Assessment of the risk of the respiratory-distress syndrome by a rapid test for surfactant in amniotic fluid. *New England Journal of Medicine*, **286,** 1077–1081 (1972)

24 COPELAND, W., JR., STEMPOL, L., LOTT, J. A. COPELAND, W., SR. and ZUSPAN, F. P. Assessment of a rapid test on amniotic fluid for estimating fetal lung maturity. *American Journal of Obstetrics and Gynecology*, **130**, 225–226 (1978)

25 COUSINS, L., HOBEL, C. J., CHANG, R. J., OKADA, D. M. and MARSHALL, J. R. Serum progesterone and estradiol 17-beta levels in premature and term labor. *American Journal of Obstetrics and Gynecology*, **127,** 612–615 (1977)

26 DOBEK, A. S., CARPENTER, J. L., LISTUS, H., GIBBS, R. Analysis of amniotic fluid taken during intrauterine fetal monitoring. *Fifteenth Interscience Conference on Antimicrobial Agents and Chemotherapy*, Washington, American Society for Microbiology (1975)

27 EDWARDS, L. E., BARRADA, M. I., HAMANN, A. A. and HAKANSON, E. Y. Gonorrhea in pregnancy. *American Journal of Obstetrics and Gynecology*, **132**, 637–642 (1978)

28 ERENBERG, A. Unpublished data.

29 FAYEZ, J. A., HASAN, A. A., JONAS, H. S. and MILLER, G. L. Management of premature rupture of the membranes. *Obstetrics and Gynecology*, **52,** 17–21 (1978)

30 FLOWERS, C. E., DONNELLY, J. F., CREADRICK, R. N., GREENBERG, B. G. and WELLS, H. B. Spontaneous premature rupture of the membranes. *American Journal of Obstetrics and Gynecology*, **76,** 761–772 (1958)

31 GOPLERUD, C. P., OHM, M. J. and GALASK, R. P. Aerobic and anaerobic flora of the cervix during pregnancy and the puerperium. *American Journal of Obstetrics and Gynecology*, **126,** 858–868 (1976)

32 GYSLER, R. Der vorzeitige Polensprung. *Zentralblatt für Gynakologie*, **100,** 1162–1172 (1978)

33 HALLMAN, M., KULOVICH, M., KIRKPATRICK, E., SUGARMAN, R. G. and GLUCK, L. Phosphatidylinositol and phosphatidylglycerol in amniotic fluid: Indices of lung maturity. *American Journal of Obstetrics and Gynecology*, **125,** 613–617 (1976)

34 HANDSFIELD, H. H., GODSON, W. A. and HOLMES, K. K. Neonatal gonococcal infection. I. Orogastric contamination with *Neisseria gonorrhaeae. Journal of the American Medical Association*, **225,** 697–701 (1973)

35 HARWICK, H. J., IUPPA, J. B., FOKETY, F. R., JR. Microorganisms and amniotic fluid. *Obstetrics and Gynecology*, **33,** 256–259 (1969)

36 HUFF, R. W. Antibiotic prophylaxis for puerperal endometritis following premature rupture of the membranes. *Journal of Reproductive Medicine*, **19,** 79–82 (1977)

37 JONES, M. D., JR., BURD, H. T. BOWES, W. A., JR., BATTAGLIA, F. C. and LUBCHENKO, L. O. Failure of association of premature rupture of membranes with respiratory distress syndrome. *New England Journal of Medicine*, **292,** 1253–1257 (1975)

38 KAPPY, K. A., CETRULO, C. L., KNUPPEL, R. A., INGARDINA, C. J., SBARRA, A. J., SEERBO, J. C. and MITCHELL, G. W. Premature rupture of the membranes: A conservative approach. *American Journal of Obstetrics and Gynecology*, **134,** 655–661 (1979)

39 KOHEN, D. P. Neonatal gonococcal arthritis: Three cases and review of the literature. *Pediatrics*, **53**, 436–440 (1974)

40 KOVAKS, D. Crystallization test for the diagnosis of ruptured membranes. *American Journal of Obstetrics and Gynecology*, **83,** 1257–1260 (1962)

41 LANIER, R. L., JR., SCARBRAUGH, R. W., FILLINGIN, D. W. and BAKER, R. E., JR. Incidence of maternal and fetal complications associated with rupture of membranes before onset of labor. *American Journal of Obstetrics and Gynecology*, **93,** 398–404 (1965)

42 LARSEN, B. and GALASK, R. P. Protection of the fetus against infection. *Seminars in Perinatology*, **1**, 183–193 (1977)

43 LARSEN, B., SNYDER, J. S. and GALASK, R. P. Bacterial growth inhibition by amniotic fluid II. Reversal of amniotic fluid bacterial growth inhibition by addition of a chemically defined medium. *American Journal of Obstetrics and Gynecology*, **119**, 497–501 (1974)

44 LARSEN, J. W., GOLDKRAND, J. W., HANSON, T. M. and MILLER, C. R. Intrauterine infection on an obstetric service. *Obstetrics and Gynecology*, **43**, 838–845 (1974)

45 LAVERY, J. P. and MILLER, C. E. Deformation and creep in the human chorioamniotic sac. *American Journal of Obstetrics and Gynecology*, **134,** 366–375 (1979)

46 LEBHERZ, T. B., HELLMAN, L. P., MADDING, R., ANCTIL, A. and ARJE, S. L. Double-blind study of premature rupture of the membranes. *American Journal of Obstetrics and Gynecology*, **87,** 218–225 (1963)
47 LEDGER, W. J. Premature rupture of membranes and influence of invasive monitoring techniques upon fetal and newborn infection. *Seminars in Perinatology*, **1,** 79–87 (1977)
48 LIGGINS, G. C. and HOWIE, R. N. A controlled trial of antepartum glucocorticoid treatment for prevention of the respiratory distress syndrome in premature infants. *Pediatrics*, **50**, 515–525 (1972)
49 MARTIN, J. E. Management of premature rupture of the membranes. *Clinical Obstetrics and Gynecology*, **14**(4). 213–225 (1973)
50 MEAD, P. B. and CLAPP, J. F. The use of betamethasone and timed delivery in management of premature rupture of the membranes in the preterm pregnancy. *Journal of Reproductive Medicine*, **19**, 3–7 (1977)
51 MELINGOS, S., MESSINIS, I., DIAKOMANOLIS, D., ARAVANTINOS, D. and KASKARELIS, D. Influence of meteorological factors on premature rupture of fetal membranes. *Lancet*, **2,** 435 (1978)
52 MILLER, J. M., PUPKIN, M. J. and CRENSHAW, C., JR. Premature labor and premature rupture of membranes. *American Journal of Obstetrics and Gynecology*, **132,** 1–6 (1978)
53 NAEYE, R. L. and BLANC, W. A. Relation of poverty and race to antenatal infection. *New England Journal of Medicine*, **283,** 555–560 (1970)
54 NAEYE, R. L., DELLINGER, W. S. and BLANC, W. A. Fetal and maternal features of antenatal bacterial infections. *Pediatrics*, **48**, 733–739 (1971)
55 PARRY-JONES, E. and PRIYA, S. A study of the elasticity and tension of fetal membranes and of the relation of the area of the gestational sac to the area of the uterine cavity. *British Journal of Obstetrics and Gynaecology*, **83,** 205–212 (1976)
56 POLISHUK, W. J., KOHANE, S. and PERANIO, A. The physical properties of fetal membranes. *Obstetrics and Gynecology*, **20,** 204–210 (1962)
57 PREVEDOVAKIS, C. N., STRINGOU-CHARALABIS, E. and KASKARELIS, D. B. Bacterial invasion of amniotic cavity during pregnancy and labor. *Obstetrics and Gynecology*, **37,** 459–461 (1971)
58 RICHARDSON, C. J., POMERANCE, J. J. CUNNINGHAM, M. D. and GLUCK, L. Acceleration of fetal lung maturation following prolonged rupture of the membranes. *American Journal of Obstetrics and Gynecology*, **118,** 1115–1118 (1976)
59 SBARRA, A. J., MICHLEWITZ, H., SELVARAJ, R. J., MITCHELL, G. W. JR., CETRULO, C. L., KELLEY, E. C., KENNEDY, J., HERSCHEL, M. J., PAUL, B. B.

and LOUIS, F. Correlations between amniotic fluid optical density and L/S ratio. *Obstetrics and Gynecology*, **48,** 613–615 (1976)

60 SCHRIEBER, J. and BENEDETTI, T. Conservative management of preterm premature rupture of the fetal membranes in a low socioeconomic population. *American Journal of Obstetrics and Gynecology*, **136,** 92–96 (1980)

61 SHUBECK, F., BENSON, R. C., CLARK, W. W., BERENDES, H., WEISS, W. and DENTSCHBERGER, J. Fetal hazard after rupture of the membranes. *Obstetrics and Gynecology*, **28,** 22–31 (1966)

62 SMITH, B. T., WORTHINGTON, D. and MALONEY, A. H. A. Fetal lung maturation. III. The amniotic fluid cortisol/cortisone ratio in preterm human delivery and the risk of respiratory distress syndrome. *Obstetrics and Gynecology*, **49,** 527–531 (1977)

63 STEWARDSON-KRIEGER, P. B. and GOTOFF, S. P. Risk factors in early onset neonatal group B streptococcal infections. *Infection*, **6,** 50–53 (1978)

64 STROUP, P. E. Amiotic fluid infection and the intact fetal membrane. *Obstetrics and Gynecology*, **19,** 736–739 (1962)

65 TAFARI, N., ROSS, S. M., NAEYE, R. L., GALASK, R. P. and ZAAR, B. Failure of bacterial growth inhibition by amniotic fluid. *American Journal of Obstetrics and Gynecology*, **128,** 187–189 (1977)

66 THIBEAULT, D. W. and EMMANOUILDES, G. C. Prolonged rupture of fetal membranes and decreased frequency of respiratory distress syndrome and patent ductus arteriosus in preterm infants. *American Journal of Obstetrics and Gynecology*, **129,** 43–46 (1977)

67 WARD, M. E., ROBERTSON, J. N., ENGLEFIELD, P. M. and WATT, P. J. Gonococcal infection: Invasion of the mucosal surfaces of the genital tract. In *Microbiology–1975*, edited by D. Schlessinger. 188–199. Washington, American Society of Microbiology, (1975)

68 WEBSTER, A. Management of premature rupture of the fetal membranes. *Obstetrical and Gynecological Survey*, **24,** 485–496 (1969)

69 WIDEMAN, G. L., BAIRD, G. H. and BALDING, D. F. Ascorbic acid deficiency and premature rupture of fetal membranes. *American Journal of Obstetrics and Gynecology*, **88,** 592–595 (1964)

70 WORTHINGTON, D., MALONEY, A. H. A. and SMITH, B. T. Fetal lung maturity. I. Mode of onset of premature labor. *Obstetrics and Gynecology*, **49,** 275–279 (1977)

71 YOON, J. J. and HARPER, R. G., Observations on relationship between duration of rupture of the membranes and the development of idiopathic respiratory distress syndrome. *Pediatrics*, **52,** 161–168 (1973)

72 ZAHL, P. A. and BJERKNES, C. Induction of deciduoplacental hemorrhage in mice by the endotoxins of certain gram-negative bacteria. *Proceedings of the Society for Experimental Biology and Medicine*, **54,** 329 (1943)

7
The case for nonintervention in preterm labor

Charles H. Hendricks

Does drug treatment do any good?

The use of tocolytic agents to suppress preterm labor has now become standard obstetric practice throughout most of the industrialized world. These tocolytic agents have not yet been studied systematically in relationship to their effectiveness and overall safety.

Much of the clinical practice in human reproduction has been derived empirically in the past only to be discarded after some period of time as treatment styles changed and as the ineffectiveness of some of the proposed treatments became apparent. For example, morphine was used in relatively large doses for many years to prevent the onset or stop the progress of preterm labor. It has been only 25 years since it was demonstrated objectively that the use of morphine even in large doses does not significantly diminish uterine contractility[10] and even less time since the demonstration that the use of another opiate, Demerol (pethidine), may even increase uterine contractility[49]. Furthermore the use of morphine in the woman who is at risk of delivering within the ensuing few hours might today be considered potentially threatening to fetal well-being should the child be born before the drug has been completely metabolized.

History of drug suppression of premature labor

Much can be learned from an examination of practices designed to control preterm labor as reported in the literature during the past quarter century. Let us examine several reports of the successful management of incipient or actual preterm labor reported between the years of 1955 and 1979 (*Table 7.1*). Abramson and Reid[1] in 1955 reported on the use of relaxin in the treatment of threatened preterm labor. Among five cases treated at 29 to 31 weeks gestation all delivered within the range of 36 to 40 weeks pregnancy, a 100 percent success rate. In 1955 Majewski and Jennings[38] reported on the use of a 'uterine

Table 7.1 Therapeutic intervention in threatened preterm labor in the past 25 years has included among other agents, relaxin, alcohol, β-mimetic agents, antiprostaglandins and acupuncture, all of which have been reported to give excellent results in uncontrolled studies.

Reference	*Agent*	*Criteria for use*	*Criteria for success*	*Number of cases*	*Success*	*Percent success*
1	'Relaxin'	Labor – 29–31 weeks	Delivery – 36–40 weeks	5	5	100
38	'Relaxin'	Preterm labor	'Labor halted'	20	16	80
39	'Relaxin'	Preterm labor	'Labor halted'	79	54	68.4
20	Alcohol	Preterm labor Membranes intact	72 hour delay	52	35	67
4	Orciprenaline	Probable preterm labor	Delivery 36 weeks or more	30	21	70
34	Salbutamol	Preterm labor	24 hour delay	88	75	85
44	Ritodrine	Threatened preterm labor	Prolong pregnancy minimum of 24 h	64	56	87.5
			1 week delay	52	42	81
15	Salbutamol	Preterm labor	24 hour delay	14	12	86
40	Salbutamol	Preterm labor (21–35 weeks)	Prolong 24 hours (all cases)	28	11	39.3
			(membranes intact)	17	8	47.1
60	Terbutaline	Labor prior to 36 weeks	Prolongation at least 72 hours	50	39	78
42	Fenoterol	Preterm labor (28–36 weeks)	Prolong pregnancy at least 1 week	47	41	87.2
63	Indomethacin	Preterm labor	Prolong pregnancy at least 1 week	50	40	80.0
59	Acupuncture	Preterm labor	Pregnancy carried to term	12	11	91.7

relaxing agent', presumably relaxin, administered for the suppression of established preterm labor. In their initial report they found that the drug would suppress labor in 16 out of 20 cases (80 percent). Two years later they reported an extended series, using the same drug, but despite a 'correction of the figures' through the removal for various reasons, of more than 10 percent of the patients in whom the medication was ineffective, the successful arrest of preterm labor dropped to 68.4 percent. The uncorrected success rate was only 61.3 percent[39].

In 1967 Fuchs *et al.*[20] published their first report concerning the use of the alcohol for the suppression of preterm labor. They found that the drug was not effective in any of the 16 cases where the membranes were intact at the onset of therapy, 35 (67 percent) had the pregnancy prolonged for at least 72 hours following initiation of therapy.

Further studies are outlined in *Table 7.1*. The great majority of studies performed during the past decade have related to the use of β-mimetic agents for the suppression of labor. Baillie, Meehan and Tyack[4] found that the use of orciprenaline in what was diagnosed as probable preterm labor was followed by delivery at 36 weeks or greater in 21 or 30 cases (70 percent).

Liggins and Vaughan[34] studied salbutamol with a view to prolonging pregnancy for at least 24 hours during the time when corticosteroids administered to the mother could work their effect upon increasing fetal lung maturation. They were successful in this endeavor in 75 of 88 cases (85 percent). Renaud *et al.*[44] used ritodrine for the treatment of threatened preterm labor. Pregnancy was prolonged at least 24 hours in 56 of 64 cases (87.5 percent) and there was a full week delay in 42 of 52 cases (81 percent). Dawson and Davies[15] in a study of various effects of salbutamol on the fetus and mother found a delay of delivery of at least 24 hours in 12 of 14 patients (86 percent). Martin and McDevitt[40] also studied salbutamol, but they found a delay from treatment to delivery of more than 24 hours in only 11 of 28 cases (39.3 percent). Of the 17 of their cases in whom the membrances were intact, eight (47 percent) carried the pregnancy for 24 hours or more, but in only three of the 11 cases (27 percent) where the membranes were already ruptured was pregnancy extended more than 24 hours.

Wallace *et al.*[60] studied terbutaline in 50 women who went into labor prior to 36 weeks. Thirty-nine of the 50 (78 percent) had the pregnancy prolonged 72 hours or more.

Ng, TambyRaja and Ratnam[42] reported on the inhibition of preterm labor with fenoterol. They were successful in extending the pregnancy at least 1 week in 41 of 47 cases (87.2 percent).

In a different pharmacologic approach Zuckerman, Reiss and Rubenstein[63] used an antiprostaglandin, indomethacin, for the treatment of premature labor. The treatment succeeded in prolonging pregnancies more than one week in 40 out of 50 cases (80 percent). There were five perinatal mortalities among these 50 patients with living fetus who were selected for the suppression of preterm labor.

A nonpharmacologic method for the control of preterm labor has been proposed by Tseui, Lai and Sharma[59] who, during the course of a study designed to induce labor by acupuncture, discovered that acupuncture electric stimulation applied at specific points will actually reduce uterine contractility. Utilizing this knowledge they then treated 12 cases of preterm labor twice daily for the first three days and then twice a week on an outpatient basis thereafter for the duration of the pregnancy. Eleven of the 12 (91.6 percent) carried to term.

Each of the above described series has the following features in common:

(1) the women were judged to be in actual or incipient preterm labor.
(2) An almost uniformly high rate of success. With the exception of one series there was a success rate of at least 67 percent and in seven of the 11 series the success rate was 80 percent or more.
(3) The series were completely uncontrolled.

There is a wide variation and poor description of how far in pregnancy were the women at the time treatment was initiated. The criteria of success varied from 24 hours delay (three series) to a minimum of 72 hours delay (two series) on to carrying the pregnancy at least to 36 weeks gestation.

Assessment of controlled clinical studies

None of the above cited series were performed with randomized selection of patients and the concomitant study of a randomly selected placebo group. Without the addition of concomitant controls to such a study it is patently impossible to make any judgment as to the effectiveness of a given drug. In an attempt to improve our understanding of this problem Hemminki and Starfield[24] made an in depth assessment of drugs which have been used for the prevention of or treatment of preterm labor. They were able to identify in the literature 18 series, reported between 1953 and 1977, where the use of tocolytic agents was compared with a control series. In eight of the controlled trials the agent was used prophylactically, i.e. it was given early in pregnancy in an attempt to prolong the pregnancy beyond what might otherwise be anticipated in a high risk group of pregnancies. In the other 10 series the intervention was therapeutic, i.e. the drug therapy was used for what was deemed to be impending or actual preterm labor. Only 13 of the trials compared the drug with placebo. The authors found a number of features which made it difficult to compare the drug versus placebo groups. Among the problems which they identified were the following.

(1) Arbitrary exclusion of some patients.
(2) Additional procedures including cerclage in patients being treated by drug therapy.
(3) A wide variety of other drugs used unsystematically in both test drug and placebo groups.
(4) Some instances of wide disparity in numbers in treatment groups comparing various drugs to each other and drug to placebo groups.

The conclusion from this summary of a quarter of a century of reported effort in the prevention or control of premature labor is scarcely encouraging. Only two of the therapeutic trials indicated that the drug was more effective than placebo. Only one of the therapeutic trials and one of the prophylactic trials gave an indication that there was some improvement in the fetal prognosis. In the total of 18 studies fetal wastage was only mentioned in 13 while the condition of the newborn was only mentioned in three. None of the studies included a follow-up done at one year of age or older. Further comment about the *prophylactic* studies evaluated by Hemminki and Starfield appears later in this chapter.

Comparative studies including placebo

A careful search is required to find any large published experience in which placebo treatment is one of the fully comparative parameters. Since 1973 there have appeared in the literature six series of cases in which alcohol, various β-mimetic agents and magnesium sulfate respectively, have been compared with the placebo in terms of effectiveness. *Table 7.2* presents a short summary of all such studies. These suffer somewhat from the fact that there is a fairly wide disparity in some of the studies between the number of drug cases versus the number of placebos, despite the fact that the series were constructed as randomized double-blind studies. Nevertheless, these represent in aggregate the information available to date which might give an indication as to the effectiveness of drug intervention over placebo in the management of preterm labor. A total of 307 drug treatment outcomes are available to be compared with 134 placebo treated outcomes.

Table 7.2 Studies where tocolytic agents were compared to placebo on a random selection double-blind basis are not numerous. The studies which meet all or most of the required criteria have been published since 1971.

Reference	*Agent*	*Number of cases*		*Success (%)*	
		Drug	*Placebo*	*Drug*	*Placebo*
61	Ritodrine	35	33	27(77.1)	17(51.5)
62	Alcohol	21	21	17(80.9)	8(38.1)
11	Nylidrin	43	41	37(86.0)	29(70.7)
	Isoxuprine	60		45(75.0)	
	Alcohol	50		35(70.0)	
26	Terbutaline	15	15	13(86.7)	4(26.7)
53	Alcohol	38	9	14(36.8)	4(44.4)
	Magnesium sulfate	31		24(77.4)	
51	Ritodrine	14	15	4(28.6)	4(26.7)
Total		307	134	216(70.4)	66(49.2)

Each of these studies addressed itself overwhelmingly to the question, ‘Does use of this drug during premature labor prolong pregnancy?’ None of the studies was designed to deal effectively with the question of improvement or lack thereof in fetal outcome. It will be noted (*Table 7.2*) that the mean effectiveness of the drug series reported was 70 percent (range 28.6–86.7 percent), while the mean effectiveness of placebo in prolonging pregnancy was 49.2 percent (26.7–70.7 percent).

From an examination of these results it is tempting to conclude that the effectiveness of drug intervention approximates only to that percentage of claimed successes by which these successes exceed the successful management by placebo alone, about 20 percent. This does indicate, however, that according to the arbitrary definition of success, there were some successes attributable to drug intervention. Nevertheless, about two-thirds of the ‘successes’ claimed in uncontrolled series are attributable to a placebo effect and/or failure to diagnose with certainty the presence of premature labor that would progress to delivery if untreated.

The meaning of such successes is somewhat difficult to fathom. The mere prolongation of a pregnancy by 72 hours might conceivably improve pregnancy outcome, but this has been by no means proven. If the criterion of success is to carry the pregnancy to 37 weeks or more, the effectiveness of the drug would be tied in to the question as to when in pregnancy the treatment was initiated. With such widely varying criteria of success in the interpretation of these results, it is impossible to assess the overall value of either drug or placebo. The most that can be claimed is that, according to the criteria arbitrarily selected by the investigators, placebo management is a 'success' in about half the cases, while drug intervention is successful in a modest additional percentage.

The effect of drug therapy upon the prematurity rate in a large population

Theoretically if sufficient effective interventions are carried out at the appropriate time is should be possible to reduce the preterm birth rate to zero. For this unlikely event to occur it would be necessary to prevent all third trimester hemorrhage from all sources, to prevent premature rupture of the membranes or to negate the effects thereof and to prevent intrauterine growth retardation, among other challenges. Granting that it would be unrealistic to expect to reduce the incidence of low birth weight so drastically, it should still be possible to demonstrate over a period of time that a sufficient application of an

Table 7.3 Incidence of children of low birth weight(< 2500 g) West Germany 1972–1975. During the years when fenoterol was coming into general use in West Germany the overall incidence of prematurely born infants remained almost constant. (From Kubli[31], courtesy of the Royal College of Obstetricians and Gynaecologists)

	1972	*1973*	*1974*	*1975*
Total number deliveries (live)	701 000	632 000	626 373	600 512
500–2500 g (live)	39 010	36 771	36 461	35 361
Incidence 500–2500 g (live) %	5.56	5.81	5.82	5.88
Incidence 500–2500 g (live and stillborn) %			6.22	6.26

effective intervention agent should bring about a reduction in the overall incidence of low birth weight. The experience in West Germany in recent years offers limited, but nevertheless, very interesting negative evidence along this line. Kubli[31] reported that in West Germany the β-mimetic drug, fenoterol, began to be used to a limited extent in 1970 and thereafter coming into general use by German obstetricians by 1974. Kubli[31] estimates the annual consumption of this drug in 1977 by pregnant German women to be at the rate of six million 5 mg tablets and one million 0.5 mg ampules. Despite this enormous dosage of fenoterol, the low birth weight incidence among the approximately 600 000 births per year has remained essentially unchanged through 1975, the latest year for which Kubli had access to the complete figures (*Table 7.3*).

Reduction of perinatal mortality

If the intervention is to be successful, presumably there must be some reduction in perinatal mortality. In all the controlled studies surveyed by Hemminki and Starfield the number of deaths in either the drug or placebo was too small to make any judgment as to the value of intervention or the lack thereof.

Fuchs[21] reported on his total experience with the use of alcohol for the arrest of premature labor in 1976. Among the 319 infants in Fuchs' total alcohol experience the overall neonatal mortality was 135 per 1000. A breakdown by birth weights is illustrated in *Table 7.4*. No information is available concerning the neonatal death rate from premature cases where intervention was not used in the same institution. In the study there had been eliminated many cases of premature rupture of the membranes and all cases of premature separation of the placenta, placenta previa if the bleeding was severe enough to necessitate intervention, dead or malformed fetus and maternal or fetal complications requiring immediate delivery.

Despite the fact that one cannot make comparisons between institutions there may be some interest in making a rough comparison between the alcohol-treated group and the figures from another hospital where with few exceptions it has not been the practice to suppress labor with either alcohol or β-mimetics. At the other hospital, (*Table 7.4*) the neonatal mortality rate for all cases (which included all cases of premature rupture of the membranes, all cases of abruptio placenta and placenta previa where intervention needed to be carried out, and all cases of congenital anomaly) was startlingly lower

Table 7.4 A comparison between neonatal mortality in a group of infants whose mothers were selected for alcohol suppression of labor versus neonatal mortality among all live born infants at another institution where suppression of labor is not commonly practiced

Weight group (g)	*Live births whose mothers were selected for ethanol suppression of labor Fuchs*[21]		*All live births over 500 g North Carolina Memorial Hospital 10/72–12/75*		*1/76–9/79*	
	Neonatal deaths	*Rate/1000*	*Neonatal deaths*	*Rate/1000*	*Neonatal deaths*	*Rate/1000*
500–750	3/3	1000.0	7/7	1000.0	23/27	851.9
751–1000	19/22	863.6	8/10	800.0	25/56	446.4
1001–1500	10/35	285.7	14/50	280.0	15/149	100.7
1501–2000	7/40	175.0	3/114	26.3	9/230	39.1
2001–2500	3/58	51.7	3/225	13.3	11/366	30.1
2500	0/153	0.0	3/2939	1.0	7/4155	1.7

in the institution which tends not to practice intervention during the period 1972–1975, which coincides with the time when a large portion of the Fuchs alcohol studies were being performed. Among infants of birth weight between 1501 and 2000 g the neonatal death rate was only one-sixth as high where intervention was not used as compared to the cases where alcohol had been employed. Among the cases of birth weight 2001–2500 g, the neonatal loss was three times as high among the alcohol treated series as compared to the results in the institution which did not practice drug intervention to any significant extent. Subsequent to 1975, a new phenomenon has appeared in the 'non-intervention' institution. This is the rapidly increasing survivorship of very low birth weight infants. From January 1976 through September 1979 the mortality among infants of the birth weight range 501–750 g dropped from 1000 per 1000 to 852 per 1000. The mortality in the 751–1000 g weight group dropped from 800 per 1000 to 446 per 1000. Among the birth weight group 1001–1500 g the mortality dropped from 280 per 1000 to 101 per 1000. It is difficult to escape the conclusion that improved pediatric expertise in dealing with severely preterm infants has played the major role in bringing about this dramatic change in neonatal mortality. None of the improvement at the institution cited can be ascribed to the use of tocolytic agents.

As a result of all these examinations we now can come up with some response to the question, 'does drug intervention do any good in the treatment of preterm labor?' It appears that what is diagnosed as preterm labor will stop by itself about half the time and/or placebo treatment will be effective about half the time. Tocolytic drug therapy does indeed acutely reduce uterine contractility when used in appropriate dosage, but the reduction in uterine contractility cannot be demonstrated to be associated with improved fetal outcome. There is as yet no evidence in the literature that the widespread use of drug intervention has altered the overall preterm birth rate in any population.

There is as yet no convincing evidence in the literature that drug intervention lowers the perinatal mortality. The recent papers of Barden, Peter and Mertkatz[5] and Merkatz, Peter and Barden[41] describe a multi-center study which was designed to resolve this issue. They did indeed find that the incidence of neonatal deaths was lower among the ritodrine treated group than among their control group. Unfortunately more than half of the control group patients received ethanol and only 66 patients received a placebo in the course of the entire study which reported the results of 223 women who received ritodrine treatment. Thus, it is impossible to compare definitively the perinatal mortality of the ritodrine group versus a placebo control group.

Does the use of drug intervention do any harm?

In order to be acceptable, a drug intervention should not carry any significant risks for the mother or fetus.

Maternal risks

The significant maternal side-effects associated with the use of alcohol for the suppression of labor relate to the inhibition of gluconeogenesis and the appearance of significant hypoglycemia. Severe lactic acidosis associated with the intravenous administration of alcohol for the suppression of premature labor has been reported by Ott, Hayes and Polin[43]. Severe aspiration pneumonia has also been observed (Greenhouse, Hook and Hehre[23]). Life threatening respiratory depression has been observed in one patient referred to our hospital from another community after having been treated with intravenous alcohol.

The most dramatic and potentially significant, untoward maternal response to tocolytic drugs of the β-mimetic type is that of pulmonary hypertension. The full-blown syndrome has been reported to date only in association with the administration of corticosteroids for the purpose of accelerating fetal lung maturation, the β-mimetic having been given as a delaying action to stave off delivery long enough for the corticosteroids to be effective. At least 27 cases have now been reported in detail or referenced in the recent literature (*Table 7.5*). Kubli[31]

Table 7.5 Pulmonary edema following upon the use of tocolytic agents combined with corticosteroids

Reference	*Location*	*Agent*	*Number of cases*	*Remarks*
31	W. Germany	Fenoterol and corticosteroids	9	All had pulmonary edema. 2 Deaths: 1 viral myocarditis, 1 congenital cardiomyopathy
17	UK	Ritodrine and betamethasone	1	Pulmonary edema and right heart failure
55	USA (Boston)	Terbutaline and corticosteroids	1	Pulmonary edema
46	USA (N. California)	Terbutaline and dexamethasone	9	Pulmonary edema
57	Netherlands	Ritodrine, indomethacin and betamethasone	1	Pulmonary edema
18	USA (S. California)	Magnesium sulfate and betamethasone	2	Pulmonary edema and congestive heart failure
27	USA (Missouri)	Terbutaline and corticosteroids	4	Pulmonary edema
Total			27	

reported eight cases of maternal pulmonary edema in West Germany in women who had been treated with fenoterol and corticosteroids. Among these there was one death which autopsy study indicated was due to a viral myocarditis. Kubli then reported a second death from his own institution where at autopsy the pathologist attributed the death to a congenital cardiomyopathy in which the primary anatomical abnormality was only a mild subvalvular pulmonary stenosis. This woman had also received fenoterol and corticosteroids. A death where ritodrine was used in a woman in the United States with a pre-existing undiagnosed idiopathic hypertension was reported by Barden, Peter and Merkatz[5] who also reported a death in Belgium in a woman who had been receiving ritodrine, corticosteroids and other drugs.

Elliott *et al.*[18] reported an additional case of pulmonary edema where ritodrine had been used in combination with betamethasone. Stubblefield[55] reported a similar case after the use of terbutaline combined with dexamethasone therapy. Rogge, Young and Goodlin[46] reported three such cases of their own and referred to six additional cases in northern California where terbutaline administration was combined with use of corticosteroids. Tinga and Aarnoudse[57] reported a case of pulmonary edema arising after treatment with ritodrine, indomethacin and betamethasone. Jacobs, Knight and Arias[27] reported four additional cases of pulmonary edema following β-mimetic and glucocorticoid therapy. That pulmonary edema in the management of preterm labor is not confined entirely to the use of β-mimetic agents is indicated by the fact that Elliott *et al.*[18] observed two patients with pulmonary edema after the use of betamethasone where magnesium sulfate was used as the tocolytic agent.

The pulmonary edema episodes often appear insidiously after repeated administration or prolonged administration of tocolytic β-mimetic agents; the process may make its appearance up to 12 hours postpartum after the drug is discontinued. Tinga and Aarnoudse[57] have suggested that the genesis of the problem may be sodium and water retention. Rogge, Young and Goodlin[46] suggested the mechanism as being due to the combination of expanded blood volume, increase of heart rate and the abrupt withdrawal of the drug.

Rogge, Young and Goodlin[46] made the additional observation that about one in six of their patients given terbutaline plus betamethasone for suppression of preterm labor have complained of substernal pain which these authors feel may be a possible prodrome of the clinical syndrome. Riess[45] has described another case where ritodrine was being used without any concomitant corticosteroid agents. This previously exceptionally healthy individual developed substernal pain radiating into the shoulder, neck and arm during the intravenous administration of ritodrine. ECG was interpreted by a cardiologist as revealing diffuse ischemia. The cardiac pain subsided two hours after discontinuing ritodrine. Chew and Lew[12], after 12 hours of low dose salbutamol given for the suppression of preterm labor, found a dramatic pattern of ventricular ectopics in association with hypokalemia. The patient had no history of any cardiac problem. The authors postulated that this may have been a woman with increased susceptibility to ECG abnormalities where the susceptibility was unmasked by the use of salbutamol.

Another drawback to the combined administration of β-mimetic drugs and dexamethasone involves alterations in glucose and insulin metabolism. It was reported by Thomas, Dove and Alberti[56] that the administration of this combination of agents causes elevated plasma glucose and insulin levels. Steel and Parboosingh[52] noted that the combination increased the insulin requirement in diabetics. Borberg *et al.*[6] in two normal patients being thus treated found that glucose and insulin levels were markedly elevated. Subsequently they observed the development of ketoacidosis in a chemical diabetic. They then noted that treatment of an insulin-dependent diabetic with dexamethasone alone was followed by a major increase of her insulin requirements. They concluded that 'the diabetogenic effect of β-sympathomimetic drugs and dexamethasone may be additive and that regular plasma glucose estimations should be made when they are used, especially on patients with impaired glucose tolerance.'

Thus one needs to be aware that tocolytic drugs do exert effects on the pregnant woman that go far beyond the mere suppression of uterine contractility. The principle culprits in the complications discussed above relate particularly to the cardiopulmonary system and carbohydrate metabolism.

In an attempt to minimize the risk of severe complications there have been listed various disease processes in pregnant women in which the use of one or more of these drug regimens is contra-indicated. The recommended contra-indications for β-mimetics have included women with diabetes, hypertension, and cardiac disease. In the case of alcohol one adds to this list women with uncompensated liver disease and previously successfully treated alcoholism. Unfortunately the great majority of complications reported to date have not been in patients previously diagnosed as having such severe conditions as diabetes and pre-existing heart disease. Most of the complications have happened to women in whom no such severe pre-existing disease has been diagnosed in advance, while in a minority of cases a latent phase of severe disease appears to be brought out by the use of these regimens in the treatment of preterm labor.

It might be reasonable for the physician who wishes to suppress preterm labor pharmacologically to ask himslf seriously the question as to whether or not any potential fetal benefit from the proposed therapy is worth the maternal risk.

Fetal risks

It has been noted that there is a statistically significant higher incidence of respiratory distress syndrome in the infants of mothers in whom the alcohol treatment failed to stop labor as compared to weight-comparable infants of mothers who were not treated at all[22]. Fetal depression of the central nervous system has been recorded in the very small preterm infant who is born after administration of alcohol[48, 13].

Concerning the fetal complications associated with the use of β-mimetic drugs, only one systematic study has been done. Brazy and Pupkin[8] studied the effects of maternal isoxsuprine administration upon preterm infants. They compared the results of preterm labor in 43 infants whose mothers received isoxsuprine with a group of 107 infants grouped by comparable stages of gestation treated over the same period of time whose mothers did not receive isoxsuprine administration. They found that among the isoxsuprine-treated pregnancies the infants had significantly more hypotension, hypoglycemia and hypocalcemia. Forty percent of the isoxsuprine-treated infants exhibited ileus as compared to 10 percent among the non-isoxsuprine-treated group. Mortality among the isoxsuprine group was 16 percent as compared to only five percent among the untreated group. The excess in both hypotension and death appeared predominantly in infants within the 26–31 week gestation range. The highest incidence of hypotension and death occurred in infants who were delivered within eight hours of the initiation of the isoxsuprine therapy. It may have been significant in relationship to the previous discussion about maternal complications that the frequency with which neonatal problems appeared was directly correlated to the time and the severity of maternal cardiovascular effects during the administration of the drug.

The neonatal complications of the β-mimetic agents are by no means confined to the use of isoxsuprine. Epstein, Nichols and Stubblefield[19]. observed 12 newborns whose mothers had received either fenoterol or terbutaline. They found a significant, and in a number of cases, sustained hypoglycemia which was particularly marked in patients where tocolytic treatment was terminated less than 24 hours prior to delivery. They also found that the cord serum insulin concentration was higher in the group that exhibited sustained hypoglycemia.

The use of magnesium sulfate as a tocolytic drug has not been reported to be associated with untoward fetal results. This drug, however, has been used for many years as an anticonvulsant agent in pre-eclamptic women. A number of case reports have appeared[7, 35, 36, 58] indicating that magnesium sulfate may be responsible for neonatal depression. Stone and Pritchard[54] found no evidence that use of the drug affected the perinatal mortality rate on their service.

There are no large-scale controlled studies demonstrating the safety of tocolytic drugs. Furthermore, other than the isoxsuprine series reported above there is a great paucity of reports comparing perinatal mortality in infants whose mothers received tocolytic agents versus those equally preterm infants whose mothers did not receive such agents.

In general it appears that fetal complications are greater if the infant delivers prematurely during or shortly after the discontinuation of the drug. It seems that the very fragile prematurely born fetus fails to benefit from being born while under the load of acute alcoholism or while under the effects of β-mimetic drugs. Those who claim 'good results' from the use of the tocolytic agents must include in their list of complications the untoward adventures of those infants whose birth is not delayed by the use of tocolytics, but who labor under the metabolic burden of toxic dosage of those tocolytic agents.

Does intervention to suppress preterm labor address the problem?

Whether or not such agents are capable of reducing uterine contractility acutely is not at issue. It has been clearly and repeatedly demonstrated that tocolytic drugs will reduce uterine contractility at any stage of labor if a sufficiently high dosage is used. Each of the suppressant drugs in current use has an appropriate pharmacologic rationale for its employment for this purpose.

What are we trying to achieve?

One should raise the question as to what one may hope to achieve if one administers tocolytic intervention at, for example, 4 cm of dilatation. Under such circumstances only a few hours of labor at best remain to be performed before parturition has been accomplished. Whether or not simply reducing uterine contractility can undo not only the previously achieved progress in labor, but also the even more remote weeks of prelabor for which there is objective evidence, is a critical question. No one has yet demonstrated that the process can be reversed to a significant extent.

Perhaps then the real issue should not be whether or not clinically active labor can be stopped, but rather why labor started in the first place, and this brings us logically to another critical point in the argument.

Identifiable groups at risk for preterm delivery
For reasons which we do not understand, but which are associated with individuals who have varying degrees of socio-economic deprivation, certain groups of people tend to deliver prematurely. It appears that extrinsic influences, perhaps acting over the entire duration of a woman's prior life, may be the critical determinants in predisposing her to deliver her offspring prematurely. (*Figure 7.1*)

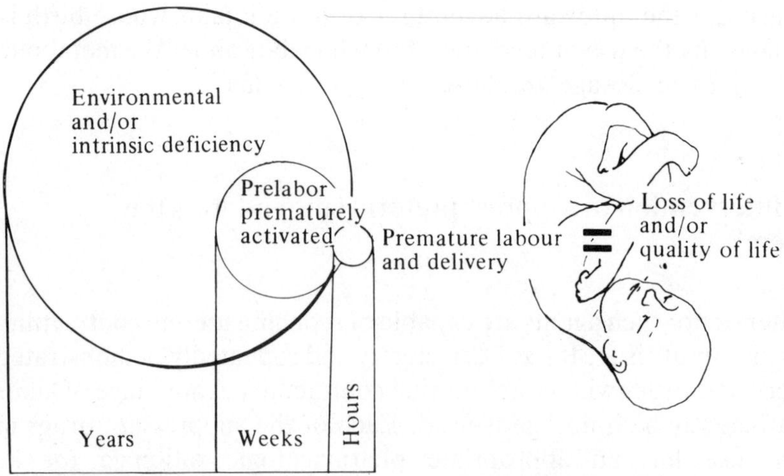

Figure 7.1 Most preterm labors occur in women who are laboring under some environmental and/or intrinsic deficiency which tends to 'preprogram' them for early termination of their pregnancy. These factors operate usually for very prolonged periods of time. After several weeks of prematurely activated prelabor, preterm labor itself appears

Extrinsic factors It has been demonstrated that people who come from poverty backgrounds have an approximately twofold incidence of preterm delivery as compared to those who come from non-poverty backgrounds[25]. The proclivity to preterm delivery is only one of a cluster of associated findings which tend to limit reproductive effectiveness: other factors are the tendency to develop infections (particularly urinary tract infections) abruptio placenta, and spontaneous abortion as well as preterm labor.

Intrinsic factors Certain individuals also appear to carry intrinsic factors which tend to produce both preterm labor and intrauterine growth retardation. A classic example is the individual with severe heart disease where one frequently anticipates both preterm delivery and appearance of an unusually small for gestational age infant. Other intrinsic factors may include such disparate items as physiologic incompetence of the lower portion of the uterus or genetic factors.

Women preprogrammed for preterm delivery

It has been observed by Keirse *et al.*[30] that women who deliver repeatedly prior to 37 weeks are at continued risk of spontaneous preterm delivery in subsequent pregnancies. Of critical importance in the study is the determination that prior first trimester abortions do *not*

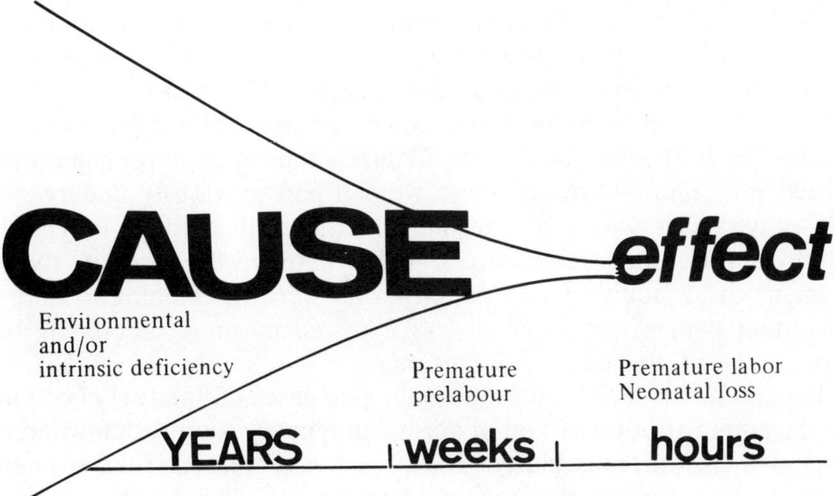

Figure 7.2 Intervention in early or established prelabor comes at a time when the factors destined to lead to premature termination of the pregnancy have been operating for long periods of time. The preterm labor is an *effect* of complex pattern of *causation*. Thus intervention may be thought of as treating an effect rather than dealing with the cause of preterm labor

serve as indicators of risk of subsequent preterm delivery, but that prior *second trimester spontaneous abortions* are indeed very strong indicators of such a risk. The Oxford study showed that a woman with one previous preterm delivery was at 37 percent risk of preterm delivery with the next pregnancy, and women with two or more preterm deliveries were at 70 percent risk of delivering early with a subsequent pregnancy. This matter is further discussed in Chapter 3.

Thus we see that there are multiple influences, some extrinsic and some intrinsic, which may be operating throughout the entire duration of pregnancy and which are destined to set forces in motion which will cause preterm parturition. Preterm delivery is thus only the effect of poorly understood causes. Intervention to stop preterm labor may be thought of as treating an *effect* rather than treating its cause (*Figure 7.2*).

Attempting to treat the cause

Through the years numerous attempts have been made to intervene early in pregnancy (prophylactically) in order to bring about an improved result. Some of these studies were nutritional. For example, in 1937 Ley[33] treated 10 women with a history of habitual abortion with what were then considered to be large doses of vitamin C administered intramuscularly during pregnancy. Nine of the pregnancies resulted in the birth of living infants – a success rate of 90 per cent. Currie[14] in 1937 gave wheat-germ oil during the course of pregnancy to 50 women. Thirty-seven of these women had previously undergone 130 pregnancies which had resulted in the birth of only 16 viable children. After the treatment, 37 living babies were born to these women. In an additional 15 patients who were threatening to abort treatment with wheat-germ oil was followed by pregnancy going to term in 14 of the cases (93 percent).

Rosenfeld[47] in 1938 reported treating 20 cases of habitual abortion by the administration of 5 ml of normal pregnancy serum administered once a week intramuscularly. The dose was increased if the woman had bleeding during the course of treatment. This treatment was followed by the birth of normal living infants in 19 out of 20 cases (95 percent).

Hormonal treatment also has been used prophylactically. For example Elden[16] in 1938 treated eight cases of habitual abortion with progesterone. Progesterone 10–44 iu in toto were administered to each of the women (1 international unit of progesterone is equal to 1 mg). The most common dosage used was 1 iu administered intramuscularly at weekly intervals. If preterm labor threatened or bleeding occurred, dosages as high as 4 iu progesterone every other day were used temporarily. Elden concluded that less than 1 iu (1 mg) per week of the progesterone might be sufficient to carry a pregnancy to term. Six out of eight cases delivered viable pregnancies – a success rate of 75 percent. The effectiveness of progesterone in 1 mg doses weekly is remarkable in view of the fact that it appears that the placenta produces progesterone at a rate as high as *1000 mg per day* during much of the time in later pregnancy.

Smith and Smith[50] reported in 1949 on the influence of diethylstilbestrol on the progress and outcome of pregnancy. They compared 387 treated primigravidas with all the other 555 primigravidas cared for during the same period of time who did not receive diethylstilbestrol. They found that among the treated patients there was a significant reduction in the incidence of toxemia of pregnancy. They found no change in the rate of spontaneous preterm delivery, but that the preterm infants were larger than in nontreated controls. None of the 43 diethylstilbestrol-treated preterm infants died, but nine of the 69 control group of preterm infants perished.

Hemminki and Starfield[24] identified eight reasonably controlled trials in which a pharmacologic agent had been used prophylactically. In only one of the prophylactic trials was there some indication of improvement of the fetal prognosis. The best result identified by the Hemminki and Starfield study was that of Johnson *et al.*[28] who used α-hydroxyprogesterone caproate in women with poor reproductive histories. Johnson *et al.* have subsequently expanded their study group from the 43 cases reported in 1975 to 64 cases reported in 1979[29]. Their results continue to appear encouraging and they are continuing their studies.

Hemminki and Starfield[24] are among those who feel that there is no longer any justification for doing an uncontrolled clinical trial. They call into question the fact that the use of tocolytic agents seems to have become part of standard obstetric practice. They add, 'As the ultimate purpose of the drugs is to improve the prognosis for the infant, it is difficult to understand how, in the absence of supportive evidence from controlled clinical trials, this practice evolved. Presumably it reflects the tendency for doctors to use a drug if it seems harmless and is based on acceptable physiological principles.'

Why is it so hard to make a critical judgment about the effectiveness of tocolytic agent intervention?

We are now in the curious position that drug intervention of unproven value has become the norm in the management of threatened and actual preterm labor in many industrialized countries without ever having been subjected to critical study. Let us examine a number of reasons which tend to act as barriers toward evaluating the usefulness of such pharmacologic approaches to the control of preterm labor.

The difficulty in recognizing preterm labor

About half of the patients clinically identified as being in preterm labor will subsequently carry the pregnancy substantially further. It is undeniable fact that many women have flurries of painful contractions in third trimester pregnancy and that many of them come to the hospital for observation. After a period of simple observation about half of such patients are sent home without having made any progress in the presumed labor. Whether or not this is a failure to diagnose accurately or some sort of placebo effect of having taken the trip to the hospital and been admitted for observation will never be known.

The difficulty in recognizing preterm labor inevitably plays a role in studies designed to control it. Steer and Petrie[53] found that when the cervical dilatation at the beginning of treatment was 1 cm or less that 83 percent would go on to successful outcome, i.e. contractions would be stopped for one day or more. The success rate among the alcohol-treated patients in this group was 73 percent, that for magnesium sulfate, 96 percent, and that for the 'placebo' management of five percent dextrose and water was 60 percent. (*Figure 7.3*) When the cervix was dilated 2 cm or more at the initiation of the treatment, however, the results were vastly different. Here only 16 percent of the pregnancies were prolonged 24 hours or more. Those treated with alcohol were successful in eight percent of the cases while those treated with magnesium sulfate and five percent dextrose and water were each successfully prolonged for one day or more in 25 percent of the cases. From these results Steer and Petrie concluded that 'Both alcohol and magnesium sulfate have some effect in stopping premature labor. This effect seems to be directly related to the degree of dilatation of the cervix at the time treatment is started. If treatment can be started before the cervix is dilated more than 1 cm, it is very likely that premature labor will stop.' An alternative interpretation might be that a women having painful contractions and with a cervix dilated at least 2 cm is more apt to be in true preterm labor than is the individual whose cervix is only dilated 1 cm or less.

Curiously enough the patient plays a very active role in making the diagnosis of preterm labor. Anderson[2] reported that at Oxford three percent of all of the prenatal patients are admitted before term apparently in labor without bleeding and with singleton pregnancies.

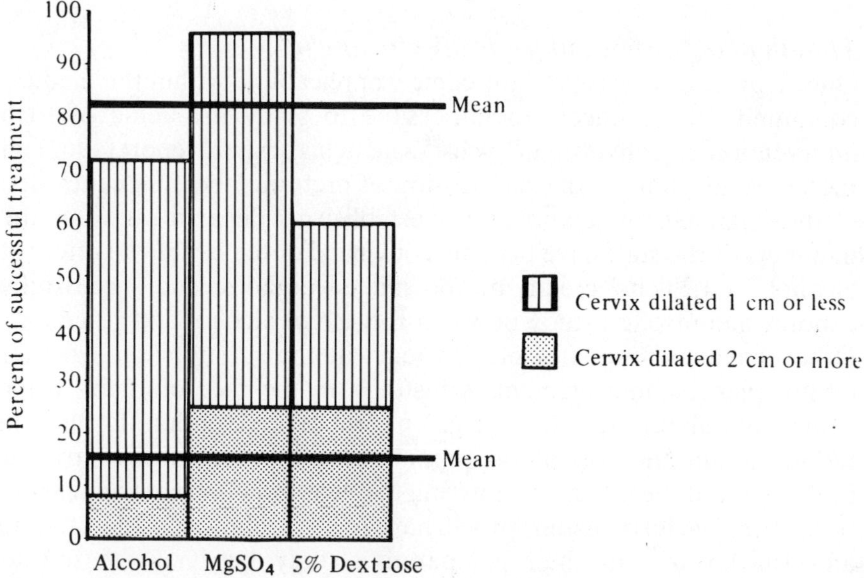

Figure 7.3 The overall effectiveness of treatment for preterm labor is determined more than anything else by the state of cervical dilatation at the time the intervention is begun. In the study cited more than 80 percent of preterm labors could be controlled when treatment was started at 1 cm or less of cervical dilatation. When the cervix had been dilated to 2 cm or more before the initiation of treatment, however, only 15 percent of the cases were successfully treated. (From data of Steer and Petrie[53])

Only half of these actually deliver before term including those with ruptured membranes. If one excludes from this group individuals with ruptured membranes, cervical effacement, or dilatation 2 cm or more only about one quarter will go on to preterm delivery. Anderson concluded that unless the membranes are ruptured it is extremely difficult to predict preterm delivery in such women unless the cervix is already well effaced and dilatation is already 4–5 cm. Patients who meet these criteria of active labor, full effacement and dilatation is already 4–5 cm, are obviously those in whom intervention, if intervention is of value at all, might possibly exert its most dramatic beneficial effect. Unfortunately when the process of preterm labor has already advanced to that degree such cases are ordinarily excluded from studies of tocolytic agents by a steadily progressing labor.

The ethics of 'withholding effective treatment'

Once a practice is accepted for clinical applicability within the medical community it is henceforth impossible to study the value of such intervention objectively. As Fuchs[20] said in his original report (1967) on the use of alcohol for the suppression of preterm labor, 'A controlled study is planned, but it is not easy to establish in a department where the members of the staff have become convinced of the beneficial effect of alcohol.' To Fuchs' credit, he did indeed organize and successfully conduct a controlled study between the use of alcohol and placebo.[62] Others have not found it so easy to deal with the question as to whether or not placebo management is justified in the face of their strong convictions about the value of a given form of intervention. Baillie[4], in talking about the use of orciprenaline said, 'A controlled trial is indicated, but the ethics of depriving the "controls" of what appears to be an effective form of therapy will have to be carefully considered.' Liu and Blackwell[37], in their comparative study between the use of aminophylline and salbutamol for the suppression of preterm labor, stated that 'Ideally, comparison should be made with an untreated control group, but that was rejected on ethical grounds.'

Despite the fact that there is no convincing evidence that any drug is effective in arresting preterm labor as compared to placebo administration there has been an increasing tendency in recent years to compare one unproven drug against another unproven drug seeking to report on which is 'superior' as a tocolytic agent. This appears to be partly because of the conviction of clinical workers that all tocolytic drugs are actually capable of improving pregnancy outcome. Another feature is that various workers feel that it would somehow be improper to study the effect of placebos. In discussing why ritodrine was compared with alcohol instead of a placebo, Fuchs[21] stated that 'It would be unreasonable to use a placebo when an effective agent, i.e. alcohol was available.' Wallace *et al.*[60] also felt that one drug should be compared to another instead of a placebo stating, 'Because previous studies had shown sympathomimetic means as effective inhibitors of uterine activity, it was considered unwise to use a placebo initially in the curtailment of uterine activity.' Consequently they offered their patients the alternative of alcohol versus terbutaline. None of the 50 patients selected alcohol, so no comparison between the terbutaline and any other agent was done at all.

The above cited examples convey the clinicians' conviction that treatment by one or more drugs is vastly to be preferred to no treatment and, by implication, the conviction that treatment of preterm labor leads to an outcome that is somehow superior to that which would follow no treatment at all. Nevertheless, despite the strength of conviction of the advocates of one or another of the tocolytic drugs, there is some interest in determining the extent to which pregnancy would continue in women treated only by placebo for preterm labor. It is difficult to find any large published experience in which placebo treatment appears to be a full partner in the comparative parameters. The feeling of many workers that it would be somehow unethical *not* to use some form of drug intervention in preterm labor might be questioned.

Is it ethical to intervene with tocolytic agents if there is no demonstrated value of such agents and when using them to intervene may prove dangerous to the health of the mother and/or the child?

The acceleration phenomenon

Wallace *et al.*[60] have made the following interesting statement: 'Overdiagnosis, and therefore overtreatment, of premature labor utilizing a *safe* tocolytic agent may not represent meddlesome obstetrics.' (The 'safe' tocolytic agent referred to was terbutaline.) That appears to be a reasonable statement. The results appearing to follow upon sufficient overdiagnosis and overtreatment, however, have a direct bearing upon the clinician's ability to keep his perspective about the efficacy of a given intervention.

The more overused is any given ineffective treatment, the higher the percentage of cases where there appears to be a good result. For example, if one is dealing with a situation where the risk of perinatal mortality in a high-risk group is 10 percent, while that of the rest of the population is zero, treatment of all the high-risk patients plus the treatment of an equal number of non-high-risk patients where there is no indication for treatment will automatically reduce the mortality among the treated group by one half. This gives a superficial indication of major improvement among those assigned to the high-risk group.

If, encouraged by this apparent reduction from 10 percent to five percent brought about by intervention, one then increases the prophylactic use to four times as many as the actual population at high risk, the results will look even better because then the mortality will be only two percent. It could be that only when, encouraged by the apparent improvement to give such noneffective intervention to the entire population, one might return to reality and recognize that one had not affected the actual results in any way whatsoever. This assumes that there were no bad results induced by the intervention itself.

A case in point was published recently. Lazar *et al.*[32] reported that they had used cervical cerclage in five percent of patients during a period of months of February 1971 and 1972. During a second period (1973 and 1974) their incidence of cervical cerclage rose to 18 percent of their total obstetric population. They did not emphasize the important fact that there was no statistically significant difference in the percentage of preterm deliveries in the *total population* between the first and second time period. They did find, however, that 23 percent of the women with cervical cerclage delivered preterm when they were doing only five percent cerclages while, when the incidence of cerclage rose to 18 percent of the total population, only 11 percent among the much larger group delivered preterm. Among the women who did not receive a suture the incidence of preterm births was 7.7 percent in the first time period and 6.2 percent in the second time period, a statistically nonsignificant difference.

Because they were so encouraged by their good results associated by the diminution of preterm deliveries among that portion of their patients who received cervical cerclage, Lazar and his coworkers felt that there was urgently needed a cooperative and randomized trial to assess the overall benefits of cerclage.

A more sober view of cervical suture comes from Oxford. In a comparative study of individuals with poor obstetric histories between those who received a cervical suture versus those with similar obstetric history in whom suture was not used, Keirse *et al.*[30] could not identify any prolongation of pregnancy or diminution of preterm delivery among those who had received cervical suture. Commenting on this problem Anderson[3] said, 'I would dispute that the rather mechanistic approach to the prevention of labor by tying the baby in will prove helpful in the prevention of preterm labor.'

One may postulate with some confidence that equal overuse of any drug intervention among a population would have a similar outcome, i.e. an improvement in good outcome among all the individuals grouped with the high-risk pregnancies in proportion to the number of low-risk individuals in the group on whom it is used and no effect on the overall perinatal mortality of the population at large. The apparent good results tend to produce steady acceleration. The more the drug is overused the 'better' the results. The better the results attributed to overuse of a drug the more confidence in the method. The more confidence developed in the method the greater the tendency to liberalize indication for the intervention modality and thus in turn the greater the reduction in perinatal mortality in the direction of, *but never better than*, the experience of the total population.

Conclusion

Perhaps the question as to whether or not intervention with drugs is warranted in preterm labor warrants thoughtful reexamination. There is a certain lack of logic in solemnly warning a pregnant woman not to drink alcohol during pregnancy, but when that woman goes into premature labor and when her fetus is at maximum risk from not being able to adapt to extrauterine existence to have that fetus subjected to levels of alcohol which make the mother maudlin drunk, occasionally combative and which put her in danger of developing aspiration pneumonia and even life-threatening acidosis. This is probably the first instance in history where it has been implied that it might be unethical to withhold from a pregnant woman the use of β-mimetic agents which as a group have been demonstrated to be capable of inducing substernal pain, documented cardiac ischemia and, when used in conjunction with corticosteroids, even pulmonary hypertension and death.

The rule of *primum non nocere* should not be repealed on behalf of an intervention which has not been shown to do any good and which in some instances has been shown to do harm to mother and fetus. If treatment does no good, there is no reason to use it. If a treatment is potentially dangerous to mother or infant it should certainly not be used.

It is not enough to say simply that all these drugs are not good for cardiac mothers and that such mothers should be screened and eliminated from the women on whom these drugs may be used. The two deaths in West Germany and one in the USA were attributed to cardiac disease. Each death occurred in association with the use of a β-mimetic drug[54].

The effects of initiating major alterations in medical practice on an illogical basis are capable of exerting a profound impact upon medical care. Once such practices are widely introduced into the body of obstetric lore it requires a long period of time to weed them out of clinical practice, even after there has accumulated convincing evidence of the ineffectiveness and/or potential dangers of such practices. For example, we used to treat threatened abortion with such agents as corpus luteum extract, estrogenic substances and/or progesterone. Even after the evidence became overwhelming that none of these agents singly or in combination was effective in salvaging pregnancies threatening to abort, the use of such practices was continued because many physicians felt it would do no harm and that it was desirable to offer some treatment as an expression to the patient and her family of the physician's concern for her pregnancy. It took a generation of education to teach physicians not to follow such a gratuitous course of management. Now it appears that we may be in the same relative position with respect to the use of the tocolytic agents in the management of preterm labor.

One may quite safely predict that the use of tocolytic agents in preterm labor will continue to be widespread during the next few years. For reasons discussed earlier in this chapter this trend to active intervention will appear falsely to produce 'good results' to the extent that it will continue to be practiced upon a progressively larger segment o the pregnant population. Overuse on larger and larger numbers of women who do not need the treatment in the first place may tend to strengthen the physician's conviction that the treatment is of value since almost always there will be a good outcome of the pregnancy. Tragically, it may be only when a sufficiently large number of maternal deaths have appeared in association with the administration of tocolytic agents that use of such agents will begin to decline. One may hazard the prediction that eventually the use of these agents may disappear without a trace and without ever having been completely studied in terms of their effect upon fetal outcome and fetal safety.

An editorial comment from the *British Medical Journal*[9] offers a thoughtful summary of the matter: 'On balance and in terms of fetal outcome the use of drugs to inhibit labour is usually unnecessary, frequently ineffective, and occasionally harmful. Indeed, when all cases of threatened and progressive preterm labour are analysed retrospectively, specific treatment to try to stop labour is found to be of potential value in only relatively few patients, either because of complicating factors indicating a need for delivery or because the patient is in advanced labour at the time of admission. Improvement in perinatal mortality and morbidity is more likely to come from concentrating efforts on the identification of high-risk pregnancies, on early admission, and on measures to ensure that infants at risk are delivered in optimum condition in centres of perinatal skill.'

References

1 ABRAMSON, A. and REID, D. E. Use of relaxin in treatment of threatened premature labor. *Journal of Clinical Endocrinology and Metabolism*, **15,** 206–209 (1955)

2 ANDERSON, A. In *Pre-term Labour* (Proceedings of the Fifth Study Group of the Royal College of Obstetricians and Gynaecologists), edited by A. Anderson, R. Beard, M. J. Brudenell, P. M. Dunn, 4. London, Royal College of Obstetricians and Gynaecologists (1977)

3 ANDERSON, A. In *Pre-term Labour* (Proceedings of the Fifth Study Group of the Royal College of Obstetricians and Gynaecologists), edited by A. Anderson, R. Beard, M. J. Brudenell, P. M. Dunn, 48. London, Royal College of Obstetricians and and Gynaecologists (1977)

4 BAILLIE, P., MEEHAN, F. P. and TYACK, A. J. Treatment of premature labor with orciprenaline. *British Medical Journal*, **4**, 154–155 (1970)

5 BARDEN, T. P., PETER, J. B., and MERKATZ, I.R. Ritodrine hydrochloride: a betamimetic agent for use in preterm labor. I.Pharmacology, clinical history, administration, side effects, and safety. *Obstetrics and Gynecology*, **56,** (1) 1–6 (1980)

6 BORBERG, C., GILLMER, M. D. G., BEARD, R. W. and OAKLEY, N. W. Metabolic effects of beta-sympathomimetic drugs and dexamethasone in normal and diabetic pregnancy. *British Journal of Obstetrics and Gynaecology*, **85,** 184–189 (1978)

7 BRADY, J. P. and WILLIAMS, H. C. Magnesium intoxication in a premature infant. *Pediatrics*, **40,** 100 (1967)

8 BRAZY, J. E. and PUPKIN, M. D. Effects of maternal isoxsuprine administration on preterm infants. *Journal of Pediatrics*, **94,** 444–448 (1979)

9 EDITORIAL. Drugs in threatened premature labour. *British Medical Journal*, **1,** 71 (1979)

10 CALDEYRO-BARCIA, R., ALVAREZ, H. and POSEIRO, J. J. Action of morphine on the contractility of the human uterus. *Archives Internationales de Pharmacodynamie et de Therapie*, **6,** (2) 171–188 (1955)

11 CASTREN, O., GUMMERUS, M. and SAARIKOSKI, S. Treatment of imminent premature labour. *Acta Obstetrica and Gynaecologica Scandinavica*, **54,** 95–100 (1975)

12 CHEW, W. C. and LEW, L. C. Ventricular ectopics after salbutamol. *Lancet*, **2** (9156–7) 1383–1384 (1979)

13 COOK, L. N., SHOTT, R. J. and ANDREWS, B. F. Acute transplacental ethanol intoxication. *American Journal of Diseases of Children*, **129,** 1075–1076 (1975)

14 CURRIE, D. Vitamin E in treatment of habitual abortion. *British Medical Journal*, **2,** 1218–1219 (1937)

15 DAWSON, A. M. and DAVIES, H. J. The effect of intravenous and oral salbutamol on fetus and mother in premature labor. *British Journal of Obstetrics and Gynaecology*, **84,** 348–353 (1977)

16 ELDEN, C. A. The treatment of habitual abortion by progesterone. *American Journal of Obstetrics and Gynecology*, **35,** 648–652 (1938)

17 ELLIOTT, H. R., ABDULLA, U., and HAYES, P. J. *British Medical Journal*, **2,** 799 (1978)

18 ELLIOT, J. P., O'KEEFFE, D. F., GREENBERG, P. and FREEMAN, R. K. Pulmonary edema associated with magnesium sulfate and betamethasone administration. *American Journal of Obstetrics and Gynecology*, **134** (6), 717–719 (1979)

19 EPSTEN, M. F., NICHOLLS, E. and STUBBLEFIELD, P. G. Neonatal hypoglycemia after beta-sympathomimetic tocolytic therapy. *Obstetrics and Gynecological Survey*, **34,** 759–761 (1979)

20 FUCHS, F., FUCHS, A. R., POBLETE, V. G., and RISK, A. Effect of alcohol on threatened premature labor. *American Journal of Obstetrics and Gynecology*, **99,** 627 (1967)

21 FUCHS, F. Prevention of prematurity. *American Journal of Obstetrics and Gynecology*, **126,** 809–817 (1976)

22 FUCHS, F. Discussion of previous reference. *American Journal of Obstetrics and Gynecology*, **126**, 820 (1976)

23 GREENHOUSE, B. S., HOOK, R. and HEHRE, F. W. Aspiration pneumonia following intravenous administration of alcohol during labor. *Journal of the American Medical Association*, **210,** 2392–93 (1969)

24 HEMMINKI, E. and STARFIELD, B. Prevention and treatment of premature labour by drugs: review of controlled clinical trials. *British Journal of Obstetrics and Gynaecology*, **85,** 411–417 (1978)

25 HENDRICKS, C. H. Delivery patterns and reproductive efficiency among groups of differing socioeconomic status and ethnic origins. *American Journal of Obstetrics and Gynecology*, **97,** 608–624 (1967)

26 INGEMARSSON, I. Effect of terbutaline on premature labor – a double-blind placebo-controlled study. *American Journal of Obstetrics and Gynecology*, **125** (4) 520–524 (1976)

27 JACOBS, M. M., KNIGHT, A. B. and ARIAS, F. Maternal pulmonary edema resulting from betamimetic and glucocorticoid therapy. *Obstetrics and Gynecology*. **56,** (1) 56–59 (1980)

28 JOHNSON, J. W. C., AUSTIN, K. L., JONES, G. S., DAVIS, G. H. and KING, T. M. Efficacy of 17 α-hydroxyprogesterone caproate in the prevention of premature labor. *The New England Journal of Medicine*, **293** (14) 675–680 (1975)

29 JOHNSON, J. W. C., LEE, P. A., ZACHARY, A. S., CALHOUN, S. and MIGEON, C. J. High-risk prematurity – progestin treatment and steroid studies. *Obstetrics and Gynecology*, **54** (4) 412–417 (1979)

30 KEIRSE, M. J. N. C., RUSH, R. W., ANDERSON, A. B. M. and TURNBULL, A. C. Risk of pre-term delivery in patients with previous pre-term delivery and/or abortion. *British Journal of Obstetrics and Gynaecology*, **85** (2) 81–85 (1978)

31 KUBLI, F. In *Pre-term Labour* (Proceedings of the Fifth Study Group of the Royal College of Obstetricians and Gynaecologists) edited by A. Anderson, R. Beard, M. J. Brudenell, P. M. Dunn, 218–220 (1977)

32 LAZAR, B. S., DREYFUS, J., GUEGUEN, S. and PAPIERNIK, E. Comparison of two successive policies of cervical cerclage for the prevention of pre-term birth. *European Journal of Obstetrics and Gynecologic Reproductive Biology*, **9** (5) 307–312 (1979)

33 LEY, L. Treatment of habitual abortion with Vitamin C. *Munchener Medizinische Wochenschrift*, **84,** 1814–1816 (1937)

34 LIGGINS, G. C. and VAUGHAN, G. S. Intravenous infusion of salbutamol in the management of premature labor. *Journal of Obstetrics and Gynaecology of the British Commonwealth*, **80,** 29–33 (1973)

35 LIPSHITZ, P. M. and ENGLISH, I. C. Hypermagnesemia in the newborn infant. *Pediatrics*, **40,** 865 (1967)

36 LIPSHITZ, P. M. The clinical and biochemical effects of excess magnesium in the newborn. *Pediatrics*, **47,** 501–509 (1971)

37 LIU, D. T. Y. and BLACKWELL, R. J. The value of a scoring system in predicting outcome of pre-term labour and comparing the efficacy of treatment with aminophylline and salbutamol. *British Journal of Obstetrics and Gynaecology*, **85,** 418–424 (1978)

38 MAJEWSKI, J. I. and JENNINGS, T. A uterine relaxing factor for premature labor. *Obstetrics and Gynecology*, **5,** 649–652 (1955)

39 MAJEWSKI, J. T. and JENNINGS, T.Further experiences with a uterine-relaxing hormone in premature labor. *Obstetrics and Gynecology*, **9,** 322–325 (1957)

40 MARTIN, D. H. and MCDEVITT, D. G. Salbutamol in the management of premature labour: a preliminary report. *Irish Journal of Medical Science*, **146,** 424–429 (1977)

41 MERKATZ, I. R., PETER, J. B., and BARDEN, T. P. Ritodrine hydrochloride: a betamimetic agent for use in preterm labor II. Evidence of efficacy. *Obstetrics and Gynecology*, **56,** (1) 7–12 (1980)

42 NG., S. C., TAMBYRAJA, R. L. and PATNAM, S. S. Inhibition of preterm labour with fenoterol. *Singapore Journal of Obstetrics and Gynaecology*, **10** (1) 17–22 (1979)

43 OTT, A., HAYES, J. and POLIN, J. Severe lactic acidosis associated with intravenous alcohol for premature labor. *Obstetrics and Gynecology*, **48** (3) 362–364 (1976)

44 RENAUD, R., IREMANN, M., GANDAR, P. and FLYNN, M. J. The use of ritodrine in the treatment of premature labor. *Journal of Obstetrics and Gynaecology of the British Commonwealth*, **81,** 182–186 (1974)

45 RIES, G. H. Kasuistische mitteilung uber dass auftreten einer myokardischamie unter medikamentoser tokolyse mit ritodrin (pre-par). *Geburtshilfe und Frauenheikunde*, **39,** 33–37 (1979)

46 ROGGE, P., YOUNG, S. and GOODLIN, R.Pulmonary edema. *Lancet*, **1** (8124) 1026–1027 (1979)

47 ROSENFELD, S.S. Habitual abortion: treatment by injection of pregnancy serum. *New York State Journal of Medicine*, **38,** 440–443 (1938)

48 SEPPALA, M., RASHA, N. C. R. and TAMMINEN, Y. Ethanol elimination in a mother and her premature twins. *Lancet*, **1,** 1188 (1971)

49 SICA-BLANCO, Y., ROZADA, H. and REMEDIO, M. R. Effect of meperdine on uterine contractility during pregnancy and labor. *American Journal of Obstetrics and Gynecology*, **97,** 1096–1100 (1967)

50 SMITH, O. W. and SMITH, G. The influence of diethylstilbestrol on the progress and outcome of pregnancy as based on a comparison of treated and untreated primigravidas. *American Journal of Obstetrics and Gynecology*, **50,** 994–1005 (1949)

51 SPELLACY, W. N. CRUZ, A. C., BIRK, S. A. and BUHI, W. C. Treatment of premature labor with ritodrine: a randomized controlled study. *Obstetrics and Gynecology*, **54** (2), p. 220–223 (1979)

52 STEEL, J. M. and PARBOOSINGH, J. Insulin requirements in pregnant diabetics with premature labour controlled by ritodrine. *British Medical Journal*, **1,** 880 (1977)

53 STEER, C. M. and PETRIE, R. H. A comparison of magnesium sulfate and alcohol for the prevention of premature labor. *American Journal of Obstetrics and Gynecology*, **129** (1) 1–4 (1977)

54 STONE, S. R. and PRITCHARD, J. A. Effect of maternally administered magnesium sulfate on the neonate. *Obstetrics and Gynecology*, **35,** 574–577 (1970)

55 STUBBLEFIELD, P. G. Pulmonary edema occurring after therapy with dexamethasone and terbutaline for premature labor: a case report. *American Journal of Obstetrics and Gynecology*, **132,** 341–342 (1978)

56 THOMAS, D. J. B., DOVE, A. F. and ALBERTI, K. G. M. M. Metabolic effects of salbutamol infusion during premature labour. *British Journal of Obstetrics and Gynaecology*, **84,** 497–499 (1977)

57 TINGA, D. J. and AARNOUDSE, J. G. Post-partum pulmonary edema associated with preventive therapy for premature labour. *Lancet*, **1** (8124) 1026 (1979)

58 TSANG, R. C. Neonatal magnesium disturbances. *American Journal of Diseases of Children*, **124**, 282–293 (1972)

59 TSUIE, J. J., LAI, Y. F. and SHARMA, S. D. The influence of acupuncture stimulation during pregnancy. *Obstetrics and Gynecology*, **50** (4) 479–488 (1977)

60 WALLACE, R. L., CALDWELL, D. L., ANSBACHER, R. and OTTERSON, W. H. Inhibition of premature labor by terbutaline. *Obstetrics and Gynecology*, **51**, 387–392 (1978)

61 WESSELIUS-DE CASPARIS, A., THIERY, M., YO LE SIAN, A., BAUMGARTEN, K., BROSENS, I., GAMISANS, O., STOLK, J. G. and VIVIER, W. Results of double-blind, multicentre study with ritodrine in premature labour. *British Medical Journal*, **3,** 144–147 (1971)

62 ZLATNIK, F. J. and FUCHS, F. A controlled study of ethanol in threatened premature labor. *American Journal of Obstetrics and Gynecology*, **112,** 610–612 (1972)

63 ZUCKERMAN, H., REISS, U. and RUBINSTEIN, I. Inhibition of human premature labor by indomethacin. *Obstetrics and Gynecology*, **44,** 787–792 (1974)

8
Preterm labor: the use of ß–mimetics

Ronald A. Chez

Introduction

There are presently four major pharmacological approaches to the arrest of preterm labor. The categories are magnesium salts, ethanol, prostaglandin synthase inhibitors and β-adrenergic stimulators. Increasingly, the β-adrenergic stimulators (also called β-agonists or β-mimetic drugs) are being used. Initially available in hospital pharmacies as bronchial dilators, they are administered to women in preterm labor as tablets, aerosols, or as subcutaneous or intravenous injections. As a group they have a variable success rate, are not specific tocolytic agents, and do have both nuisance and adverse side-effects. In my judgment, they will be the primary drugs offered to patients by most obstetricians for several years. It is also my judgment that as a group of agents they eventually will be replaced by more highly selective tocolytic drugs.

β-Adrenergic responses

Relaxation of the myometrial cell is a β-2-adrenergic phenomenon. There are other β-2-adrenergic related events and there are also β-1-, α-1-, α-2- and dopaminergic-mediated responses. The rapid accumulation of knowledge about adrenergic receptors is reviewed by Exton[16] and Steer[46]. Receptor research is now explored at the molecular level; identifiable physiological changes are being related to *in vitro* kinetic phenomena; species variations are being identified and resolved. The result of this progress is the reexamination of the accepted categorization of biochemical and biophysical response to agonist and antagonist stimulation of receptors. Although divisions are more fuzzy and occasionally overlap, an appreciation by the clinician of the standard classification of β-adrenergic receptors can help in anticipating nonuterine systemic responses from the use of β-mimetics.

Ahlquist[1] classified adrenergic receptors according to the effects of a series of catecholamines – epinephrine, norepinephrine and isoproterenol. He thereby differentiated an α- and β-group by order of potency. Isoproterenol had the most potent effect on the β-receptors and norepinephrine on the α-receptors. Lands *et al.*[27] further subdivided the receptors into β-1 and β-2, again on their relative responsivity to sympathomimetic amines. We now know more about the molecular nature of the receptors on the cell surface, and that the binding of agents to the receptor is rapid and reversible.

Sutherland, Robison and Butcher[48] discovered the cell membrane enzyme adenylate cyclase and this provided the link between the β-adrenergic receptor and biochemical changes in the cell. These take place via the cascade of cyclic AMP formation to dependent protein kinase activation to phosphorylation of metabolic enzymes to effects on cytosolic calcium ion concentration. The latter is an important regulator of enzyme activation, and modification of calcium efflux and influx into the cytosol is considered a common pathway for many cell processes.

The interaction of actin and myosin filaments determines contractility. An essential regulatory process is myosin light-chain phosphorylation by a calcium-influenced, light-chain kinase activity. Cyclic AMP inhibits myosin light-chain kinase activity. β-Mimetics stimulate the production of cyclic AMP.

The mechanism of action of a β-mimetic is most likely mediated by the drug binding to a β-receptor on the myometrial cell. The resultant stimulation of adenylate cyclase results in the production of cyclic adenosine monophosphate from its precursor. Subsequent protein kinase activation and then other enzyme actions result in storing mechanisms and a reduction of free circulating calcium ion in the cytosol. Lowering the concentration of calcium ion results in a noncontracted cell or a relaxed myometrium. The β-mimetics are therefore tocolytic agents.

β-Receptors are a part of the adrenergic system ubiquitous throughout the body. There is no evidence that the β-receptor on the myometrial cell is unique from β-receptors elsewhere in the body. Uterine relaxation is a β-2 response. β-2-adrenergic stimulation also is associated with bronchodilation, liver and muscle glycogenolysis, pancreatic beta cell insulin release, and peripheral arteriolar dilation.

β-1-Adrenergic responses include ionotropic and chronotropic effects on the myocardium, lipolysis, and small bowel relaxation.

The β-mimetics

The β-mimetics that are used for the treatment of preterm labor are pharmacologically sympathomimetic amines. Innes and Nickerson[24] provide detailed information on this topic. In general, this group of drugs has the capacity to provoke peripheral, cardiac, and central nervous system excitatory actions, peripheral inhibitory actions, and metabolic changes. No drug has a single effect nor do all the drugs share all multiple actions. There is no selective activation of either β-1- or β-2-receptors exclusive of the other. The clinical appearance of exclusive actions in a patient is a function of dose. The potency does vary in those drugs that share similar actions. Finally the endocrine and other physiologic changes of pregnancy may provide a milieau that enhances or decreases receptor responsivity.

Phenylethylamine is the parent compound of the sympathomimetic amines. The subset of tocolytic agents tend to have hydroxy substitutions on the three, four and/or five portions of the benzene ring. The two carbon atoms and the terminal amino group of the ethylamine group side-chain all lend themselves to other substitutions. The extent or the size of the substitution on the amino group as well as the presence of hydroxy groups in the three and five position favor selective β-2-receptor stimulation. The drugs presently being used clinically to treat preterm labor – orciprenaline, terbutaline, fenoterol, isoxsuprine, ritodrine and salbutamol all fall into this category.

Other pharmacological considerations include the presence of a 5-hydroxy group which tends to decrease the effectiveness of the drug when ingested because of increased gastrointestinal metabolism. Another is the fact that substitution on the carbon atoms of the aliphatic portion modifies the susceptibility to monoamine oxidation and the extent of peripheral versus central stimulation. Optical isomerism of the two carbons also can affect the extent of both peripheral and central action.

There is no pure β-2 stimulant. However, such drugs are suggested in advertising copy and in some medical articles. This probably comes about because of differences in dosage schedules for different therapeutic goals. Some of the β-mimetics that are used for the treatment of preterm labor are marketed for the treatment of bronchial asthma because of their bronchodilatory action. The doses given by aerosol or orally or subcutaneously for the treatment of bronchial asthma show a relative lack of β-1 activities. However, with the large intravenous doses used for the treatment of preterm labor the potential β-1 actions are frequently revealed. These drugs are free of direct α-activity.

The tocolytic agents are not metabolized by monoamine oxidase or catechol methyltransferase. The exact metabolic route for these drugs in the myometrial cells is not certain. According to route of administration they are excreted from the kidneys either unaltered or as conjugates, the latter through actions of the liver and gastrointestinal tract. The intravenous route provides much greater bioavailability than does the oral route. Although the data is scant in pregnant women, the half-life of the drugs is measured in minutes when administered intravenously, and up to four hours when ingested. There is no evidence of tissue accumulation of the agents, and the majority of excretion is usually complete by 12 hours[2].

Clinical experience: efficacy

Most reports of the use of a β-mimetic for there treatment of preterm labor describe success. Further, when compared to the therapeutic alternatives in the control population, the β-mimetic is usually better. Some examples of favorable outcome include ritodrine versus ethanol[28, 35], terbutaline versus placebo[23], ritodrine versus placebo[53], isoxsuprine and nylidrin versus ethanol and placebo[11], and isoxsuprine versus placebo[12, 13]. Examples of unfavorable reports include salbutomol versus ethanol[42], and ritodrine versus placebo[44].

The validity of the comparisons and the definition of success can be questioned. The clinical questions are how much better is the β-mimetic than the alternative and what does 'successful' mean? I am unwilling to provide percentages extracted from the literature although I am 'certain' from the literature and personal experience that the β-mimetics are better and more successful than bed rest and hydration alone, ethanol, and magnesium sulfate for the treatment of preterm labor.

Consider the medical literature on the subject. Ignoring the lack of a standard definition of preterm labor, the multiple etiologies that result in preterm labor, and the presence or absence of such variables as premature ruptured membranes, the definition of success still is not consistent. Some, but not all of the following criteria have been labelled success: number of days gained before delivery; number of deliveries delayed at least to 36 weeks; incidence of neonatal death; incidence of fetal weights greater than 2499 g; incidence of respiratory distress syndrome; and gestational age at delivery. A criterion for successful treatment could also be the number of newborns weighing more than 1250 or 1500 g or delivered after 33 weeks gestational age since survival of these infants is now so frequent in most neonatal centers. In a more restricted sense, success could be the proportion of deliveries that were delayed by at least 48 hours while other therapeutic measures such as the use of corticosteroid induction of surfactant could be accomplished. It is appropriate to deduce from the literature that for each of these criteria, the result of the β-mimetic treatment group has usually been found to be significantly better than that for the control group.

There are five β-mimetics that have been frequently used. There have been studies comparing one to another both with regard to their β-2 selectivity and associated lack of side-effects as well as their efficacy in diminishing both the frequency and the intensity of uterine contractions[11,31,32,38,39,40].

Neither studies of one agent, nor studies comparing agents are comparable in terms of control populations and use of placebo; the use of bed rest, hydration, other concurrent medications; route of administration; dose schedules including amount and number of days used; extent of bed rest and ambulation; or the gestational age at which the therapy was started. In multicenter populations, there can be wide differences in (1) the etiology of preterm labor between one subset and another, (2) the rate of recruitment of subjects, (3) length of time necessary to obtain numbers adequate for comparison, (4) number of completed cases, and (5) the reasons for subject dropouts. When the overall results are combined, important differences may be diluted or lost.

Further, although the credo of the research clinician is random selection of patients, prospective collection of data, use of placebo, and double-blind design, the reality of clinical practice dictates otherwise. For instance, double-blind and placebo can be negated by clues from drug-induced physiological changes. There is also the psychological pressure exerted by staff on the clinical investigator once they believe that a drug is effective and they are also certain as to which agent the patient is receiving. A recent study of ritodrine highlights many of these issues[3,35].

β-Mimetics can be effective tocolytic agents in the treatment of preterm labor. The recent FDA approval of ritodrine for the treatment of preterm labor in the United States will provide a standard against which other non-approved tocolytic agents can be more readily tested. Differences in specificity for uterine muscle and absence of other β-receptor stimulation may emerge, and additional clinical trials with appropriate scientific methodology are essential[19].

Clinical experience: side-effects, maternal

The side-effects of the β-mimetics are due to their action on both β-1 and other β-2-receptors at sites other than the uterus. All of the presently available agonists produce some of the side-effects. There is individual patient variation. The incidence and intensity are reduced when the medication is ingested as opposed to injected, a function of bioavailability.

Stimulation of β-1-adrenergic receptors results in chronotropic and ionotropic effects. The combination of the two results in increased cardiac output; a 50 percent increase has been directly measured by Bieniarz, Ivankovich and Scommenga[5]. The heart rate may increase by 15–50 beats per minute; this appears to be dose-related. Adrenergic stimulation increases conduction velocity through the atria, shortens the refractory period at the AV node, and increases conduction through the His-Purkinje system. The time of onset and the degree of tachycardia have been correlated with the time of onset and the degree of effectiveness upon uterine contractions[32]. There is no evidence that metabolic substrate and oxygen requirements for the heart can be exceeded with this degree of tachycardia and no evidence of myocardial damage was found in one study in which creatine kinase isoenzyme MB was measured[34]. Patients experience palpatations, sternal and substernal pressure pain, reaching a degree of discomfort that may require a reduction in drug dose.

Stimulation of β-2-receptors results in arteriolar dilation of coronary, skeletal muscle, abdominal visceral, and renal circulation. There is increased peripheral blood flow[37]. This can result in relative hypotension with diastolic levels decreasing by 20 mmHg (20 torr). Systolic levels may not change, may increase, or may decrease 20 mmHg[2, 12, 28, 32, 39]. The resultant mean arterial pressure is either not changed or decreased. There is little or no change in pulse pressure. Hypotension will stimulate baroreceptors and this can result in increased cardiac output and relative hypertension. Patients manifest symptoms of restlessness, face flushing and sensations of warmth, and occasionally dizziness. Purposeful intravenous hydration with crystalloid solution prior to infusion of the β-mimetic, and maintaining the patient in a left lateral decubitus position minimizes the frequency and intensity of hypotension.

There does not appear to be a specific sensitivity to either hypotension or hypertension in β-mimetic-treated patients with pregnancy-induced hypertension. Miller *et al.*[36] found an increase in fetal hypoxia and acidemia when patients with pregnancy-induced hypertension received β-mimetics.

Pulmonary edema has been reported from single case studies and from small groups of patients[2, 14, 41, 47, 51]. Associations include sudden stopping of the drug post partum without appropriate weaning and particularly when corticosteroids were used concurrently for the purpose of accelerating fetal surfactant production. There was no apparent pre-existing cardiovascular disease in these patients and no evidence of excess fluid loading. Expansion of blood volume and low colloid osmotic pressure have been suggested, but not confirmed as the cause of the pulmonary edema. Prompt reversal has been achieved each time by discontinuing the drug.

The extent of redistribution of blood flow through dilated peripheral vascular beds and the possibility of increased uterine blood flow has been examined in women[10], [25, 30]. Indirect measurements with radioactive materials are required in humans; one investigator using xenon has not found evidence of increased flow and one using indium has found such evidence. A different question is whether utero-placental arteries are sensitive to β-mimetic stimuli. Huszar and Bailey's report[22] that the smooth muscle in placental anchoring villi and vessels contains actin and myosin seems pertinent. Their interaction is regulated by phosphorylization, the regulatory pathways for which are influenced by calcium levels. Calcium flux is effected by cyclic AMP production. β-Adrenergic receptors are found in membrane fractions of human placenta[54]. Therefore, the theoretical possibility that utero-placental blood flow could be modified by adrenergic mimetics and antagonists in the human must be considered.

The β-mimetics are marketed as bronchodilators; they are associated with an increased peak expiratory flow rate, a decreased expiration flow resistance, and increased vital capacity. It is theoretically possible that an excess dose of a β-mimetic in a patient receiving this medication on a chronic basis could result in a paradoxical bronchoconstrictive response due to the development of drug tolerance.

Sympathomimetic amines stimulate the central nervous system. Patients who receive these drugs will manifest trembling, nervousness, restlessness, tremor, sleepiness, and dizziness. Whether these are

A hyperadrenergic state is one sign of hyperthyroidism. A patient with poorly controlled thyrotoxicosis could experience thyroid crisis with use of these drugs.

Other phenomena that have been reported with the use of β-mimetics include allergic dermatitis[21], effects on the bladder detrusor reflex, and a decreased platelet count at high doses secondary to the effect of the drugs on human platelet adenylate cyclase activity[26].

Many patients experience nausea, and some vomiting. The etiology could be central nervous system excitatory reflex or a direct β-1 effect on small bowel, stomach, and gallbladder with decreased motility and tone.

There can be a decrease in the number of β-adrenergic receptor sites after exposure to excess catecholamine stimulation and other environmental changes[46]. Tachyphylaxsis has been reported when these drugs have been used in the treatment of preterm labor[29,56].

When labor begins after a course of therapy there has been no identified prolongation of labor, increased incidence of dystocia, or increased occurrence of postpartum atony.

For reasons that are unclear, the peripheral concentrations of progesterone have been found to be decreased in two studies and increased in one study[4,12,55]. Estradiol-17β has both increased or not changed[4,55]. Placental lactogen has not been found to change[4,43,55].

Stimulation of cyclic AMP production results in phosphorylization of liver glycogenolytic enzymes with consequent maternal hyperglycemia. Increased peripheral insulin resistance has also been described. The duration of hyperglycemia with parenteral administration β-mimetics of has not been studied. However, with long-term oral dosage, there is no abnormal glucose tolerance and no hyperglycemia[6]. The degree of hyperglycemia and its duration may be a diagnostic clue to the unsuspected presence of gestational diabetes, but it could also be a function of the state of maternal nutrition.

There is a hyperinsulinemia both from a response to hyperglycemia and from direct stimulation of the β-2-receptor on the pancreatic islet cell. Increased C-peptide levels occur as a function of this polypeptide's presence in proinsulin. It is not clear whether there is a direct effect on the alpha cell of the pancreas or whether those cases in which increased glucagon has been found are secondary to hyperglycemia in a patient with a relative lack of insulin[2,6,8,17,33,43,45,49,50].

Diabetes mellitus is considered to be a contra-indication to the use of the drug by many investigators. However, if the clinician recognizes that hyperglycemia can occur and uses hourly monitoring of blood glucose levels and appropriately increased amounts of exogenous insulin, maintenance of euglycemia should be possible. Ketoacidosis has been reported in pregnant diabetics and the possibility is that the metabolic changes are exaggerated in the diabetic because of relative lack of insulin[45,50]. When concurrent dexamethasone has been given for the purposes of lung maturation, the β-mimetic-induced hyperglycemia can be exaggerated in the diabetic but this may not be so in the normal woman.

There is an increased influx of potassium into the cell as a reflection of the insulin-related movement of glucose into the cell and also as a direct effect on sodium–potassium translocation and possibly muscle cell permeability. Hypokalemia results[52], but electrocardiogram changes usually do not occur and there is no identified adverse effect. Since this is not a true depletion of body potassium stores, but a transfer from the extracellular to the intracellular compartment, replacement therapy is not necessary. Correction occurs rapidly upon stopping the infusion. Changes in blood levels of magnesium, calcium, and phosphate have not been found[49].

Through β-1-stimulated lipolysis there is mobilization of free fatty acids and glycerol. The high concentration of free fatty acids results in the increased production of acetetoacetyl-ÇoA, and then β-hydroxybutyrate and acetoacetate. Increased muscle glycogenolysis is associated with increased circulating lactate levels. There is a suggestion that gluconeogenesis is increased in the presence of increased substrate. The fixed organic acids from increased ketogenesis and increased muscle glycogenolysis can result in lowering of pH of the maternal blood.

A question of overriding importance is 'How safe is the drug?' In animal data, the LD_{50} far exceeds the normal therapeutic range, and this relationship probably applies in humans. Hundreds of thousands of women have received these agents. Maternal mortality is very rare, although at least two maternal deaths have been reported[2]. In one, underlying viral myocarditis and in the other congenital cardiomyopathy was found. There is always the concern that the β-1 effects on the heart will result in the diagnosis of previously unrecognized myocardial disease or the precipitation of such disease. A patient with pulmonary hypertension or obstruction to left ventricular output such as with hypertrophic subaortic stenosis could be at particular risk as cardiac output increases. If electrocardiograms were used more frequently in women treated for preterm labor, it would be likely that the presence of arrhythmias might be noted. The adverse effect of general anesthesia with halogenated hydrocarbons for an obstetrical emergency in a patient who has a cardiac arrhythmia is of particular concern. The potential for concurrent hypokalemia to exaggerate this condition has also to be considered.

The extent of these biochemical and biophysical changes in any one patient is not predictable. Further, there is lack of uniform β-1 responses or uniform β-2 responses from patient to patient. In addition to the properties of the individual drug itself, there appears to be marked differences in patient sensitivity and therefore probably the number of β-1 or β-2-receptors in any one organ or tissue site. Because there is not a specific uterine relaxing agent, it is necessary to be aware of these changes, to look for their occurrence, and to modify dose and treatment schedules accordingly.

Clinical experiences: fetal/neonatal effects

The β-mimetics cross the human placenta. There is scant data as to the kinetics of transfer, the volume of distribution, and equilibrium constants.

There are β-receptors in the human fetus but the stimulating effect of the drug on fetal cells, or fetal drug sensitivity, is related to the gestational age of the fetus and the ability of the fetus to metabolize the agent through excretion and conjugation. The presence of placental and fetal catechol methyltransferase and monoamine oxidase is not pertinent to the metabolism of β-mimetics because of their chemical structures. When fetal changes are observed, it is not always clear whether these are direct or secondary to pharmacologically induced changes in the mother. Examples include changes in fetal heart rate, fetal plasma glucose levels, and fetal pH.

In general, changes in fetal heart rate are inconsistent, occur later, and return sooner to baseline than those of the mother. The fetal heart rate has been reported to increase up to 20 beats per minute after administration of the drug to the mother[52]. These changes may be within normal beat-to-beat variability. Also, an increase is defined as a function of the initial fetal heart rate used as base line. This rate may already have been modified by existing maternal disease. The rate may also change as a function of β-mimetics related to maternal effects such as induced hypotension. β-Mimetics injected into the fetal scalp showed a direct effect of the drug on fetal heart rate[2].

After the mother has received a β-mimetic, fetal blood gases have been shown to increase, decrease, or not change. Through β-receptor stimulated lipolysis and muscle glycogenolysis there will be an increase in fixed organic acids in the mother; this may result in a decreased maternal pH. In addition to this potential indirect source of decreased fetal pH, organic acids produced in the mother will cross the placenta and thereby directly influence pH in the fetus. The possibility also exists that the agonist will, by producing fetal lipolysis and muscle glycogenolysis, produce organic acids in the fetus. The studies on fetal blood gases and fetal pH obtained from patients who have received β-mimetics for the treatment of preterm labor must be differentiated from those clinical trials in which bolus injection of the drug has been used to treat or prevent acute fetal distress on an emergency basis. In those instances a compromised fetus may already exist. The arrest of labor is intended to provide an environment in which the values can return to the normal range through physiologic mechanisms.

Fetal hyperglycemia has been documented with the use ofmimetics in the mother, secondary to maternal hyperglycemia through a transplacental diffusion gradient and/or from a direct effect on fetal liver glycogenolysis and gluconeogenesis. Theoretically, induced fetal hyperglycemia in the presence of pre-existing hypoxia secondary to maternal disease may intensify a tendency toward fetal acidemia and acidosis.

Compared to controls, birth weight has been observed to increase in pregnancies in which β-mimetics were given[10, 53]. However, if the fetus initially is appropriate size for gestational age, the birth weight may not increase. In contrast, it is more likely to do so if the fetus manifested intrauterine growth retardation prior to treatment. Both chronic fetal hyperglycemia and a chronically increased uterine blood flow with concurrent transfer of substrates and gases have been suggested as the cause; there is no confirmatory data. Moreover, many women in preterm labor are placed at bed rest, which may be sufficient to result in an enhanced rate of fetal growth in previously small for dates fetuses.

There is usually a significant decrease in the incidence of respiratory distress syndrome in those infants born after β-mimetic therapy given during pregnancy[7], but a causal relationship is not clear. Accelerated induction of surfactant in the presence of chronic intrauterine stress has been demonstrated. Many causes of preterm labor are associated with chronic intrauterine stress. Another related variable is the number of days achieved with effective tocolysis during which time normal surfactant production could occur. As opposed to the laboratory animal, there is no direct evidence in the human that β-mimetics have a direct effect on surfactant production.

Epstein, Nicholls and Stubblefield reported eight newborns with hypoglycemia persisting for several hours after being delivered from mothers treated with β-mimetics[15]. Relative hyperinsulinemia was found. The problem was accentuated if delivery occurred soon after the mother received large doses of the drug. Brazy and Pupkin[9] retrospectively analyzed 43 infants born of β-mimetic-treated mothers. Compared to controls, there was an increased incidence of hypotension, hypocalcemia, hypoglycemia, hyperbilirubinemia and an increased incidence of ileus and excess gastric aspirates.

Specific hyperadrenergic reactive states in the newborns have not been reported. Some clinical signs of such states cannot be differentiated from the normal immature homeostatic mechanisms that exist in preterm infants. For perspective, there have been literally hundreds of thousands of women who have received this drug in varying doses including up to the time of delivery. Many of these women have delivered in settings in which newborns have been cared for by capable clinicians in a neonatal intensive care unit. The paucity of reports of adverse effects suggest strongly that the drugs are relatively safe in the perinatal period.

Infants have been studied up to two years after delivery by Freysz *et al.*[18]. Their growth and development appeared normal. There are more long-term, on-going studies mentioned in various papers and reviews, none of which apparently show evidence of mental or physical developmental abnormalities. There is always the theoretical question of subtle changes difficult to identify because of the large numbers of subjects needed to compensate for the variables that influence the development of the infant born preterm. However, considering the metabolism of the drug, the nature of the binding sites and receptors, and the types of biophysical and biochemical changes that are associated with adrenergic stimulation, there is no reason there should be subsequent problems in the infant and child. Although it is not appropriate to extrapolate the data, it may be reassuring to recognize that no unusual effects from extremely high doses have been found in experiments done on rats, mice, rabbits, guinea-pigs, dogs, and pregnant ewes.

Clinical experience: the Penn. State protocol

This protocol is the one presently use on our service. It was designed by Dr J. J. Botti to standardize use of the β-mimetic agent terbutaline

terbutaline in treating premature labor. It is applicable to any β-mimetic agent that the clinician wishes to use in a consistent way. It is presented in a format that allows the preparation of an information–instruction document for nursing personnel, physicians-in-training, and other obstetricians.

Diagnosis of preterm labor

The diagnosis of preterm labor is made at a gestational age of less than 37 weeks if uterine contractions occur at least every 7–10 min, last at least 30 s, and are present for at least 30 min. The presence of contractions and their frequency should be documented by recording with an external tocodynamometer.

A single pelvic examination is performed to determine the dilation and effacement of the cervix, the presentation, and the status of the membranes. In the following instances, treatment should be expedited.

(1) The primigravida at 2 cm or more or the multigravida at 3 cm or more cervical dilatation.
(2) Any patient with ruptured membranes. Documentation of ruptured membranes is made by finding vaginal pooling of fluid with a positive nitrazine reaction, the presence of ferning on a smear, or the presence of fetal cells on a smear with nile blue sulfate.
(3) Any patient with cervical effacement of 75 percent or more.
(4) Any patient with progressive cervical dilatation or effacement.

Patient eligibility

A patient is eligible for treatment if the gestation is between 20 0/7 and 36 6/7 weeks with intact membranes, or the gestation is between 27 0/7 and 33 6/7 weeks with ruptured membranes.

Exclusions

Patients may be excluded for medical or obstetrical reasons. However, the clinical range of disease and the individualization of care make the more usual contra-indications relative rather than absolute.

(1) Pregnancy-induced hypertension.
(2) Abruptio placenta or vaginal bleeding from unknown cause. Patients with stable documented placenta previa may be treated.

(3) Fetal anomaly incompatible with life.
(4) Dead fetus.
(5) Chorioamnionitis.
(6) Benign essential hypertension – blood pressure 150/90 or greater.
(7) Heart disease – including patients with rheumatic or congenital disease.
(8) Hyperthyroidism.
(9) Diabetes mellitus – insulin-dependent or gestational.
(10) Fetal distress.
(11) Maternal febrile illness or hypoxia.
(12) Cervix dilated 5 cm or more.

Treatment objectives

The overall objective in patients with intact membranes is to maintain pregnancy until at least 37 0/7 weeks gestation. In patients with ruptured membranes, pregnancy may be continued unless there are maternal or fetal indications for immediate delivery. A patient can be retreated with this drug throughout pregnancy if repeated episodes of threatened preterm labor occur.

During the drug infusion, the objective is to reduce uterine contractions to a frequency of less than one every 15 min. If, after two hours of therapy, contractions persist at greater than one every 15 min, then an alternative protocol may be started.

Side effects of drug

The following are some of the side-effects that may occur with the drug's infusion. The patient should be informed of the associated symptoms.

(1) Maternal tachycardia – an increased heart rate up to 120–130 beats per minute is expected with the highest infusion rates. A high heart rate requires physician notification. Excessive tachycardia may require discontinuing the infusion.
(2) Fetal tachycardia – heart rates up to 170 beats per minute are not uncommon, but short and long term variability of the heart rate should not be affected. Periodic changes indicative of fetal distress are still valid. The infusion rate of the drug may require reduction if the fetal heart rate exceeds 180–200 beats per minute.
(3) Maternal hypertension – an increase of more than 20 mmHg (20 torr) systolic is uncommon.

(4) Maternal hypotension – diastolic blood pressure should not fall more than 20 mmHg (20 torr) nor systolic blood pressure more than 35 mmHg (35 torr). Change of maternal position and/or infusion of crystalloid solution should ameliorate the problem.
(5) Maternal palpitations, chest tightness, angina and shortness of breath – all of these must be carefully evaluated since the drug can cause pulmonary edema and ventricular tachycardia, particularly in patients with unrecognized cardiac disease. The infusion may need to be reduced gradually or even discontinued if such symptoms appear. An irregular heart rhythm may also be an indication to discontinue the infusion.
(6) Maternal headache – it is not significant as a single symptom and if blood pressure is not increased.
(7) Maternal hyperglycemia – mild, reversible hyperglycemia may be seen. Values greater than 200 mg/dl may be treated with 5 units of regular (soluble) insulin, but the infusion rate need not be reduced.
(8) Maternal acidemia or ketoacidosis – hyperglycemia and an increase in lactate and free fatty acids may cause both maternal and fetal acidemia. It can be treated by decreasing or discontinuing the drug infusion or, if necessary, by administering insulin.
(9) Hypokalemia – this may occur as a consequence of insulin-mediated glycogen deposition into cells. If present, it should not be treated with replacement therapy.

Dosage

This is our present regimen for terbutaline. The patient receives an initial intravenous bolus of terbutaline 250 μg in 5 ml N saline over 3 min via the intravenous tubing.

Terbutaline 10 mg is added to 500 ml ½N saline, providing a concentration of 20 μg/ml. The infusion is started at 10 μg/min and is increased by 5 μg/min at 30 min intervals. If an infusion rate of 30 μg/min for 30 min has had no apparent effect on uterine contractions, the physician decides either to stop treatment, to increase the infusion rate or to use another tocolytic agent.

Effective tocolysis is considered to be present when uterine contractions are reduced to a frequency of less than one every 15 min. Once this level of suppression is achieved, the infusion is maintained for six hours. The infusion rate may then be decreased by 5 μg/min at 30 min intervals so long as excessive contractility does not reappear. When the infusion rate has been decreased to 10 μg/min, subcutaneous and oral terbutaline administration are started simultaneously. The subcutaneous dose is 250 μg every six hours; it is stopped at 72 hours. The oral dose is 5 mg every six hours. This dosage is maintained or decreased at the physician's discretion. Generally, oral therapy is continued for at least five days after contractions have ceased.

The infusion is considered ineffective if tocolysis is not achieved after two hours at the maximum rate chosen by the obstetrician. The infusion rate should then be decreased gradually by 10 μg/min at 30 min intervals until the infusion is stopped.

A dosage plan for ritodrine recommended and tested by Barden, Peter, and Merkatz[3] includes an initial dose of 100 μg/min which is increased in 50 mg/min increments every 10 min until contractions stop or a maximum dose of 350 μg/min is reached. The infusion is continued at the effective rate for at least 12 hours once tocolysis is achieved, after which the intravenous dose is gradually reduced. Thirty minutes before stopping the infusion, ritodrine 10 mg is given orally. This dose is repeated every two hours for 12 doses. Then 10–20 mg amounts are given orally every four to six hours (maximum 120 mg per day) until further treatment is not considered necessary.

Fenoterol has been investigated in a multicenter study in the United States. Treatment is initiated with an infusion at 1.0 μg/min for 10 min. Increments are 0.5 μg/min at 10 min intervals until uterine contractions are inhibited or intolerable side-effects occur or greater than 4.0 μg/min levels are necessary. The infusion is continued for 11 hours once an effective level is reached. Half an hour before stopping the infusion, 5 mg of the drug is taken orally. This dose is given every four hours for 12 doses and then every six hours until an acceptable gestational age is reached.

Patient management during infusion

(1) Uterine activity – continuous readjustment of the tocodynamometer to assess contractions is mandatory, particularly during the period of drug infusion.

(2) Pelvic examination – this is repeated if the maximum infusion rate has no apparent effect on uterine contractions.

(3) Other medications – medications which have antagonistic effects such as propranolol or which may contribute to side-effects, such as large doses of analgesics are used with precautions or avoided. An anti-emetic may be ordered for nausea as necessary.

(4) Diet and activity – activity is limited to bed rest. Because an event at delivery may result in the need for anesthesia, nothing is given by mouth except ice chips.

Patient management after infusion

(1) Subcutaneous and oral doses are administered per protocol.
(2) The patient is transferred to a hospital room if no evidence of uterine activity is present six hours after cessation of the infusion.
(3) Electrophysiologic monitoring of the fetal heart rate and uterine activity may be discontinued eight hours after the end of the infusion.
(4) Vital signs, fetal heart rate and uterine activity should be measured every four hours for 24 hours, then every shift.
(5) Diet, patient activity and other medications are at the discretion of the physician.
(6) After subcutaneous therapy is finished, patient discharge from the hospital may be considered.
(7) In patients with ruptured membranes, a policy of nonintervention may be preferred in the absence of evidence of infection or fetal distress.
(8) If discharged home, the patient may resume usual daily activity. Douching, enemas, and coitus are proscribed.
(9) If labour recurs after discharge, she may be retreated with the drug.

Physicians orders

These written orders pertain to intravenous administration of the drug.

(1) Bed rest in left lateral tilt or decubitus.
(2) NPO during intravenous infusion except for ice chips; lip/mouth care.
(3) Maternal heart rate, blood pressure, and respiratory rate every 10 min during intravenous infusion; all vital signs every 30 min during control and weaning periods. Call physician if diastolic pressure decreases 20 mmHg (20 torr) from control, if systolic pressure is decreased 35 mmHg (35 torr) or if maternal heart rate exceeds 120 beats per minute.
(4) Temperature every four hours (every two hours, with ruptured membranes).

(5) Apply external fetal monitor with tocodynamometer.
(6) Input and output during the intravenous infusion.
(7) CBC and differential every 24 hours if no evidence of infection, bleeding, or ruptured membranes; every six hours with premature ruptured membranes or vaginal bleeding.
(8) Blood type and antibody screen.
(9) Urine microscopic and culture.
(10) Blood sugar prior to infusion, then every four hours during infusion.
(11) Serum potassium prior to infusion, then every four hours during infusion.
(12) 1000 ml of ½ N saline to run at 500 ml in 30 min, then 2 ml/min.
(13) Administer β-mimetic with infusion pump according to the dosage schedule.

Neonatal assessment

The following is done with infants delivered from patients who received a β-mimetic.

(1) Cord serum glucose, potassium and calcium; repeat tests at one and two hours of age.
(2) Cord blood gases – pH, P_{CO_2}, P_{O_2}, base excess.
(3) Appropriate observations for hyperbilirubinemia, ileus, and hypotension.

A checklist

(1) Perform complete physical examination including pelvic exam.
(2) Obtain a 30 minute segment of tocodynamometer-documented uterine contractions.
(3) Make diagnosis of preterm labor.
(4) Ascertain whether patient is a candidate for tocolysis with a β-mimetic.
(5) Explain use of drug to patient.
(6) Write orders.
(7) Obtain maternal blood work.
(8) Start ½N saline intravenous infusion.
(9) Start intravenous drug dose regime by infusion pump.

Comment and conclusions

Isoxsuprine was first used for the treatment of premature labor two decades ago[20]. It is assumed that the β-mimetics will be the dominant pharmacological agent for the treatment of preterm labor for a number of years, and that they are more efficacious than bed rest. They can be used over a longer period of time and by a variety of routes compared to alcohol and magnesium salts, and do not have the potentially harmful effects on the fetus of the presently available prostaglandin synthase inhibitors. There is no specific β-2 uterine relaxing agent free of other β-2 effects or even of β-1 effects. Thus, the clinician can expect to be confronted with published data and advertising copy about various β-mimetics that make percentage point comparisons between either the tocolytic benefits or the apparent lack cf adverse side-effects.

The clinical benefit/risk ratio is an important way to compare drugs but this is not always easy to calculate. What are the benefits of treatment? Are they the number of days of pregnancy gained, the size of the infant, newborn morbidity and mortality, or the ability to use the agent recurrently? The adverse effects, whether they be changes in maternal heart rate, blood pressure, or maternal biochemistry also cause discussion. Moreover, there are other variables which make these comparisons difficult, including the lack of standardization as to the highest dose that can be used, whether the drug was used by the proper route and maintained for enough time, the manner in which the route of administration was altered to maintain therapeutic levels, and particularly the characteristics of the woman treated in terms of the etiology of the preterm labor and other aspects of her overall medical care. There is also the unresolved issue as to whether breakthrough of labor, also called drug failure, is an important clinical indication that any further attempt at tocolysis is inappropriate.

My suggestion is that the clinician learns to use one of these drugs. In the United States, ritodrine will have FDA sanction, but terbutaline and fenoterol appear to be satisfactory alternates. These three drugs are available in other countries, as are salbutamol and orciprenaline.

I believe the drugs should be used on a protocol so that there will be a consistent approach to dosage, route of administration, and length of time. The individual clinician will have to wait for large enough series to be published showing significant differences in outcome or other important variables before changing medications. The agents cannot be considered a panacea both because of the physiological mechanisms which result in labor and the multiple etiologies of the process of preterm labor[57].

(*Note*: I was unable to include articles not written in English and those materials quoted from various European proceedings, workshops, and symposia related to the use of β-mimetics in pregnant women. The latter are only fortuitously available in the United States. I regret that I was unable to benefit from additional insights and supporting data from these materials. However, it is my belief that the opinions and conclusions in this chapter reflect the consensus of clinician-investigators at this time.)

References

1 AHLQUIST, R. P. A study of the adrenotropic receptors. *American Journal of Physiology*, **153,** 586–600 (1948)

2 ANDERSON, A., BEARD, R., BRUDENELL, J. M. and DUNN, P. M. (editors). *Pre-term Labour* (Proceedings of the 5th Study Group of the Royal College of Obstetricians and Gynaecologists). London, Royal College of Obstetricians and Gynaecologists (1977)

3 BARDEN, T. P., PETER, J. B. and MERKATZ, I. R. Ritodrine hydrochloride: a betamimetic for use in preterm labor. Part I: Pharmacology, clinical history, administration, side effects, and safety. *Obstetrics and Gynecology*, **56,** 1–6 (1980)

4 BIBBY, J. G., HIGGS, S. A., KENT, A. P., FLING, A. P. F., MITCHELL, M. D., ANDERSON, A. B. M. and TURNBULL, A. C. Plasma steroid changes in preterm labour in association with salbutamol infusion. *British Journal of Obstetrics and Gynaecology*, **85**, 425–430 (1978)

5 BIENIARZ, J., IVANKOVICH, A. and SCOMMENGA, A. Cardiac output during ritodrine treatment in premature labor. *American Journal of Obstetrics and Gynecology*, **118,** 910–920 (1974)

6 BLOUIN, D., MURRAY, M. A. F. and BEARD, R. W. The effect of oral ritodrine on maternal and fetal carbohydrate metabolism. *British Journal of Obstetrics and Gynaecology*, **83,** 711–715 (1976)

7 BOOG, G., BEN BRAHIM, M. and GANDAR, R. Beta-mimetic drugs and possible prevention of respiratory distress syndrome. *British Journal of Obstetrics and Gynaecology*, **82,** 285 (1975)

8 BORBERG, C., GILLMER, M. D. G., BEARD, R. W. and OAKLEY, N. W. Metabolic effects of beta-sympathomimetic drugs and dexamethasone in normal and diabetic pregnancy. *British Journal of Obstetrics and Gynaecology*, **85,** 184–189 (1978)

9 BRAZY, J. E. and PUPKIN, M. J. Effects of maternal isoxsuprine administration on preterm infants. *Journal of Pediatrics*, **94,** 444–448 (1979)

10 BRETTLES, J. P., RENAUD, R. and GANDAR, R. A double-blind investigation into the effects of ritodrine on uterine blood flow during the third trimester of pregnancy. *American Journal of Obstetrics and Gynecology*, **124,** 164–168 (1976)

11 CASTRÉN, O., GUMMERUS, M. and SAARIKOSKAI, S. Treatment of imminent premature labor – a comparison between the effects of nylidrin chloride and isoxsuprine chloride as well as of ethanol. *Acta Obstetrica et Gynecologica Scandinavica*, **54,** 95–100 (1975)

12 CSAPO, A. I. and HERCZEG, J. Arrest of premature labor by isoxsuprine. *American Journal of Obstetrics and Gynecology*, **129,** 482–491 (1977)

13 DAS, R. K. Isoxsuprine in premature labor. *Journal of Obstetrics and Gynaecology of India*, **19,** 566–575 (1969)

14 ELLIOT, H. R., ABDULLAH, U. and HAYES, P. J. Pulmonary oedema asociated with ritodrine infusion and betamethasone administration in premature labor. *British Medical Journal*, **2,** 799–800 (1978)

15 EPSTEIN, M. F., NICHOLLS, E. and STUBBLEFIELD, P. G. Neonatal hypoglycemia after beta-sympathomimetic tocolytic therapy. *Journal of Pediatrics*, **94,** 499–453 (1979)

16 EXTON, J. H. Mechanisms involved in alpha adrenergic phenomena: role of calcium ions in action of catecholamines in liver and other tissues. *American Journal of Physiology*, **238,** 83–812 (1980)

17 FREDHOLM, B. B., LUNELL, N. O., PERSSON, B. and WAGER, J. Actions of salbutamol in late pregnancy: Plasma cyclic AMP, insulin, and C-peptide, carbohydrate and lipid metabolites in diabetic and nondiabetic women. *Diabetologia*, **14,** 235–242 (1978)

18 FREYSZ, H., WILLARD, D., LEHR, A. and MESSER, J. A long term evaluation of infants who received a beta-mimetic drug while in utero. *Journal of Perinatal Medicine*, **5,** 94–99 (1977)

19 HEMMINKI, E. and STARFIELD, B. Prevention and treatment of premature labor by drugs: review of controlled clinical trials. *British Journal of Obstetrics and Gynaecology*, **85,** 411–417 (1978)

20 HENDRICKS, C. H., CIBILS, L. A., POSE, S. V. and ESKES, T. K. A. B. The pharmacologic control of excessive uterine activity with isoxsuprine. *American Journal of Obstetrics and Gynecology*, **82,** 1064–1078 (1961)

21 HOROWITZ, J. J. and CREASY, R. K. Allergic dermatitis associated with administration of isoxsuprine during premature labor. *American Journal of Obstetrics and Gynecology*, **131,** 225–226 (1978)

22 HUSZAR, G. and BAILEY, P. Relationship between actin-myosin interaction and myosin light chain phosphorylation in human

placental smooth muscle. *American Journal of Obstetrics and Gynecology*, **135,** 718–726 (1979)

23 INGEMARSSON, I. Effect of terbutaline on premature labor: a double-blind placebo-controlled study. *American Journal of Obstetrics and Gynecology*, **125,** 520–524 (1976)

24 INNES, I. R. and NICKERSON, M. Norepinephrine, epinephrine, and the sympathomimetic amines. In *The Pharmacologic Basis of Therapeutics*, edited by L. S. Goodman and A. Gilman. New York, MacMillan (1975)

25 KAUPPILA, A., KUIKKA, J. and TUIMALA, R. Effect of fenoterol and isoxsuprine on myometrial and intervillous blood flow during late pregnancy. *Obstetrics and Gynecology*, **352,** 558–562 (1978)

26 KUTTI, J., OLSSON, L. B., LUNDBORG, P. and FREDEN, K. The peripheral platelet count in response to intravenous infusion of salbutamol. *Acta Medica Scandinavica*, **201,** 515–517 (1977)

27 LANDS, A. M., ARNOLD, A., MCAULIFF, J. P., LUDUENA, F. P. and BROWN, T. G., JR. Differentiation of receptor systems activated by sympathomimetic amines. *Nature*, **214,** 597–598 (1967)

28 LAUERSEN, N. H., MERKATZ, I. R., TEJANI, N., WILSON, K. H., ROBERSON, A., MANN, L. I. and FUCHS, F. Inhibition of premature labor: a multicenter comparison of ritodrine and ethanol. *American Journal of Obstetrics and Gynecology*, **127,** 837–845 (1977)

29 LIGGINS, G. C. and VAUGHAN, G. S. Intravenous infusion of salbutamol in the management of premature labor. *Journal of Obstetrics and Gynecology of the British Commonwealth*, **80,** 29–33 (1973)

30 LIPPERT, T. H., DEGRANDI, P. B. and FRIDRICH, R. Actions of the uterine relaxant, fenoterol on uteroplacental hemodynamics in human subjects. *American Journal of Obstetrics and Gynecology*, **125,** 1093–1098 (1976)

31 LIPSHITZ, J., BAILLIE, P. and DAVEY, D. A. A comparison of the uterine β-2 adrenergic selectivity of fenoterol, hexoprenaline, ritodrine, and salbutamol. *South African Medical Journal*, **50,** 1969–1972 (1976)

32 LIPSHITZ, J. and BAILLIE, P. Uterine and cardiovascular effects of beta-2 selective sympathomimetic drugs administered as an intravenous infusion. *South African Medical Journal*, **50**, 1973–1977 (1976)

33 LUNNELL, N. O., JOELSSON, I., LARSSON, A. and PERSSON, B. The immediate effect of a beta-adrenergic agonist (salbutamol) on carbohydrate and lipid metabolism during the third trimester of pregnancy. *Acta Obstetrica et Gynecologica Scandinavica*, **56,** 475–478 (1977)

34 MEINEN, K., BREINL, H., SCHMIDT, E. W. and WELLSTEIN, A. Study to confirm the lack of severe cardiac side-effects following treatment with the beta-adrenergic drug fenoterol. *Gynecologic and Obstetric Investigation*, **9,** 319–324 (1978)

35 MERKATZ, I. R., PETER, J. B. and BARDEN, T. P. Ritodrine hydrochloride: a betamimetic agent for use in preterm labor. Part II: Evidence of efficacy. *Obstetrics and Gynecology*, **56,** 7–12 (1980)

36 MILLER, F. C., NOCHIMSON, D. J., PAUL, R. H. and HON, E. H. Effects of ritodrine hydrochloride on uterine activity and the cardiovascular system in toxemic patients. *Obstetrics and Gynecology*, **47,** 50–55 (1976)

37 RAGNI, N., PINT, P. F., BENTIVOGLIO, G., REPETTI, F., PELUCCO, D. and DIMUZIO, M. Poly-plethysmographic study on the effects of ritodrine on the cardiovascular system of patients in labor. *British Journal of Obstetrics and Gynaecology*, **86,** 866–872 (1979)

38 RICHTER, R. Evaluation of success in treatment of threatening premature labor by betamimetic drugs. *American Journal of Obstetrics and Gynecology*, **127,** 482–486 (1977)

39 RICHTER, R. and HINSELMANN, M. J. The treatment of threatened premature labor by betamimetic drugs: a comparison of fenoterol and ritodrine. *Obstetrics and Gynecology*, **53,** 81–87 (1979)

40 RYDEN, G. The effect of salbutamol and terbutaline in the management of premature labor. *Acta Obstetrica et Gynecologica Scandinavica*, **56,** 293–296 (1977)

41 ROGGE, P., YOUNG, S. and GOODLIN, R. Postpartum pulmonary edema associated with preventive therapy for premature labor. *Lancet*, **1,** 1026–1027 (1979)

42 SIMS, C. D., CHAMBERLAIN, G. V. P., BOYD, I. C. and LEWIS, P. J. A comparison of salbutamol and ethanol in the treatment of preterm labor. *British Journal of Obstetrics and Gynaecology*, **85,** 761–776 (1978)

43 SPELLACY, W. N., CRUZ, A. C., BUHI, W. C. and BIRK, S. A. The acute effects of ritodrine infusion on maternal metabolism: measurements of levels of glucose insulin, glucagon, triglycerides, cholesterol, placental lactogen, and chorionic gonadotropin. *American Journal of Obstetrics and Gynecology*, **131,** 637–642 (1978)

44 SPELLACY, W. N., CRUZ, A. C., BIRK, S. A. and BUHI, W. C. Treatment of premature labor with ritodrine: a randomized controlled study. *Obstetrics and Gynecology*, **54,** 220–223 (1979)

45 STEEL, J. M. and PARBOOSINGH, J. Insulin requirements in pregnant diabetics with premature labour controlled by ritodrine. *British Medical Journal*, **1,** 880–881 (1977)

46 STEER, M. L. Adrenergic receptors. *Clinics in Endocrinology and Metabolism*, **6,** 577–598 (1977)

47 STUBBLEFIELD, P. G. Pulmonary edema occurring after therapy with dexamethasone and terbutaline for premature labor: a case report. *American Journal of Obstetrics and Gynecology*, **132,** 341–342 (1978)

48 SUTHERLAND, E. W., ROBISON, G. A. and BUTCHER, R. W. Some aspects of the biological role of adenosine 3, 5′-monophosphate (cyclic AMP). *Circulation,* **37,** 279–306 (1968)

49 THOMAS, D. J. B., DOVE, A. F. and ALBERTI, K. G. M. M. Metabolic effects of salbutamol infusion during premature labor. *British Journal of Obstetrics and Gynaecology*, **84,** 497–499 (1977)

50 THOMAS, D. J. B., GILL, B., BROWN, P. and SUBBS, W. A. Salbutamol-induced diabetic keto-acidosis. *British Medical Journal*, **2**, 438 (1977)

51 TINGA, D. J. and AARNOUDSE, J. G. Postpartum pulmonary edema association with preventive therapy for premature labor. *Lancet*, **1**, 1026 (1979)

52 UNBEHAUN, V. Effects of sympathomimetic tocolytic agents on the fetus. *Journal of Perinatal Medicine*, **2,** 17–29 (1974)

53 WESSELIUS-DE CASPARIS, A., THIERY, M., YO LE SIAN, A., BAUMGARTEN, K., BROSENS, I., GAMISSANS, O., STOLK, J. G. and VIVIER, W. Results of a double-blind multicenter study with ritodrine in premature labor. *British Medical Journal*, **3,** 144 (1971)

54 WHITSETT, J. A., JOHNSON, C. L., NOGUCHI, A., DAROVEC-BECKERMAN, C. and COSTELLO, M. Beta adrenergic receptors and catecholamine-sensitive adenylate cyclase of the human placenta. *Journal of Clinical Endocrinology and Metabolism*, **50,** 27–32 (1980)

55 YLIKORKALA, D., KAUPPILA, A., TUIMALA, R., HAAPOLAHTI, J., KARPPANEN, H. and VIINIKKA, L. Effects of intravenous isoxsuprine and ritodrine, with and without concomitant dexamethasone, on feto-placental and pituitary hormones and cyclic adenosine monophosphate during late pregnancy. *American Journal of Obstetrics and Gynecology*, **130,** 302–306 (1978)

56 ZILIANTI, M. and ALLER, J. Action of orciprenaline on uterine contractility during labor, maternal cardiovascular system, fetal heart rate, and acid-base balance. *American Journal of Obstetrics and Gynecology*, **109,** 1073–1078 (1971)

57 ZLATNICK, F. J. The applicability of labor inhibition to the problem of prematurity. *American Journal of Obstetrics and Gynecology*, **113,** 704–706 (1974)

9
Preterm labour: other drug possibilities including drugs not to use

Nils Wiqvist

The choice of drugs for the pharmacological treatment of preterm labour is limited. The β-mimetic compounds are by far the dominating, not to say the only type of drugs that are currently used in clinical practice. As has been outlined earlier in this volume there are a number of reasons for this policy. It is, on the other hand, well known that β-mimetics in the acute situation sometimes fail to accomplish uterine quiescence. If the clinical conditions are such that the process must be arrested by any means to give the fetus a chance of survival there may be a demand for some alternative or additional pharmacological agent.

The present survey aims to discuss the possible usefulness of various alternative drugs. However, major emphasis will be given to drugs which inhibit prostaglandin synth(et)ase in view of the rationale behind their use as tocolytic agents and their controversial nature with regard to fetal hazards.

Progestogens

The significance of progesterone in the maintenance of pregnancy and in the initiation of labour has been clearly demonstrated in several animal species but its role in this respect in man remains obscure[54, 56]. It has not been possible to demonstrate consistent changes in the peripheral circulating concentrations of progesterone prior to the onset of labour in the human. In the absence of such changes, Csapo[11] introduced the local myometrial block hypothesis, which states that the myometrial concentration of progesterone is significantly higher in uterine segments adjacent to the placenta than at other sites. The hypothesis is supported by the results of Barnes, Kumar and Goodno[3], and Runnebaum and Zander[47] who found the concentration of progesterone to be higher in myometrium underlying the placenta than in that of other segments of the uterus. These results could, however, not be confirmed in the recent studies of Batra and Bengtsson[4]. The myometrial block hypothesis has been criticized on several grounds[12]. Firstly, the myometrium underlying the placenta is permeated by venous sinuses draining the retro-placental space, that is filled with blood containing very high concentrations of progesterone. The values for myometrial progesterone concentration in the biochemical studies were not corrected for the steroid in this blood. Secondly, it is not certain how the progesterone diffuses away from the retro-placental space. Thirdly, the uterus is able to concentrate progesterone from plasma using specific receptor proteins, so some gradient from plasma to myometrium might be expected, and finally if the inhibitory effect of progesterone on the myometrium depends on its interaction with cytoplasmic receptor protein, then it is not the concentrations of the steroid in the muscle which are important, but the degree to which the receptors are occupied. It seems possible that saturation of receptors may occur at relatively low progesterone concentrations.

Kumar, Goodno and Barnes[31] administered high doses of progesterone intravenously to women in preterm labour resulting in a transient decrease in uterine activity mainly in terms of a decrease in the frequency of contractions. However, the dose was so high that non-specific effects may have occurred, and the results are therefore hardly of any physiological significance. A number of different investigators[5, 13, 28, 41], have administered progesterone or synthetic gestagens in cases of preterm labour but were unable to show any inhibitory effect on uterine contractions.

Although progesterone binds very rapidly to its cytoplasmic receptors it takes many hours for its effect on myometrial activity to develop. It is too late, therefore, to try to reinforce the progesterone level once the uterus has begun to contract. There is, however, some evidence that progestogens may forestall the onset of preterm labour if given earlier in pregnancy[44, 51]. This possibility was reinvestigated a few years ago by Johnson *et al.*[29] in a prospective, double-blind, randomized study. The drug used was 17α-hydroxyprogesterone caproate (17α OHP-C) and only women at high risk for preterm labour, as judged from their past obstetric history, were included in the series. The mean duration of pregnancy for the patients treated with 17α OHP-C was 38.6 ± 1.4 weeks (± SD), this being significantly greater than that for the placebo group which was 35.2 ± 6.2 weeks ($P < 0.025$). Striking differences were found between the drug and placebo groups in terms of birth weight. The perinatal mortality rate in the group given the progestational agent (0 per cent) was significantly less than that observed in the placebo group (27 per cent). However, concern as to the validity of the results relates to differences between the groups such as the incidence of cervical cerclage, treatment with β-mimetics and some other details. Despite these drawbacks, this is probably one of the few controlled trials that have been published on this subject. There were no maternal or fetal complications attributable to the progestational drug but the study population is too small to confirm the efficacy of this medication as well as to delineate the precise maternal and fetal risks associated with its administration. For the time being there are hardly enough basic or clinical data at hand to justify routine use of progestational agents either in the treatment or in the prevention of preterm labour.

Ethanol

Opinions regarding the involvement of neurohypophyseal hormones in parturitional physiology have varied over the years. Recent observations indicate, however, that maternal oxytocin may be of some importance for both the initiation and the course of labour (reviewed by Swaab and Boer[53]). During pregnancy circulating levels of oxytocin are within the low picogram range and the values seem to increase before the beginning of normal labour at term. During labour there is a further increase so that maximum values are generally found during the second stage of labour. There is some controversy regarding the occurrence of a pulsatile pattern of secretion or a tonic release giving stable levels of oxytocin. By and large, administration of ethanol has been shown to inhibit the release of oxytocin from the neurophysis[15].

Following their first reports in 1965 a series of experimental and clinical publications have originated from F. Fuchs *et al.*[14] and A. R. Fuchs *et al.*[16], the principle advocates of this type of therapy. Since then more than 450 patients in preterm labour have been treated with ethanol in their institution and the method has been widely adopted, particularly in the United States, where no β-mimetic compounds of the β_2-type was approved for use in preterm labour until 1980. A loading dose of ethanol of 7.5 ml/kg body weight per hour as a 10 per cent solution is administered during a two-hour period followed by a lower maintenance dose of 1.5 ml/kg body weight per hour for a further 10 hours. In patients admitted with intact membranes the overall success rate, defined as arrest of labour or postponement of delivery for at least 72 hours, has been consistently around 65 per cent. A retrospective study of 165 live-born infants matched with controls showed, however, that infants weighing between 1000–1500 g whose mothers had received ethanol had significantly lower one-minute Apgar scores, and a higher neonatal mortality rate than the control infants[16]. There was also a higher incidence of respiratory distress in the ethanol group, significantly so in infants weighing over 2000 g. The respiratory distress problem seemed to be concentrated in infants born after failure of the treatment when a certain amount of ethanol still remained in the circulation. The authors concluded that if it appears that ethanol is unable to arrest labour the treatment should be discontinued at an early stage to permit the mother to eliminate as much ethanol as possible before delivery.

The same group of investigators have also conducted a comparative trial of ethanol and ritodrine showing that the β-mimetic agent gave better results than ethanol. Spearing[52] has completed a similar trial comparing ethanol and salbutamol. Labour was arrested for 48 hours or more in 32 per cent of the former and in 60 per cent of the latter group. However, the difference was not significant as only 22 and 20 cases respectively were studied. Salbutamol was more acceptable to the patients and to the staff than ethanol. Graff[19] was unable to confirm any difference between ethanol and glucose infusion for the inhibition of labour. Complications of ethanol such as lactic acidosis, aspiration pneumonia, and metabolic acidosis[40] and nervous system depression following ethanol have also been reported[18]. Common, but less harmful side effects of an intravenous infusion of ethanol are nausea, vomiting, headache and restlessness.

In summary, although ethanol has been shown to have some efficacy in arresting labour, β-mimetics are more acceptable to the patient and are perhaps associated with less neonatal morbidity than ethanol. It may be argued that ethanol has a mechanism of action that is different from β-mimetics and that a combination of the two treatments would increase the efficacy. However, in Europe, where β_2-adrenergic stimulants are freely available, there are few, if any, departments that advocate alcohol treatment as a routine. Whatever attitude the individual obstetrician may have it is self-evident that alcohol, always available, still can be useful in emergency situations when β-mimetics are not available.

Calcium antagonists

Calcium ions are of fundamental importance for the activation of contractile proteins and drugs that inhibit the passage of extracellular calcium through excitable membranes into the cell have a relaxing effect on smooth muscle contractility both *in vitro* and *in vivo*[62]. Calcium antagonists are mainly used in the treatment of ischaemic heart disease but are also potentially useful as tocolytics. A dose-limiting factor is the drug-induced impairment of the atrio-ventricular conduction. Verapamil is the most widely used drug of this type and has been tried in combination with β-mimetics to reduce cardiovascular side effects of the latter compound[36]. In the doses that verapamil can be used there is, however, little if any effect on the myometrium.

Nifedipine has fewer effects on atrio-ventricular conduction and has more specific effects on myometrial contractility. When given orally in doses of 10–30 mg there is significant inhibition of uterine activity both in non-pregnant and pregnant women[1]. Nifedipine has been found to reduce the amplitude of uterine contractions.

Andersson[1] tried nifedipine in 10 women with significant uterine contractions between the 28th–35th week of pregnancy. The initial oral dose was 20 or 30 mg followed by 10 or 20 mg every sixth to eighth hour. This treatment was sufficient to produce a reduction in, or complete inhibition of, uterine activity in all women. Maternal side-effects included transient facial flushing and moderate tachycardia, rarely exceeding an increase of 25 beats per minute. There was little change in fetal heart rate and all neonates were in good condition after delivery. These preliminary data are of great interest, but as the effectiveness and side-effect rate of the drug are incompletely known it can hardly be recommended for routine use until further animal experiments and clinical trials have been completed. Theoretically, there is a possibility of negative influence on fetal myocardial performance during labour.

Prostaglandin synthase inhibitors

Irrespective of the cause and nature of the pathophysiological process of preterm labour, there seems to be one common denominator or link in the chain of events that plays a crucial role in its initiation. This is the local release of substantial quantities of prostaglandins from uterine epithelium, fetal membranes and other tissues[22] (reviewed by Keirse[31]). These compounds not only activate the myometrium but are

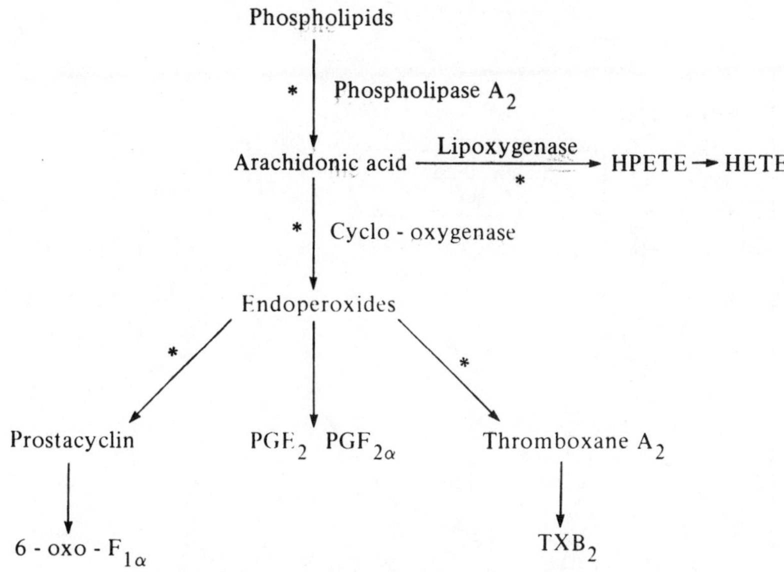

Figure 9.1 Pathways of arachidonic acid metabolism. Pathways marked (*) represent enzymatic stages which can be selectively inhibited. HETE = 12-hydroxy-arachidonic acid, HPETE = the corresponding hydroperoxide. (From Whittle[63], courtesy of Dr A.Ingelman-Sundberg, Scandinavian Association of Obstetricians and Gynecologists)

also thought to have an action on the connective tissue causing softening of the cervix and even weakening of the fetal membranes[21].

$PGF_{2\alpha}$ and PGE_2 have a potent stimulatory action on the uterus and represent the only endogenously synthesized prostaglandins that have been studied to any degree in the context of preterm labour. However, metabolites from arachidonic acid include also the unstable prostaglandin endoperoxides, PGD_2, prostacyclin (PGI_2), thromboxane A_2 and other compounds which may play a role in the process in one way or the other. Anti-inflammatory drugs such as aspirin, indomethacin, fenamates, naproxen and others inhibit the synthesis of prostaglandins[60]. This inhibition occurs by an action on the enzyme cyclo-oxygenase and affects the primary step in the metabolic conversion of arachidonic acid (*Figure 9.1*). This means that adminis-

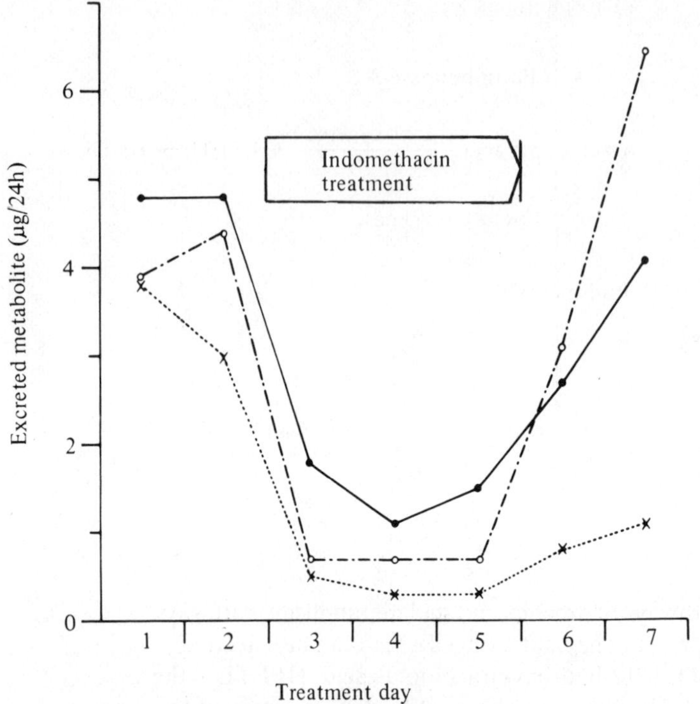

Figure 9.2 Excretion of the major urinary metabolite of PGE_1 and PGE_2, 7α-hydroxy-5,11-diketotetranor-prostane-l,16dioic acid, in three females receiving indomethacin (4 × 50 mg per 24 hours) on day 3–5 of the experiment. (From Hamberg[25], courtesy of the Editor and Publishers, *Biochemical and Biophysical Research Communications*)

tration of prostaglandin synthase inhibitors decreases the formation of almost all subsequent compounds, which generally results in partial or complete inhibition of uterine contractility[61]. Substances with selective effects on the particular pathways within the metabolic chain are available. However, these compounds are toxic and can only be used in *in vitro* systems. Drugs which act by inhibition at the cyclo-oxygenase step, resulting in an overall suppression of the prostaglandin synthesis are therefore the only substances, at the present time, that can be used in clinical practice (*Figure 9.2*).

Prostaglandin levels and preterm labour

The involvement of prostaglandins in the physiology of labour is discussed elsewhere in this volume. In this context it should only be emphasized that there is minimal evidence that PGF and PGE concentrations in blood, urine or amniotic fluid tend to increase during the last few days prior to the onset of normal labour at term, whereas there are clear indications that there is a significant elevation of these levels at the beginning of active labour(reviewed by Keirse[30]). Details as to the corresponding data in connection with preterm labour are for obvious reasons more difficult both to obtain and to interpret. Under these circumstances it is for ethical reasons not possible to collect amniotic fluid obtained by transabdominal amniocenteses, and prostaglandin levels in amniotic fluid collected from the cervix or the vagina are increased as a result of the membrane rupture.

There remains the possibility of measuring concentrations of prostaglandins in the circulation but these measurements do not discriminate between general reactions and uterine disorders, nor do they reflect details as to the nature of the intrauterine events. Uterine haemorrhage or necrotic fibroids represent pathological events with possible specific effects on prostaglandin synthesis and release[66]. Another problem relates to the methods of determining prostaglandins in plasma. The fact that the primary prostaglandins are formed and released from platelets during blood sampling invalidates the results of many investigations aimed at determining levels of the primary prostaglandins in plasma. Measurement of the main metabolite, 13, 14-dihydro-15-keto-$PGF_{2\alpha}$ (PGFM), eliminates the errors due to sampling and allows some conclusions to be reached.

Preterm labour is by definition a situation in which labour-like contractions are present and one would consequently expect the prostaglandin levels to be increased as in normal term labour[31]. Wiqvist,Lundström and Gréen[66] analyzed the plasma concentration of PGFM, which is not formed during sampling, using the gas-liquid chromatography mass spectrometry method in five cases admitted in preterm labour. Four of these patients had levels which were consistent with normal pregnancy (40–60 pg/ml), whereas one case in a more advanced stage of labour had values similar to those found during normal labour at term (450 pg/ml). Oral administration of indomethacin in a dose of 100 mg/day suppressed the PGFM values to undetectable or low levels except in the advanced case where labour rapidly proceeded to delivery. Schwartz *et al.*[50] determined the PGFM

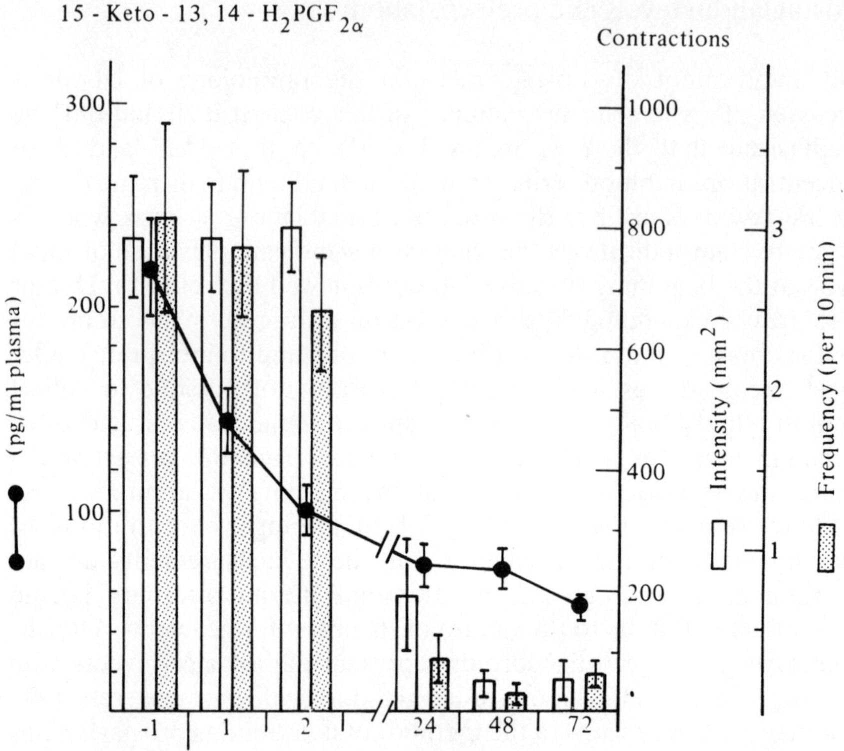

Figure 9.3 The effect of flufenamic acid on plasma levels of 15-keto-13,-14-dihydro $PGF_{2\alpha}$ and uterine contractions in patients with preterm labour. (From Schwartz *et al.*[50], courtesy of the Editor and Publisher, *Gynecologic and Obstetric Investigation*)

concentration in the plasma of 18 women in preterm labour using a radioimmunoassay. They found that the average level of the metabolite was 200 pg/ml which is far above the normal levels of the metabolite at this stage of pregnancy. Administration of flufenamic acid in a dose of 0.8–1.2 g/day resulted in a decrease in the average concentration of the metabolite so that values in the order of 40–70 pg/ml were present after one day of the treatment (*Figure 9.3*). It seems probable that the concentration of prostaglandins in the circulation is proportional to the level of uterine activity and cervical involvement. Normal or low values are present in cases of early preterm labour whereas the levels are high in advanced preterm labour.

Tocolytic effect

One of the difficulties in an objective evaluation of the effect of tocolytic agents in preterm labour is the criteria of selecting patients. A significant number of women admitted with symptoms of preterm labour are patients with so-called false labour. In other women there is a rapid spontaneous decrease in the uterine contractility immediately following hospitalisation. It is therefore questionable whether or not a reduction in uterine contractility should be attributed to the effect of the tocolytic drug or to hospitalisation and bed rest.

Evidence for the tocolytic efficacy of prostaglandin synthase inhibitors may, however, be obtained from various experimental situations. Waltman, Tricomi and Palav[58] studied the effect of indomethacin on the duration of the abortion process in saline-induced second trimester abortions. It was found that indomethacin in doses of 200 mg/day prolonged the average duration of abortion from normally 36 hours to 68 hours, a difference that was statistically significant.

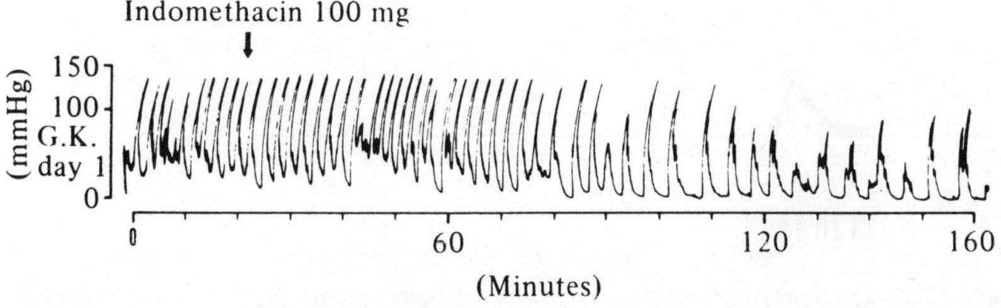

Figure 9.4 The effect on uterine contractility of rectal administration of 100 mg of indomethacin. First day of menstruation in a woman with dysmenorrhoea. (From Lundström, Green and Wiqvist[33], courtesy of the Editor and Publishers, *Prostaglandins*)

Moreover, intense frequent and spastic uterine contractions are typical during menstruation in women with dysmenorrhoea. This contractility pattern remains constant for many hours and significant alterations are easy to identify. *Figure 9.4* represents a tracing recorded by an intrauterine microballoon from such a case. Rectal administration of 100 mg indomethacin resulted in a definite decrease in the amplitude and frequency of contractions as well as abolishing the pain[33]. The pathophysiological mechanisms of dysmenorrhoea are of course completely different from those in preterm labour. However, this tracing, among many others, illustrates that commonly used doses of drugs which inhibit prostaglandin synthesis reach the uterus in effective concentrations and that uterine relaxation is evident as early as 60–90 min following administration of the drug.

Objective information about the effect of these inhibitors on the reduction of uterine contractions in preterm labour may also be obtained by external, standardized monitoring of the frequency of contractions before, during and after therapy. Particularly informative in this context are cases with long standing uterine hypercontractility of moderate degree, when treatment periods may be compared with treatment-free intervals. *Figure 9.5* illustrates the frequency of uterine contractions in a patient admitted to hospital for preterm labour.

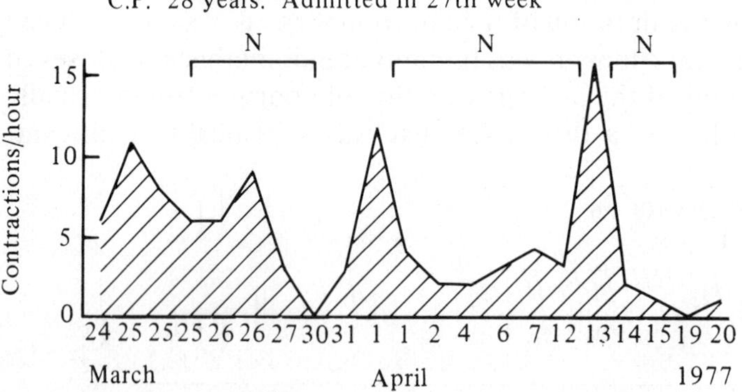

Figure 9.5 Frequency of preterm uterine contractions per hour recorded by external tocometry in the presence and absence of oral administration of naproxen (N)

Uterine contractility was monitored by external tocometry for at least one hour on most days during a period of one month. Naproxen was administered during three periods of time. The decrease in frequency during treatment was obvious as was the recurrence of uterine contractions between the treatment periods[65]. Ten women with preterm labour admitted to our department and monitored repeatedly in the same way had an average frequency of 17 contractions per hour which decreased to nine within the hour following oral administration of naproxen 500 mg. After two hours there was a further decrease of contractions to five per hour. Therapy with naproxen was continued at a dose regimen of 275 mg q.i.d. and the contractions were reduced to two to four per hour within 24 hours and remained at this level for the next few days. In the study by Schwartz *et al.*[50] on 18 women in preterm labour given flufenamic acid there was a similar reduction in contractility (*Figure 9.3*).

The tocolytic effect of prostaglandin synthase inhibitors has also been demonstrated in connection with normal labour at term. Reiss *et al.*[45] administered indomethacin as a single 100 mg suppository to 16 women, 14 of whom were in the active phase of labour. There was complete cessation of uterine activity in seven cases, marked prolongation of labour in seven and no effect on the progression of labour in two women. However, these two women delivered within one hour following administration of indomethacin.

It may be concluded that prostaglandin synthase inhibitors when given in adequate doses may decrease or inhibit preterm uterine contractions provided that therapy is not started too late in labour. It should, however, be emphasized that the tocolytic effect differs widely in individual cases. Sometimes there is no appreciable decrease in uterine activity while at other times there are dramatic effects reducing uterine tone to normal, with complete inhibition of all contractions and even reversion of the effacement of the cervix. The reason for the variability of the effect of these drugs may be that prostaglandins are by no means the only myometrial stimulants and that the inhibition of prostaglandin synthesis is only partial. The net effect may be related to the dose of drug used and the patient's weight, as well as to the rate and degree of absorption of these compounds from the gastrointestinal tract or rectal mucosa.

Clinical efficacy

Although there seems to be convincing evidence of the tocolytic effect of prostaglandin synthase inhibitors, this is of course not the same as the clinical efficacy in terms of a significant prolongation of pregnancy. The first clinical report was published in 1974 by Zuckermann, Reiss and Rubinstein[67] and at least 15 studies have subsequently appeared (*Table 9.1*). Most of these trials are open studies in which prostaglandin synthase inhibitors were administered orally or rectally. However, principles for including or excluding patients in the trials such as the degree of cervical dilatation, intact or ruptured membranes, duration of treatment (range 1–80 days), the need for supplementary therapy (β-mimetics, ethanol) as well as the criteria for the evaluation of success have been highly variable. It seems therefore meaningless to try to compare the success rates of different open studies. However,

Table 9.1 Administration of prostaglandin synthase inhibitors in preterm labour.

Drug	*Dose (mg)/day*	*Duration of therapy (days)*	*Gestational period (weeks)*	*Number of cases*	*Reference*
Indomethacin	200–300	1–42	28–35	50	7
Indomethacin	150	14	20–36	69	17
Indomethacin	100	5	26–37	29	20
Indomethacin	100–200	10	27–36	42	23
Indomethacin	150	1	26–35	15	37
Indomethacin	100	2 days after contractions ceased	26–35	20	52
Indomethacin	100–200	1–84*	20–34	51	59
Indomethacin	200–300	1 day after contractions ceased	24–36	300	68
Flufenamic acid	800–1200	4	28–36	18	50
Naproxen	1000	5–7	24–32	10	65

*7–21 days in the majority of cases

nearly all authors of the individual papers seem to be of the opinion that their attempts to postpone preterm delivery with prostaglandin synthase inhibitors have been reasonably successful.

A few studies represent controlled trials with adequate randomization of the patients and these studies may yield some objective information as to the efficacy of prostaglandin synthase inhibitors. Gamissans *et al.*[17] compared two alternative treatment regimes where the patients were randomly given either indomethacin plus ritodrine or placebo plus ritodrine (*Table 9.2*). The two treatment groups were matched with regard to gestational age, parity and tocolytic index. There were significantly better results with regard to gain in gestational age, neonatal weight and incidence of recurrences of preterm labour crises in the indomethacin plus ritodrine group compared with the placebo plus ritodrine group.

Spearing[52] conducted a comparative trial using ethanol (22 cases), ethanol plus indomethacin (20 cases) and salbutamol (20 cases). Labour was arrested for 48 hours or more in 32, 70 and 60 per cent respectively and delayed for 14 days or more in 36, 50 and 60 per cent of the cases. The results with ethanol and indomethacin were significantly better than those with ethanol alone. However, the author considered the tests of statistical significance to be of doubtful value in view of the small number of cases. No fetal complications were observed but the trial was interrupted as a consequence of literature reports on fetal cardio-pulmonary hazards such as premature closure of the ductus arteriosus. Niebyl *et al.*[37] at Johns Hopkins have completed a controlled clinical trial in 30 women randomly assigned to either a 24 hour course of indomethacin 25 mg × 6, or placebo. Only 1 of 15 in the indomethacin group failed to stop labour for 24 hours while 9 of 15 in the placebo group failed.

From a statistical point of view this is not convincing evidence as to the clinical efficacy of prostaglandin synthase inhibitors. It should, however, be kept in mind that the situation is rather similar to that of the β-mimetics where objective proof of their efficacy is difficult to provide. Individual cases may sometimes yield more information than groups of a highly heterogenous nature.

Fetal hazards

Cardio-pulmonary circulation

Disturbance of the fetal cardio-pulmonary circulation is not only the most serious complication associated with treatment by prostaglandin synthase inhibitors but also one of the few complications of significance that has been definitely documented in clinical literature. The most striking effect of these drugs is a premature constriction of the ductus arteriosus, and marked increase in pulmonary arterial pressure.

Table 9.2 Results of treatment of preterm labour in a controlled trial. I = indomethacin, R = ritodrine, P = placebo. After Gamissans *et al.*[17]

	Intact membranes		*Ruptured membranes*	
	R + P (n = 44)	*R + I (n = 41)*	*R + P (n = 27)*	*R + I (n = 28)*
Gain in days	25.7	44.2	18.7	22.8
Delivery before 37 weeks	27	15 ($P < 0.0125$)	22	21
Recurrences	23	10 ($P < 0.005$)	17	18
Fetal and postnatal deaths	5	2	2	2
Newborn weight (g)	2550	2799	2149	2215
Meconium in amniotic fluid	5	2	2	1
Apgar score less than seven	15	7	8	8
Umbilical artery pH	7.29	7.32	7.28	7.28
Respiratory distress syndrome	1	1	0	1
Pulmonary hypertension	0	0	0	1
Follow up of newborn (6–24 months)				
EEG grossly abnormal	2	1		
Psychometric test (Brunet-Lezine)	100.59%	100.66%		

These alterations may cause an increase in pulmonary resistance due to the development of pulmonary vascular smooth muscle and difficulties in maintaining adequate pulmonary blood flow. However, this increase in pulmonary resistance could be limited by a compensatory increased shunting of blood into the left atrium across the foramen ovale. Thus contraction of the ductus arteriosus is not necessarily or even generally associated with severe fetal morbidity. At birth the rise in blood oxygen tension is the prime stimulus to closure of the ductus arteriosus, although the mechanism of action of oxygen remains unclear. This dramatic alteration as well as the maintenance of a normal postnatal circulation may also be disturbed by the action of prostaglandin synthase inhibitors and may result in a syndrome of persistent pulmonary hypertension with the paradoxical situation of patent ductus arteriosus and persistent fetal circulation (reviewed by Coceani and Olley[8]).

There is by now clear evidence that endogenous prostaglandins are involved in maintaining prenatal patency of the ductus arteriosus. These prostaglandins are mainly formed intramurally in the vessel but possibly also brought to the ductus through the circulation. Judging from the relative potencies of the different prostaglandins, PGE_2 is the most probable candidate for maintaining the ductus in a relaxed state. However, there is evidence that prostacyclin (PGI_2), which has a vasodilatory effect, is the major product of arachidonic acid metabolism in the ductus and the problem is whether prenatal patency is determined by the more active PGE_2 or the more abundant PGI_2. It has been suggested that PGE_2 plays the major role in this context and that PGI_2 may complement the action on the muscle cells and prevent mechanical obstruction of the vessel by its anti-aggregatory effect on platelets[9]. It should, however, also be emphasized that PGH_1 and its metabolites are as potent as PGH_2 derivatives in relaxing ductal tissue[9].

Studies in animals

Details as to the consequences of administration of prostaglandin synthase inhibitors during pregnancy have so far been obtained principally from animal experiments. Biochemical studies have shown that prostaglandin synthetic activity is fully developed in the ductus of fetal lambs[42] at 0.7 and in calves[43] at 0.4 gestation. Administration of prostaglandin synthase inhibitors for instance in sheep during the early third trimester consequently results in constriction of the ductus. Studies in rats using the whole body freezing technique indicate, on the other hand, that these compounds have little or no effect on the diameter of the ductus until term pregnancy[48]. These results indicate that considerable species differences exist and that data from animal experiments cannot be applied to the human situation without reservation.

Novy[38] administered indomethacin intravenously over a 24 hour period in pregnant rhesus monkeys. No important changes in fetal oxygenation occurred despite levels of indomethacin in fetal cord blood that were sufficient to cause substantial inhibition of prostaglandin synthesis. There were no significant changes in the fetal heart rate or fetal arterial blood gas parameters suggesting that partial or complete constriction of the ductus, if present, had little acute effect on fetal oxygenation and also that the utero–placental and umbilical circulations were not adversely affected by these doses of indomethacin. If it is assumed that constriction of the ductus arteriosus occurred, effective cardiac output could probably be maintained by shunting across the foramen ovale. Support for this view is obtained from the work of Olley *et al.*[39] who demonstrated that in fetal sheep there was a 60 per cent reduction of the diameter of the lumen of the ductus arteriosus exposed to indomethacin, compared with the fact that there was no effect on carotid arterial P_{O_2}[39]. Similar findings were reported by Heyman and Rudolph[27], who administered aspirin to lamb fetuses *in utero*. Furthermore, despite marked constriction and shortening of the ductus in the study of Heyman and Rudolph, and a substantial increase in the calculated ductal vascular resistance, flow across the ductus arteriosus decreased by only 16 per cent. Even complete occlusion of the ductus, as by surgical ligation, is compatible with continued fetal survival *in utero*. However, under these circumstances there is progressive thickening of the free wall of the right heart ventricle and subsequent ventricular hypertrophy. If occlusion of the ductus persists *in utero* beyond two weeks, there is evidence of ventricular failure[24].

In the study by Novy[38], chronic oral administration of indomethacin to pregnant rhesus monkeys in a daily dose of 15–30 mg/kg, started on day 150 of gestation, resulted in 50 per cent fetal mortality and marked oligohydramnios. It should, however, be emphasized that this dose is 3–6 times higher than that used in pregnant women and also that administration in the monkey experiments was continued until 2–3 weeks post term (normal gestational period 168 days). Only one of eight fetuses had a ventricular weight greater than expected. There was also continued fetal and placental growth.

A problem of concern refers to possible differences in pharmacokinetics of prostaglandin synthase inhibitors between the maternal and fetal compartments. The half life of indomethacin in plasma has been shown by Traeger, Noschel and Zaumseil[55] to be 2.5 hours in young women and 14.7 hours in newborns. However, Mannaugh and Novy[34] found that the indomethacin levels in cord blood of rhesus monkey fetuses were in the same range as those of their mothers following prolonged oral administration of the drug, indicating that indomethacin crosses the placenta and that equilibrium is probably established between maternal and fetal plasma compartments during chronic administration of the drug. Similar concentrations of prostaglandin synthase inhibitors in fetal and maternal compartments were also obtained by Turner and Collins in women taking salicylates[57].

The human fetus and newborn

An association between pulmonary hypertension in the neonate and the inhibition of prostaglandin synthesis has been documented in a number of case reports from different neonatal units[2, 32, 35]. Wilkinson, Aynsley-Green and Mitchell[64] recently reported the presence of persistent pulmonary hypertension and abnormal prostaglandin E levels in three preterm infants after maternal treatment wth naproxen. One set of twins and one singleton were delivered at 30 weeks gestation although naproxen had been given to the mothers in an attempt to delay parturition. Inhibition of prostaglandin synthesis was shown by very low plasma concentrations of prostaglandin E in the fetal circulation. The ductus arteriosus remained closed despite signs of pulmonary hypertension with severe hypoxaemia. It was of interest to note that the concentration of $PGF_{2\alpha}$ and its metabolite remained at levels which were normal for this gestational age which is indicative of a differential action of prostaglandin synthase inhibitors in these cases (*Figure 9.6*).

Clinical experiences as to the incidence of fetal cardio-pulmonary complications following treatment with these drugs in preterm labour have accumulated particularly during the last few years. Some of these studies represent trials on limited numbers of patients actually in preterm labour, while others are retrospective analyses of the outcome of pregnancy and labour in large numbers of chronic users of salicylates, or are case reports describing single instances of fatality to the fetus. It is possible that unreported use of prostaglandin synthase inhibitors during pregnancy is rather common at least in western

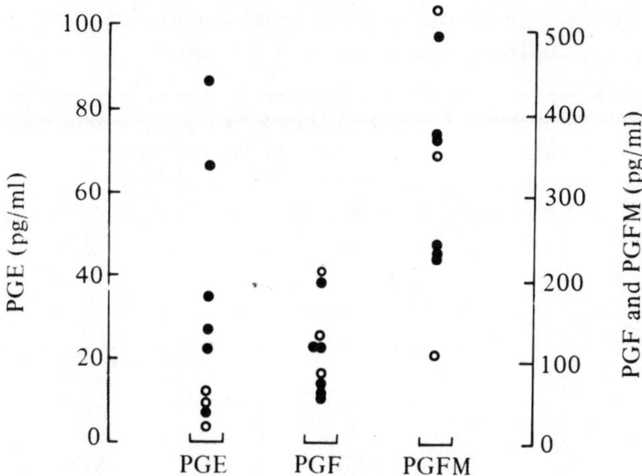

Figure 9.6 Plasma concentration of PGE, PGF and the metabolite of PGF (pg/ml) in three infants with persistent pulmonary hypertension (open circles), compared with concentrations in six premature infants without cardiopulmonary disease (closed circles). (From Wilkinson *et al.*[64], courtesy of the Editor and the British Medical Association)

Europe and case reports from a paediatric units are therefore not particularly useful in evaluating the incidence of this complication. Pulmonary hypertension can occur among preterm infants, with or without respiratory distress syndrome, who have not been exposed to prostaglandin synthase inhibitors. Its incidence increases with prematurity.

The best estimate as to occurrence of cardio-pulmonary disorders following treatment with prostaglandin synthase inhibitors is probably obtained by compiling reports from different clinical trials in which careful paediatric examination of the newborn has been carried out. *Table 9.3* represents a summary of experiences from such trials and includes a total of 730 mothers who had received these drugs during pregnancy. Seventeen babies were born with symptoms and signs of pulmonary hypertension. This means that somewhat more than two per cent of the newborns of such mothers suffered from this complication. However, 14 of the 17 neonates recovered usually within a few days, which reduces neonatal mortality due to this disorder to less than 0.5 per cent. Total perinental loss among the 730 mothers was 52 infants including those with intrauterine death and

Table 9.3 Cardio-pulmonary complications in the newborn following administration of prostaglandin synthase inhibitors to the mother.

Drug	*Number of cases*	*Persistent pulmonary hypertension in the newborn*		*Reference*
		Morbidity	*Neonatal death*	
Indomethacin	50	0	0	7
Indomethacin	10	5	2	10
Indomethacin	69	1	0	17
Indomethacin	29	4	0	20
Indomethacin	42	0	0	23
Indomethacin	15	0	0	37
Indomethacin	14	0	0	45
Indomethacin	29	5	1	46
Indomethacin	20	0	0	52
Indomethacin	51	0	0	59
Indomethacin	9	0	0	66
Indomethacin	300	0	0	68
Salicylate	64	0	0	57
Flufenamic acid	18	1	0	50
Naproxen	10	1	0	65
Total	730	17	3	

neonatal deaths. This gives a total perinatal mortality of seven per cent. These estimates are of course very crude in that details as to type and dose of the drugs, stage of pregnancy, interval between last drug dose and delivery, and birth weight, are widely variable.

The incidence of pulmonary hypertension as reported by different authors is also highly variable not to say confusing. Csaba, Sulyok and Ertl[10] administering indomethacin in a dose regimen of 100–200 mg/day for 1–2 days near term found that 5 of 10 women delivered neonates with symptoms of pulmonary hypertension, whereas Reiss *et al.*[45] were unable to identify any cases among 14 women given indomethacin 100 mg at the beginning of normal term labour. Grella and Zanor[20] reported 4 cases of pulmonary hypertension in 29, Rubatelli *et al.*[46] 5 cases in 29 and Zuckerman and Harpag-Kerpel[68] no cases in 300 women given prostaglandin synthase inhibitors for the treatment of preterm labour.

The data given in *Table 9.3* are difficult to evaluate in view of the fact that most results are based on uncontrolled trials. The study of Gamissans *et al.*[7] describes a trial, using indomethacin and ritodrine compared with placebo and ritodrine. No incident of pulmonary hypertension occurred among the babies of 71 mothers given placebo whereas one baby of 69 women had signs of the disease in the indomethacin group. This case appeared among 26 women who delivered their baby during ongoing indomethacin treatment. There was no difference between the groups with regard to meconium staining of amniotic fluid, Apgar score, umbilical artery pH, incidence of respiratory distress syndrome, postnatal EEG or psychometric test performed 6–24 months after delivery.

Niebyl *et al.*[37] have published a randomized study on 30 women given a 24 hours course of indomethacin or placebo. There was no case of pulmonary hypertension in the indomethacin treated group and there was no difference between the groups with regard to fetal wastage or neonatal morbidity or mortality. Van Kets *et al.*[59] have recently published a carefully studied, uncontrolled trial, where indomethacin was administered to 51 women with preterm labour between the 20th and 34th week of gestation. The patients received indomethacin 25 mg three to four time per day for up to three weeks or more. No single instance of cardio-pulmonary disorder could be documented. Birth weight averaged approximately 2500g and there were eight perinatal losses. In three of the eight fatal cases it could not be definitely excluded that the drug administration might have had some relation to the fatality. One of these women had gone through nine spontaneous midtrimester abortions and received two five-day courses of indomethacin beginning in the 24th week of pregnancy. Fetal heart sounds disappeared approximately 30 min before delivery; autopsy was not carried out. The second case had signs of cervical incompetence and cerclage was applied on two occasions. The patient developed an intrauterine infection and delivered a 300 g, severely macerated fetus. In the third case there were preterm labour contractions in the 30th week followed by spontaneous rupture of the membranes and fetal death due to intraventricular haemorrhage.

It may be concluded that the use of prostaglandin synthase inhibitors seems to be associated with an increased risk of cardio-pulmonary disorders. The risk of the neonate developing symptoms of this disease is probably of the order of one to three per cent and neonatal death occurring as a consequence of the complication is less than 0.5 per cent. Whether or not there is an increased incidence of intrauterine fetal death due to ductal closure following treatment with these drugs cannot be definitely answered on the basis of available reports. Preterm labour itself includes too many unknown factors.

It is also difficult to assess whether the risk of inducing pulmonary hypertension is increased when treatment with prostaglandin synthase inhibitors is undertaken in late as opposed to early pregnancy. A similar difficulty is encountered in assessing the risk for the fetus born under the influence of these drugs. It takes generally 48 hours for the endogenous prostaglandin levels to return to normal following the last dose. Whether or not normal patency of the ductus arteriosus may be re-established within the same period of time is not definitely known. The duration of treatment is probably of importance in view of the fact that such treatment may induce irreversible pulmonary vascular changes.

Other fetal disorders

Fetal hazards mainly observed in animal experiments following administration of prostaglandin synthase inhibitors include a number of different complications. Indomethacin has been shown to increase the number of areas of neuronal micro-necrosis in the fetal brain of the rat[49]. This observation of course raises serious questions and there is clearly a need for more animal work on this problem.

Novy[38] has observed that pregnant rhesus monkeys developed oligohydramnios following treatment with indomethacin. This drug is known to cause renal vasoconstriction and has an antidiuretic effect associated with decreased renal PGE_2 synthesis. It is believed that the decrease in amniotic fluid volume is related to an impairment of fetal urine excretion. However, the duration of therapy was considerable in these experiments and the dose of indomethacin very high. Oligohydramnios following treatment with prostaglandin synthase inhibitors has not been observed in the human.

Prostaglandins and thromboxanes affect platelet and vascular functions. Thromboxane A_2 is synthesized by platelets and has pro-aggregatory and pro-adhesive properties, whereas prostacyclin (PGI_2) formed by the vascular endothelium, has the opposite effect (reviewed by Vane[61]). Haslam, Ekert and Gillam[26] have found that platelet aggregation is inhibited and they have reported babies with serious bleeding manifestations associated with maternal salicylate ingestion. Turner and Collins[57] studied a similar group of 144 women who were regularly taking salicylates during pregnancy. In their series there was no clinical evidence of clotting deficiencies in the neonate despite the fact that some babies were born with raised cord-blood levels of salicylate. They concluded that, even if such a complication should occur, it must be uncommon. Van Kets *et al.*[59] observed one case of intraventricular haemorrhage among 51 fetuses whose mothers had been treated with indomethacin. Even though an iatrogenic effect could not be excluded, the authors were of the opinion that the dose of indomethacin given was small and that the haemorrhagic incident was more likely to have related to the course of labour and delivery than to the drug administration.

In the pregnant rabbit indomethacin has been found to delay fetal biochemical pulmonary maturation[6]. The levels of lecithin phosphorous in alveolar washes were less than 50 per cent of those in the control group on day 29 and 30 of pregnancy. A similar pattern of cortisol levels in fetal serum has been noted indicating that indomethacin may have an inhibitory action on the hypothalamic-pituitary-adrenal axis. The daily dose (20 mg/kg) was, however, high and further studies are clearly needed using a wider range of doses and including other species. In the human there is increasing cortisol production during pregnancy but evidence as to any fetal contribution to the cortisol pool is uncertain. Data obtained from rabbit experiments can therefore not be applied to the human situation without reservation. There is at any rate no evidence in the clinical literature as to any increased incidence of the respiratory distress syndrome following treatment with prostaglandin synthase inhibitors.

Conclusion

None of the drugs discussed in this chapter is a self-evident alternative to β-mimetics. Their efficacy is incompletely documented and there are too many side-effects or potential fetal hazards. Whether or not prevention of preterm labour can be accomplished by 17α-OHP-C injections needs to be confirmed by further studies. Ethanol has limited efficacy, can only be administered over a short period of time, has obvious side-effects and may be accompanied by an increased risk of respiratory distress syndrome in the newborn. Although administration of calcium antagonists represents an interesting approach to the problem, there is insufficient clinical documentation as to their usefulness in the treatment of preterm labour.

The prostaglandin synthase inhibitors present more of a problem. As judged from animal experimental data, there are reasons to adopt a negative attitude to their use. The results in clinical practice are not as bad as animal experimental data might suggest, in that cardiopulmonary disorders seem to be rare (one to three per cent) and fetal or neonatal death still more infrequent (less than 0.5 per cent). Other fetal hazards have hardly been documented in clinical literature. The efficacy of these drugs in arresting preterm labour may be variable.

However, there are some statistically significant results from controlled trials showing their efficacy. The traditional approach expressed in the literature is to warn against routine use of these drugs. Such a warning is probably still valid. However, it should be kept in mind that the death rate of neonates under 1000 g birth weight is high, perhaps around 80 per cent, and that of newborns between 1000–1500g is about 20 per cent. The risk of neonatal death if delivery takes place within the 20th to 30th week of pregnancy is therefore substantially higher than the estimated risk of iatrogenic death due to treatment with prostaglandin synthase inhibitors. The impression from the most recent reports within the field tend to support the view that these drugs may be useful in cases of very early preterm labour if β-mimetics fail to arrest the process. Expanded carefully controlled clinical trials are therefore clearly needed. Considering the risk of irreversible pulmonary smooth muscle vascular hyperplasia, it seems advisable to restrict the treatment to comparatively short periods of time, probably not exceeding one week.

References

1 ANDERSSON, K. E. Inhibition of uterine activity by the calcium antagonist Nifedipine. In *Pre-term Labour.* (Proceedings of the Fifth Study Group of the Royal College of Obstetricians and Gynaecologists), edited by A. Anderson, R. Beard, J. M. Brudenell, P. M. Dunn, 101–114. London, Royal College of Obstetricians and Gynaecologists (1977)

2 ARCILLA, R. A., THILENIUS, O. G. and RANNIGER, K. Congestive heart failure from suspected ductal closure *in utero. Journal of Pediatrics*, **75,** 74–78 (1969)

3 BARNES, A. C., KUMAR, D. and GOODNO, J. A. Studies in human myometrium during pregnancy. V. Myometrial tissue progesterone analysis by gas-liquid phase chromatography. *American Journal of Obstetrics and Gynecology*, **84,** 1207–1210 (1962)

4 BATRA, S. and BENGTSSON, L.-PH. 17β-estradiol and progesterone concentrations in the myometrium of pregnancy and their relationships to the concentrations in the peripheral plasma. *Journal of Clinical Endocrinology and Metabolism*, **46,** 622 (1978)

5 BRENNER, W. E. and HENDRICKS, C. H. Effect of medroxyprogesterone acetate upon duration and characteristics of human gestation and labor. *American Journal of Obstetrics and Gynecology*, **82,** 1094 (1962)

6 BUSTOS, R., BALLEJO, G., GIUSSI, G., ROSAS, R. and ISA, J. C. Inhibition of fetal lung maturation by indomethacin in pregnant rabbits. *Journal of Perinatal Medicine*, **6,** 240–245 (1978)

7 CABALLERO, A., TEJERINA, A. and DOMINGUEZ, A. L'indométacine dans la prévention de l'accouchement prématuré. *Revue Française de Gynecologie et d'Obstetrique*, **73,** 45–54 (1978)

8 COCEANI, F. and OLLEY, P. M. Prostaglandins, their synthesis inhibitors and ductus arteriosus. In *Practical applications of prostaglandins and their synthesis inhibitors*, edited by S. M. M. Karim, 53–75. Lancaster, MTP (1979)

9 COCEANI, F., BISHAI, I., BODACH, E. P., WHITE, E. P. and OLLEY, P. M. On the evidence implicating PGE_2 rather than PGI_2 in the patency of the foetal ductus arteriosus. In *Workshop on Prostacyclin and its analogues*, edited by S. Bergström, J. R. Vane. New York. Raven (in press)

10 CSABA, I. F., SULYOK, E. and ERTL, T. Relationship of maternal treatment with indomethacin to persistence of fetal circulation syndrome. *Journal of Pediatrics*, **92,** 484 (1978)

11 CSAPO, A. I. Progesterone block. *American Journal of Anatomy*, **98,** 273–291 (1956)

12 FLINT, A. P. F. In *Human Parturition* (Boerhaave Series, vol. 15), edited by M. J. N. C. Keirse, A. B. M. Anderson, J. Bennebroek Gravenhorst, 85. The Hague, Martinus Nijhoff (1979)

13 FUCHS, F. and STAKEMAN, G. Treatment of threatened premature labor with large doses of progesterone. *American Journal of Obstetrics and Gynecology*, **79,** 172 (1960)

14 FUCHS, F., FUCHS, A. R., POBLETE, JR., V. F. and RISK, A. Effect of alcohol on threatened premature labor. *American Journal of Obstetrics and Gynecology*, **99,** 627 (1967)

15 FUCHS, A. R. and FUCHS, F. The possible mechanisms of labor inhibition by ethanol. In *Uterine Contraction*, edited by J. D. Josimovich, 287. New York, Wiley (1973)

16 FUCHS, F., FUCHS, A. R., LAURSEN, N. H. and ZERVOUDAKIS, I. A. Treatment of pre-term labour with ethanol. *Danish Medical Bulletin*, **26**, 123–124 (1979)

17 GAMISSANS, O., CANAS, E., ESCOFET, J., FIGUERAS, J., LECUMBERRI, J. and JIMENEZ, R. Prostaglandin synthetase inhibitors in the management of premature labour. *Proceedings of the Ninth World Congress of Gynecology and Obstetrics* (Tokyo, 1979). Amsterdam, Excerpta Medica (in preparation)

18 GREENHOUSE, B. S., HOOK, B. and HEHRE, F. W. Aspiration pneumonia following intravenous administration of alcohol during labor. *Journal of the American Medical Association*, **210,** 2393 (1969)

19 GRAFF, G. Failure to prevent premature labor with ethanol. *American Journal of Obstetrics and Gynecology*, **110,** 878 (1971)

20 GRELLA, P. and ZANOR, P. Premature labor and indomethacin. *Prostaglandins*, **16,** 1007–1017 (1978)

21 GRIÈVES, S. and LIGGINS, G. C. Phospholipase A activity in human and ovine uterine tissue. *Prostaglandins*, **12,** 229–241 (1976)

22 GUSTAVII, B. Release of lysosomal acid phosphatase into the cytoplasm of decidual cells before the onset of labour in humans. *British Journal of Obstetrics and Gynaecology*, **82,** 177–181 (1975)

23 HALLE, H. and HEUGST, P. Zusatztokolyse durch Prostaglandinsynthetase hemmung mit Indomethacin. *Zeitschrift für Geburtshilfe und Perinatologie*, **182,** 367–370 (1978)

24 HALLAR, J. A., MORGAN, W., RODGERS, B., GENGOS, D. and MARGULIES, S. Chronic hemodynamic effects of occluding the fetal ductus ateriosus. *Journal of Thoracic and Cardiovascular Surgery*, **54,** 770–776 (1967)

25 HAMBERG, M. Inhibition of prostaglandin synthęsis in man. *Biochemical and Biophysical Research Communications*, **49,** 720 (1972)

26 HASLAM, R. R., EKERT, H. and GILLAM, G. L. Hemorrhage in a neonate possibly due to maternal ingestion of salicylate. *Journal of Pediatrics*, **84,** 556–557 (1974)

27 HEYMAN, M. A. and RUDOLPH, A. M. Effects of acetylsalicylic acid on the ductus arteriosus and circulation in fetal lambs *in utero*. *Circulation Research*, **38,** 418–422 (1976)

28 HILL, L. M., JOHNSON, C. E. and LEE, R. A. Prophylactic use of hydroxyprogesterone caproate in abdominal surgery during pregnancy. *Obstetrics and Gynecology*, **46,** 287 (1975)

29 JOHNSON, J. W. C., AUSTIN, K. I., JONES, G. S., DAVIS, G. H. and KING, T. M. Efficacy of 17α-hydroxyprogesterone acetate in the prevention of premature labor. *New England Journal of Medicine*, **293,** 675–680 (1975)

30 KEIRSE, M. J. N. C. Endogenous prostaglandins in human parturition. In *Human Parturition.* (Boerhaave Series, vol. 15), edited by M. J. N. C. Keirse, A. B. M. Anderson and J. Bennebroek Gravenhorst, 101–142, The Hague, Martinus Nijhoff (1979)

31 KUMAR, D., GOODNO, J. A. and BARNES, A. C. In vivo effects of intravenous progesterone infusion on human pregnant uterine contractility. *Bulletin of the Johns Hopkins Hospital*, **113,** 53–56 (1963)

32 LEVIN, D. L., FIXLER, D. E., MORRISS, F. C. and TYSON, J. Morphologic analysis of the pulmonary vascular bed in infants exposed *in utero* to prostaglandin synthetase inhibitors. *Journal of Pediatrics*, **92,** 478–483 (1978)

33 LUNDSTRÖM, V., GRÉEN, K. and WIQVIST, N. Prostaglandins, indomethacin and dysmenorrhea. *Prostaglandins*, **11,** 893–904 (1976)

34 MANAUGH, L. C. and NOVY, M. J. Effect of indomethacin on corpus luteum function and pregnancy in rhesus monkeys. *Fertility and Sterility*, **27,** 588–598 (1976)

35 MANCHESTER, D., MARGOLIS, H. S. and SHELDON, R. S. Possible association between maternal indomethacin therapy and primary pulmonary hypertension of the newborn. *American Journal of Obstetrics and Gynecology*, **126,** 467 (1976)

36 MASLER, K. H. and RASENBOOM, H. G. Neuere Möglichkeiten einer tokolytischen Behandlung in der Geburtshilfe. *Zeitschrift für Geburtshilfe und Perinatologie*, **176,** 85–96 (1972)

37 NIEBYL, J. R., BLAKE, D. A., WHITE, R. D., KUMOR, K. M., DUBIN, N. H. ROBINSON, J. C. and EGNER, P. G. The inhibition of premature labor with indomethacin. *American Journal of Obstetrics and Gynecology*, **136,** 1014–1019 (1980)

38 NOVY, M. J. Effects of indomethacin on labor, fetal oxygenation, and fetal development in rhesus monkeys. In *Advances in Prostaglandin and Thromboxane Research*, vol. 4, edited by F. Coceani and P. M. Olley, 285–300, New York, Raven (1978)

39 OLLEY, P. N., BODACH, E., HEATON, J. and COCEANI, F. Further evidence implicating E-type prostaglandins in the patency of the lamb ductus arteriosus. *European Journal of Pharmacology*, **34,** 247–250 (1975)

40 OTT, A., HAYES, I. and POLIN, J. Severe lactic acidosis associated with intravenous alcohol for premature labor. *Obstetrics and Gynecology*, **48,** 362 (1976)

41 OVLISEN, B. and IVERSEN, J. Treatment of threatened premature labor with 6α-methyl-17α-acetoxy-progesterone. *American Journal of Obstetrics and Gynecology*, **86,** 291 (1963)

42 PACE-ASCIAK, C. R. and RANGARAJ, G. Distribution of prostaglandin biosynthetic pathways in organs and tissues of the foetal lamb. *Biochimica et Biophysica Acta*. **592,** 13 (1978)

43 POWELL, W. S. and SOLOMON, S., Formation of 6-oxoprostaglandin $F_{1\alpha}$ by arteries of the foetal calf. *Biochemical and Biophysical Research Communications*, **75,** 815 (1977)

44 REIFENSTEIN, E. C. Clinical use of 17α-hydroxyprogesterone 17-n-caproate in habitual abortion. *Annals of the New York Academy of Sciences*, **71,** 762–786 (1958)

45 REISS, U., ATAD, J., RUBINSTEIN, I. and ZUCKERMAN, H. The effect of indomethacin in labor at term. *Journal of Obstetrics and Gynecology*, **14,** 369 (1976)

46 RUBALTELLI, F. F., CHIOZZA, M. L., ZANARDO, V. and CANTARUTTI, F. Effect on neonate of maternal treatment with indomethacin. *Journal of Pediatrics*, **94,** 161 (1979)

47 RUNNEBAUM, B. and ZANDOR, J. Progesterone and 20α-dihydroprogesterone in human myometrium during pregnancy. *Acta Endocrinologica*, Supplement 150 (1971)

48 SHARPE, G. L., LARSSON, K. S. and THALME, B. Studies on closure of the ductus arteriosus. XII. *In utero* effect of indomethacin and sodium salicylate in rats and rabbits. *Prostaglandins*, **9,** 585 (1975)

49 SHARPE, G. I., KRONS, H. and ALTSCHULER, G. Perinatal use of indomethacin. *Lancet*, **2,** 87 (1977)

50 SCHWARTZ, A., BROOK, I., INSLER, V., KOHEN, F., ZOR, U. and LINDNER, H. R. Effect of flufenamic acid on uterine contractions and plasma levels of 15-keto-13,14-dihydroprostaglandin $F_{2\alpha}$ in preterm labor. *Gynecologic and Obstetric Investigation*, **9,** 139–149 (1978)

51 SHERMAN, A. I. Hormonal therapy for control of the incompetent os of pregnancy. *Obstetrics and Gynecology*, **28,** 198–205 (1966)

52 SPEARING, G. Alcohol, indomethacin, and salbutamol. A comparative trial of their use of preterm labor. *Obstetrics and Gynecology*, **53,** 171–174 (1979)

53 SWAAB, D. F. and BOER, K. Function of pituitary hormones in human parturition–a comparison with data in the rat. In *Human Parturition*, (Boerhaave Series, vol. 15), edited by M. J. N. C. Keirse, A. B. M. Anderson, J. Bennebroek Gravenhorst, 49–71. The Hague, Martinus Nijhoff (1979)

54 THORBURN, G. D. and CHALLIS, J. R. Y. Endocrine control of parturition. *Physiological Reviews*, **59,** 863–918 (1979)

55 TRAEGER, V. A., NOSCHEL, H. and ZAUMSEIL, J. Zur Pharmakokinetik von Indomethazin bei Schwangeren, Kreissenden und deren Neugeborenen. *Zentralblatt für Gynakologie*, **95**, 635 (1973)

56 TURNBULL, A. C., ANDERSON, A. B. M., FLINT, A. P. F., JEREMY, J. Y., KEIRSE, M. J. N. C. and MITCHELL, M. D. Human parturition. In *The Fetus and Birth*, edited by J. Knight, M. O'Connor, Ciba Foundation Symposium no. 47 (new series), 427–452, Amsterdam, Elsevier (1977)

57 TURNER, G. and COLLINS, E. Fetal effects of regular salicylate ingestion in pregnancy. *Lancet*, **2,** 338–339 (1975)

58 WALTMAN, R., TRICOMI, V. and PALAV, A. Aspirin and indomethacin: Effect on instillation/abortion time of midtrimester hypertonic saline induced abortion. *Prostaglandins*, **3,** 47 (1973)

59 VAN KETS, H., THIERY, M., DEROM, R., VAN EGMOND, H. and BAELE, G. Perinatal hazards of chronic antenatal tocolysis with indomethacin. *Prostaglandins*, **18,** 893–907 (1979)

60 VANE, J. R. Inhibition of prostagladin synthesis as a mechanism of action for aspirin-like drugs. *Nature (New Biology)*, **231,** 232 (1971)

61 VANE, J. R. Inhibitors of prostaglandin, prostacyclin and thromboxane synthesis. In *Advances in Prostaglandin and Thromboxane Research*, vol. 4 edited by F. Coceani and P. M.Olley, 27–44, New York, Raven (1978)

62 VASSORT, G. Voltage-clamp analysis of trans-membrane ionic currents in guinea-pig myometrium: evidence for an initial potassium activation triggered by calcium influx. *Journal of Physiology*, (London), 252, 713–734 (1975)

63 WHITTLE, B. J. R. Prostaglandin synthetase inhibitors. Drugs which affect arachidonic acid metabolism. *Acta Obstetrica et Gynecologica Scandinavica*, Supplement 87, 21–26 (1979)

64 WILKINSON, A. R., AYNSLEY-GREEN, A. and MITCHELL, M. D. Persistent pulmonary hypertension and abnormal prostaglandin E levels in premature infants after maternal treatment with naproxen. *Archives of Disease in Childhood*, **29,** 3 (1979)

65 WIQVIST, N. The use of inhibitors of prostaglandin synthesis in obstetrics. In *Human Parturition*, (Boerhaave Series, vol. 15), edited by M. J. N. C. Kierse, A. B. M. Anderson, J. Bennebroek Gravenhorst 189–200, The Hague, Martinus Nijhoff (1979)

66 WIQVIST, N., LUNDSTRÖM, V. and GRÉEN, K. Premature labour and indomethacin. *Prostaglandins*, **10,** 515 (1975)

67 ZUCKERMAN, H., REISS, U. and RUBINSTEIN, I. Inhibition of human premature labor by indomethacin. *Obstetrics and Gynecology*, **44,** 787–792 (1974)

68 ZUCKERMAN, H. and HARPAG-KERPEL, S. Prostaglandins and their inhibitors in premature labour. In *Practical applications of prostaglandins and their synthesis inhibitors*, edited by S. M. M. Karim, 411–435. Lancaster, MTP (1979)

10
Corticosteroids: the case for their use

Mary Ellen Avery

What are the questions that require answers before a new intervention to prevent or modify disease becomes accepted and recommended therapy? I think the obvious questions are as follows:

(1) What is the seriousness of the disorder to be treated? More aggressive approaches to therapy are appropriate if the disease can be fatal or has a significant morbidity rather than a benign self-limited course.
(2) Are effective alternate approaches available?
(3) Is the proposed remedy rational? Does a body of evidence exist to document its efficacy in animals? What is known of its mechanism of action?
(4) How effective is it in controlled trials? What is known of acute or chronic toxicity?
(5) Does the putative benefit outweigh economic and other costs?
(6) When are the data adequate?

Controversies in medicine usually arise when evidence is conflicting or incomplete. Sometimes they persist because all the data available have not been presented in a way that permits the casual student of a subject to feel comfortable with the information at hand. The editors of this volume feel that enough controversy persists with respect to the use of glucocorticoids prenatally to prevent hyaline membrane disease (HMD) to justify a 'pro' and 'con' style of presentation. As the author of the 'pro' presentation, I shall try to answer the general questions just posed; my conclusion will be that the benefits outweigh the risks.

What is the seriousness of respiratory distress syndrome (hyaline membrane disease)?

The question deserves a careful answer in 1980 because both incidence and morbidity differ now in comparison to the 1950s and 1960s, when many of the classic descriptions were written. In the early 1960s we estimated the incidence of fatal hyaline membrane disease in the USA to be 3.8 per 100 births under 2500 g, or a national figure of 12 000 deaths per year[1]. In 1968, Wood and Farrell[44] found from national statistics that there were 8273 deaths from HMD/RDS and another 2624 in which it was a contributing factor, or a total of 10 897 deaths which was 19 percent of all neonatal deaths for that year. The incidence of the disease was estimated at 40 000 cases per year, or 1 percent of all births.

The next decade saw the introduction and wide availability of better methods of treatment, in particular ventilators and the use of continuous distending airway pressure. Neonatal mortality fell country-wide from 15.9 per 1000 live births in 1968 to 9.4 per 1000 in 1978.[43] Deaths from HMD decreased in larger infants, but more low birth weight infants lived long enough to manifest respiratory distress and its complications. For example, Tooley[41], reporting from the University of California, San Francisco, noted 276 infants born with HMD from 1969 through 1978. No deaths due to HMD occurred in infants weighing over 1500 g, and the proportion of survivors under 1500 g increased steadily. Most dramatic was the change in the under 1000 g group, from no survivors in 1969–71 to about 50 percent survivors in 1978.

Reports from perinatal centers would lead us to the view that RDS continues to occur in about 10–15 percent of infants under 2500 g, which is about 1 percent of live births, but deaths are rare over 1500 g. Overall mortality from HMD remains of the order of 3–4 per 100 births under 2500 g or about 7000 deaths per year, assuming that there are 3.3 million live births annually in the USA. The major change from the 1950s and 1960s is in the much larger number of very small infants who now receive intensive care and survive. Such infants did not enter our statistics of the '50s, when only infants over 1 kg birth-weight were reported.[1]

A 'new' syndrome of chronic pulmonary insufficiency after treatment of HMD, bronchopulmonary dysplasia was described in 1967, and in 1979 this was the subject of a workshop sponsored by the National Heart, Lung and Blood Institute[30], so prevalent and so vexing was the problem. This chronic lung dysfunction follows severe HMD, after use of high inspired oxygen mixtures and mechanical ventilation. Debate continues as to the role of barotrauma and/or oxygen toxicity in the pathogenesis of the pulmonary injury. The changes include interstitial fibrosis, sloughing of epithelial cells, squamous metaplasia of bronchial lining, loss of cilia, and subsequent pooling of secretions and a predisposition to secondary infection[14].

Estimates of incidence of bronchopulmonary dysplasia depend on the population under study, since the problem is more common in very low birth weight infants, who are seen in relatively larger numbers in neonatal centers that receive referrals from many nurseries[45]. In Bancalari's[6] experience in Miami, the diagnosis was made in 14.5 percent of infants who required mechanical ventilation for more than 3 days and who survived for more than 30 days, the time usually required for the chronic changes to be clinically and radiographically evident. The infants in this series were between 27 and 35 weeks and weighed between 920 and 1560 g. In tertiary centers where more 600–1000 g infants are treated, bronchopulmonary dysplasia is even more common, so that some feel that about one-third of infants under 1 kg show some chronic pulmonary changes for the first months of life[9]. Nearly all infants under 1000 g birth weight who require mechanical ventilation have pulmonary changes that persist for some weeks or even months.

Bronchopulmonary dysplasia is only one of the complications of HMD. Persistent patent ductus arteriosus has been recognized more often as more small premature infants survive their initial respiratory distress, only to develop pulmonary edema and increasing oxygen requirements several days later[23]. The association between patent ductus arteriosus and bronchopulmonary dysplasia was noted by a number of authors, and has raised the possibility of the role of chronic pulmonary edema in the pathogenesis of bronchopulmonary dysplasia.[9,10].

Other problems associated with severe HMD are intracranial hemorrhage and the complications of umbilical artery catheters, which are required for careful monitoring of blood pressure and blood gases. Some feel that necrotizing enterocolitis is a consequence of catheter complications or hypotension in association with infection. Not all these problems will be overcome if respiratory distress is prevented. Surely some of them will be avoided since we cannot blame them on prematurity *per se*.

The question of whether prevention of RDS will lead to less chronic lung problems remains open. It seems probable that avoidance of the need for mechanical ventilation and high inspired oxygen will at the least reduce the problem of air leak, which occurs in about 25 percent of ventilated infants[28]. A reduction of chronic pulmonary changes seems likely. No reasonable argument can be mounted against the desire to prevent a disorder of the prevalence and severity of HMD.

Are effective alternative methods of treatment available?

Each year we see evidence of more effective treatment of infants with respiratory distress. Ventilators, monitors, blood-gas micro-analyses, and importantly a cadre of experienced neonatologists and nurses have brought about this improvement. Nonetheless, some infants continue to die despite vigorous supportive therapy, while others will be hospitalized for months with bronchopulmonary dysplasia, which may then be fatal during the first year of life, or they may suffer the lifelong sequelae of intracranial hemorrhage. The treatment at hand is not effective enough. Promising reports of an artificial surfactant administered to sick infants may alter our views about treatment; but at present these interventions are still experimental[20].

Is it rational to use glucocorticoids? How do they work?

To summarize an extensive literature, we can list the following relevant observations.

(1) The stage is set for normal birth by fetal glucocorticoid production. Blood and amniotic fluid cortisol levels rise at about 34–36 weeks gestation[18, 37]. Birth before then is abnormal in the sense of cortisol deprivation.
(2) Glucocorticoids induce enzymes necessary for the synthesis of those phospholipids which are components of the pulmonary surfactant. They also induce other functions important in postnatal adaptations, such as liver and gut enzymes[17].
(3) Surfactant deficiency is the necessary predisposing condition for development of atelectasis and hyaline membranes[17].
(4) Glucocorticoid-specific receptors have been found in the nucleus and cytoplasm of alveolar type II pneumocytes, the cells that are the site of synthesis and storage of the pulmonary surfactant[3, 22].
(5) Extensive studies[2] in monkeys, lambs, goats, rabbits and rats have shown precocious lung maturation (increased distensibility and stability) after prenatal glucocorticoids given at least 24 hours

Table 10.1 Clinical studies of RDS prophylaxis (reviewed by Taeusch[39])

Author	*Steroid and doses*	*RDS % incidence (n)*		*% Mortality*	
		Control	*Treated*	*Control*	*Treated*
Liggins and Howie[27]	Betamethasone 12 mg IM q 24h ×2	24 (156)	9 (182)	23	9*
Caspi *et al.*[11]	Dexamethasone 4 mg IM q 8h up to delivery or 7 days	35 (62)	8 (55)	38	7†
Dluholucky, Babic and Taufer[13]	Hydrocortisone 100 mg IM ×1	45 (40)	16 (31)	35	10†
Ballard *et al.*[5]	Betamethasone 12 mg IM q 12–24h ×2	51 (138)	25 (56)	22	9†
Fargier *et al.*[16]	Betamethasone 12 mg IM q 24h ×2	20 (375)	4.4 (35)	16	7†
Block, Kling and Crosby[7]	Betamethasone 12 mg IM q 24h ×2	23 (53)	9 (57)	14	8*
Kleinschmidt *et al*[25]	Dexamethasone 12 mg PO qD ×3	12 (86)	3 (66)		
Vercherat, Thomè and Bovier-Lapierre[42]	Betamethasone 12 mg IM q 24h ×2	11 (412)	1 (79)	10	1*
Morrison *et al.*[29]	Hydrocortisone 500 mg IV q 12h ×4	24 (59)	9 (67)	12	4*
Papageoriou *et al*[32]	Betamethasone 12 mg IM q 24h ×2; then weekly	59 (32)	21 (29)	19	0†
Taeusch *et al.*[40]	Dexamethasone 4 mg IM q 8h ×6	14 (69)	2 (30)	15	14†

*total perinatal mortality
†neonatal mortality

before delivery. Alveolar cells in culture show increased uptake of radiolabeled precursors of the surfactant in the presence of glucocorticoids[36].

(6) All the reported prospective controlled clinical trials have shown a reduction in the incidence of RDS in infants whose mothers received glucocorticoids more than 24 hours and less than 7 days before delivery. It is striking and unexplained that even after a full course, of treatment some of the infants have classic RDS (*Table 10.1*).

(7) Glucocorticoid levels are elevated in infants with the disease during the hours after birth, presumably in response to stress[33]. The endogenous cortisol levels are about the same as that achieved prenatally by maternal administration[4]. It seems probable that the usual recovery from the disorder in 3–5 days depends on enzyme

induction of surfactant synthesis. Thus treatment prenatally to prevent the disease depends on the same mechanism as postnatal recovery when it occurs. The major difference is that clinical trials have evaluated synthetic analogues of cortisol, betamethasone or dexamethasone, and only a few studies have been carried out with hydrocortisone[13,29]

(8) The thymus of infants with severe RDS is larger in the first hours of life than in those without the disease. This is further evidence that RDS-afflicted infants have been in a relatively glucocorticoid-deficient environment before birth[19,21].

(9) Infants of diabetic mothers, when delivered before 37 weeks, have about a sixfold greater likelihood of developing respiratory distress syndrome as compared with infants of like gestational age in non-diabetic mothers[34]. Studies on alveolar cells in tissue culture demonstrate that insulin antagonises the enzyme-inducing effect of cortisol[35]. Presumably the hyperinsulinism of the infant of the diabetic mother leads to a delay in the normal cortisol induction of surfactant synthesis.

How effective are prenatal glucocorticoids in humans?

Prospective controlled clinical trials have all showna reduction in the incidence of RDS when glucocorticoid is given to the mother more than 24 hours and less than 7 days before birth. The first systematic use of betamethasone was reported by Liggins and Howie in 1972[27]. Betamethasone was chosen because it is long-acting and is protein-bound to a lesser extent than is hydrocortisone. It is known to cross the human placenta[27,31]. Dexamethasone-specific receptors have been found in type II alveolar cells. Two trials have shown the efficacy of hydrocortisone (*see Table 10.1*).

What is known of acute or chronic toxicity?

Glucocorticoids have been used to treat maternal illness in pregnancy for many years. Pregnant patients with asthma, rheumatoid arthritis, sarcoidosis, systemic lupus erythematosis and other illnesses have been on large doses of glucocorticoids and have given birth to normal infants. The problem has been to assemble a large series of such individuals and to follow their children over a number of years. The possibility of adverse effects of the illness itself or other medications further complicates the problem. Koppe, Smolders-de Haas and Kloosterman[25] have published a series of 34 pregnancies in 17 mothers treated with glucocorticoids. No effect on duration of pregnancy or the incidence of congenital malformations was found even when glucocorticoids were used throughout the whole of pregnancy in 18 instances. They noted a slight decrease in birth weight and placental weight as well as in the length of the infant. However, catch-up growth was found in all except one. Neurological and mental development was normal in all except for the one with delayed growth, but this infant had also been severely asphyxiated.

Given the lack of long-term studies in the literature, and the scarcity of short-term ones, the question has to be raised about possible late adverse effects on the child. The only information at hand is from the follow-up of human infants in the New Zealand trial published in 1972[24], and the preliminary follow-up of the Boston trial in 1979[8]. No abnormalities distinguish the steroid treated from the control infants in the first year after treatment. Careful neurologic assessment after school entry will be needed, since the short-term administration of glucocorticoids has been shown to affect brain histology in the monkey[15]. Most of the toxicity studies have been done with large doses of glucocorticoids given to small animals with short gestation[39]. These seem less pertinent than the studies in monkeys and the findings in human trials. The question of masking or predisposing to infection arose from clinical trials by Taeusch *et al.*[38,40] and deserves further evaluation. To date, none of the reported adverse effects have been as serious as the consequences of severe HMD.

The present situation leaves no room for either complacency or a defensive posture on behalf of dexamethasone. The best of all worlds would be the avoidance of premature birth. Since some babies will continue to be born precipitously prematurely, better treatment for surfactant deficiency would be desirable. Replacement with an artificial surfactant looks promising. Prenatal therapy continues to have a role, but we need not be restricted to glucocorticoids alone. Thyroxine deficiency is also documented in these infants[12], and induction of surfactant synthesis with thyroxine analogues is an intriguing idea. Perhaps hydrocortisone, rather than synthetic analogues, would seem more ‘physiological’ if glucocorticoids are to be given. Finally, we must search for an explanation for the failure of some infants to respond to prenatal glucocorticoids. Would they perhaps respond to other enzyme inducers, or is their problem an inhibition of surfactant?

As in any rapidly moving field of science, the list of questions usually exceeds the number of answers. It is important for the investigator to focus on the questions; it is equally important for the clinician to know about the answers at hand. In the case of prenatal glucocorticoid administration, more answers are at hand than is often the case before many new therapies are adopted. Even so, some well-informed obstetricians and pediatricians are reluctant to recommend glucocorticoids. The question I cannot answer I leave with you: when are the data adequate to achieve acceptance of a new intervention?

References

1 AVERY, M. E. and OPPENHEIMER, E. H. Recent increase in mortality from hyaline membrane disease. *Journal of Pediatrics*, **57**, 553–559 (1960)

2 AVERY, M. E. Pharmacological approaches to the acceleration of fetal lung maturation. *British Medical Bulletin*, **31**, 13–17 (1975)

3 BALLARD, P. L. and BALLARD, R. A. Cytoplasmic receptor for glucocorticoids in lung of human fetus and neonate. *Journal of Clinical Investigation*, **53**, 477–486 (1974)

4 BALLARD, P. L., GRANBERG, P. and BALLARD, R. A. Glucocorticoid levels in maternal and cord serum after prenatal betamethasone therapy to prevent respiratory distress syndrome. *Journal of Clinical Investigation*, **56**, 1548–1554 (1975)

5 BALLARD, R., BALLARD, P. L., GRANBERG, J. P. and SNIDERMAN, S. Prenatal administration of betamethasone for prevention of respiratory distress syndrome. *Journal of Pediatrics*, **94**, 97–101 (1979)

6 BANCALARI, E., ABDENOUR, G. E., FELLER, R. and GANNON, J. Bronchopulmonary dysplasia: clinical presentation. *Journal of Pediatrics*, **95**, 819–823 (1979)

7 BLOCK, M. F., KLING, O. R. and CROSBY, W. M. Antenatal glucocorticoid therapy for the prevention of respiratory distress syndrome in the premature infant. *Obstetrics and Gynecology*, **50**, 186–190 (1977)

8 BROWN, E., ZOLLINGER, E., SCHNELL, R. and TAEUSCH, H. W., JR. Normal growth and development after antenatal treatment with dexamethasone. *Pediatric Research*, **13**, 491 (abstract) (1979)

9 BROWN, E. R. Increased risk of bronchopulmonary dysplasia in infants with patent ductus arteriosus. *Journal of Pediatrics*, **95**, 865–866 (1979)

10 BROWN, E. R., STARK, A., SOSENKO, I, LAWSON, E. E. and AVERY, M. E. Bronchopulmonary dysplasia: possible relationship to pulmonary edema. *Journal of Pediatrics*, **92**, 982–984 (1978)

11 CASPI, E., SCHREYER, P., WEINTRAUB, Z., REIFI, R., LEVI, I. and MUNDEL, G. Prevention of RDS in premature infants by antepartum glucocorticoid therapy. *British Journal of Obstetrics and Gynaecology*, **83,** 187 (1976)

12 CUESTAS, R. A., LINDALL, A. and ENGEL, R. R. Low thyroid hormones and respiratory distress syndrome of the newborn. Studies on cord blood. *New England Journal of Medicine*, **295,** 297–302 (1976)

13 DLUHOLUCKY, S., BABIC, J. and TAUFER, I. Reduction of incidence and mortality by RDS by administration of hydrocortisone to mother. *Archives of Diseases of Childhood*, **51,** 420–423 (1976)

14 EHRENKRANZ, R. A., ABLOW, R. C. and WARSHAW, J. B. Prevention of bronchopulmonary dysplasia with vitamin E administration during the acute stages of respiratory distress syndrome. *Journal of Pediatrics*, **95,** 873–877 (1979)

15 EPSTEIN, M. F., FARRELL, P. M. SPARKS, J. W., PEPE, G., DRISCOLL, S. G. and CHEZ, R. A. Maternal betamethasone and fetal growth and development in the monkey. *American Journal of Obstetrics and Gynecology*, **127,** 261–263 (1977)

16 FARGIER, P., SALLE, B., BAUD, N., GAGNAIRE, J. C., ARNAUD, P. and MAGNIN. P. Prevention du syndrome de détresse respiratoire chez le prématuré. *Nouvelle Presse Médicale*, **3,** 1595–1957 (1974)

17 FARRELL, P. and AVERY, M. E. State of the art: hyaline membrane disease. *American Review of Respiratory Diseases*, **111,** 657–688 (1975)

18 FENCL, M. and TULCHINSKY, D. Total cortisol in amniotic fluid and fetal lung maturation. *New England Journal of Medicine*, **292,** 133–136, (1975)

19 FLETCHER, B. D., MASSON, M., LISBONA, A., RIGGS, T. and PAPAGEORGIOU, A. N. Thymic response to endogenous and exogenous steroids in premature infants. *Journal of Pediatrics*, **95**, 111–114 (1979)

20 FUJIWARA, T., TANAKA, Y. and TAKEI, T. Surface properties of artificial surfactant in comparison with natural and synthetic surfactant lipids. *IRCS Medical Science*, **7,** 311 (1979)

21 GEWOLB, I. H., LEBOWITZ, R. L. and TAEUSCH, H. W., JR. Thymus size and its relationship to the respiratory distress syndrome. *Journal of Pediatrics*, **95,** 108–111 (1979)

22 GIANNOPOULOS, G., MULAY, S. and SOLOMON, S. Glucocorticoid receptors in lung. II. Specific binding of glucocorticoids to nuclear components of rabbit fetal lung. *Journal of Biological Chemistry*, **248,** 5016–5023 (1973)

23 HEYMANN, M. A. and RUDOLPH, A. M. (Editors). *The Ductus Arteriosus.* (Report of the 75th Ross Conference on Pediatric Research), 1–108. Columbus, Ohio, Ross Laboratories (1978)

24 HOWIE, R. N. Clinical trial of antepartum betamethasone therapy for prevention of respiratory distress syndrome in pre-term infants. In *Pre-term Labour* (Proceedings of the 5th Study Group of Royal College of Obstetricians and Gynaecologists) edited by A. B. M. Anderson, R. Beard, J. M. Brudenell, P. M. Dunn, 281. London, Royal College of Obstetricians and Gynaecologists (1977)

25 KLEINSCHMIDT, V. R., SCHRÖDER, M., PREIBSCH, W., MATTHEUS, R., and HOFMANN, D. Zur Induktion der Lungenreife bei drohender Frühgeburt und geplanter vorzeitiger Entbindung. *Zentralblatt Gynaekologie*, **99,** 147–154 (1977)

26 KOPPE, J. G., SMOLDERS-DE HAAS H. and KLOOSTERMAN, G. J. Effects of glucocorticoids during pregnancy on the outcome of the children directly after birth and in the long run. *European Journal of Obstetrics, Gynecology and Reproductive Biology*, **7,** 293–299 (1977)

27 LIGGINS, G. C. and HOWIE, R. N. A controlled trial of antepartum glucocorticoid treatment for prevention of the respiratory distress syndrome in premature infants. *Pediatrics*, **50,** 515–525 (1972)

28 MADANSKY, D. L., LAWSON, E. E., CHERNICK, V. and TAEUSCH, H. W., JR. Pneumothorax and other forms of pulmonary air leak in newborns. *American Review of Respiratory Diseases*, **120,** 729–739 (1979)

29 MORRISON, J. C., WHYBREW, W. D., BUCOVAZ, E. T. and SCHNEIDER, J. M. Injection of corticosteroids into mother to prevent neonatal respiratory distress syndrome. *American Journal of Obstetrics and Gynecology*, **131,** 358–366 (1978)

30 NORTHWAY, W. H., ROSAN, R. C. and PORTER, D. Y. Pulmonary disease following respiratory therapy of hyaline membrane disease: bronchopulmonary dysplasia. *New England Journal of Medicine*, **276,** 357–368 (1967)

31 OSATHANONDH, R., TULCHINSKY, D., FENCL, M. and TAEUSCH, H. W., JR. Dexamethasone levels in treated pregnant women and newborn infants. *Journal of Pediatrics*, **90,** 617–620 (1977)

32 PAPAGEORGIOU, A. N., DESGRANGES, M. F., MASSON, M., COLLE, E., SHATZ, R. and GELFAND, M. M. The antenatal use of betamethasone in the prevention of respiratory distress syndrome: A controlled double blind trial. *Pediatrics*, **63,** 73–79 (1979)

33 REYNOLDS, J. W. Serum total corticoid and cortisol levels in premature infants with respiratory distress syndrome. *Pediatrics*, **51,** 884–890 (1973)

34 ROBERT, M. T., NEFF, R. K., HUBBELL, J. P., TAEUSCH, H. W., JR. and AVERY, M. E. The association between maternal diabetes and the respiratory distress syndrome. *New England Journal of Medicine*, **294,** 357–360 (1976)

35 SMITH, B. T., GIROUD, C. J. P., ROBERT, M. and AVERY, M. E. Insulin antagonism of cortisol action on lecithin synthesis by cultured fetal lung cells. *Journal of Pediatrics*, **87,** 953–955 (1975)

36 SMITH, B., TORDAY, J. and GIROUD, C. Evidence for different gestation-dependent effects of cortisol on cultured fetal lung cells. *Journal of Clinical Investigation*, **53,** 1518–1526 (1974)

37 SMITH, B. T., WORTHINGTON, D. and MALONEY, A. H. A. Fetal lung maturation. III. The amniotic fluid cortisol/cortisone ratio and the risk of respiratory distress syndrome. *Obstetric and Gynecology*, **49,** 527–531 (1977)

38 TAEUSCH, H. W. JR., WONG, Y. L., TORDAY, J. S. and EPSTEIN, M. Maternal glucocorticoid treatment and reduction of risk from respiratory distress syndrome. *Journal of Reproductive Medicine*, **23,** 252–256 (1979)

39 TAEUSCH, H. W., JR. Glucocorticoid prophylaxis of respiratory distress syndrome: A review of potential toxicity. *Journal of Pediatrics*, **87,** 617–623 (1975)

40 TAEUSCH, H. W., JR., FRIGOLETTO, F., KITZMILLER, J., AVERY, M. E., HEHRE, A., FROMM, B., LAWSON, E. and NEFF, R. K. Risk of respiratory distress syndrome after prenatal dexamethasone treatment. *Pediatrics*, **63,** 64–72 (1979)

41 TOOLEY, W. H. Epidemiology of bronchopulmonary dysplasia. *Journal of Pediatrics*, **95,** 851–855 (1979)

42 VERCHERAT, M., THOMÉ, J. and BOVIER-LAPIERRE, M. Fréquence de la détresse respiratoire idiopathique de prématuré. *Revue Française de Gynécologie et d'Obstétrique*, **72,** 183–187 (1977)

43 WEGMAN, M. E. Annual Summary of Vital Statistics–1978. *Pediatrics*, **64,** 835–842 (1979)

44 WOOD, R. E. and FARRELL, P. M. Epidemiology of respiratory distress syndrome (RDS). *Pediatric Research*, **8,** 452 (1974)

45 WUNG, J. T., KOONS, A. H., DRISCOLL, J. M., JR. and JAMES, S. Changing incidence of bronchopulmonary dysplasia. *Journal of Pediatrics*, **95,** 854–847 (1979)

11
Corticosteroids: the contrary view

Louis Gluck

Steroid therapy, as advocated for the acceleration of fetal lung maturity, produces a classical dilemma of benefit versus harm. In perinatal medicine this dilemma is perpetual; the benefits are evident long before harm becomes obvious.

Administration of steroids to accelerate fetal lung maturation is widespread throughout the world. The incidence of respiratory distress syndrome (RDS) is lessening and we are getting better at managing it. Despite a reduction from 50 000 to fewer than 9000 neonatal deaths from RDS per year in the USA, it is the most important of all newborn lung problems, and its incidence still remains significant.

Historical background

In 1968, Buckingham[7] first suggested from tissue culture studies that steroids might induce lung maturation analogous to their differentiating effects on gut. About one year later, Liggins[21] published the first evidence of pulmonary stability in lambs after steroid administration. He was studying the role of corticosteroids and corticotropin in inducing parturition in sheep whose gestations are about 150 days. By 130 days, lambs' lungs are mature enough to allow survival. At 117 to 120 days, even should they be born and breathe air, their lungs collapse since they lack stability from surfactant. However, in the offspring of ewes in whom parturition was induced by corticosteroids as early as 117 days, there was partial lung stability, although all the lambs expired. Liggins suggested that steroids had induced to some degree the accelerated maturation of the fetal lung. This was verified subsequently in rabbits, sheep and monkeys[10,11,27]. Giannopoulis[15] and Ballard[4] later showed that the fetal lung has glucocorticoid receptors. Such receptors in lung tissue means that those compounds have functions in the lung and that development is in part under hormonal control. However, receptors also are found in virtually all fetal tissue, including kidney, heart, muscle, jejunum, liver, brain, and thymus, suggesting that the steroids will bind to any fetal tissue in the body that is growing rapidly. This becomes one of the problems of the therapy.

Initiation of human applications

Following verification of acceleration of fetal lung maturation with steroids in animals, Liggins and Howie[22–24] studied approximately 1000 pregnant patients in labor prior to 37 weeks gestation. Patients initially were given alcohol and then, later in the study, salbutamol to stop labor. The study was double-blind, one group being given betamethasone, and the other group a placebo. Unfortunately the placebo was cortisone, because it had foaming characteristics similar to betamethasone; this shows the dangers of making assumptions from animal species like the sheep, whose placenta is not crossed by cortisone, while cortisone does cross the human placenta. Liggins and Howie found a particularly significant difference between the groups from 30 to 32 weeks of gestation, in which 8.7 percent of the treated group had RDS compared to 56 percent in the control group. The numbers on which these data are based were very small, being only 25 patients in one group and 23 patients in the other. This calls for caution in too literal an interpretation of these findings, especially since the incidence of RDS in the control group is extraordinarily higher than the 30–40 percent normally to be expected. To see an effect of corticosteroids required more than one and fewer than seven days from administration to the delivery of the baby.

Overall they showed a difference among all gestational ages studied, with the incidence of RDS in the betamethasone treated group being 10 percent, while in the control group, this was 15 percent. This 5 percent difference represented a one-third reduction in RDS, not its elimination, even in the treated patients. Possibly only female babies responded to steroids[33] and this is being currently evaluated.

However, there is another paramount issue. If there was only a 5 percent reduction in RDS due to treatment with steroids, this means that 20 patients would need to be treated for every one who would benefit[1]. There have been no studies reported in which the only patients treated were those in whom the fetuses had immature lungs. Not a single study has been reported where a susceptible group was defined other than by the notoriously inaccurate gestational age. Some studies have treated even more than 20 patients for every one in whom there was the potential for producing a beneficial effect. Most studies besides Liggins' and Howie's have been uncontrolled and retrospective. The study by Taeusch *et al.*[32] is one of the few controlled studies. This demonstrated a slight drop in RDS but no decrease in mortality between control and treated groups. They also found an increase in maternal infections, particularly with ruptured membranes. A very important recent controlled study by Quirk *et al.*[28] showed no difference in the incidence of RDS between a group treated with corticosteroids and the control group when all were delivered very carefully so as to avoid asphyxia.

Danger of inappropriate use

The way steroids are now being used in obstetric practice is similar to the inappropriate use of prophylactic antibiotics in the 1950s or to the probably excessive current use in West Germany of fenoterol to stop premature labor[20]. This tocolytic was initially thought to be entirely safe. About one million ampules plus 6 million oral doses were prescribed yearly for 600 000 annual deliveries, on the basis that this should significantly reduce the incidence of preterm labor. During three years of this therapy, the prematurity rate rose from 5.2 percent to 5.8 percent. Additionally there were several cases of acute pulmonary edema and at least 2 deaths after the drug was taken.

In similar fashion, the extravagant use of steroids is illustrated in the following quotation from Juan Stocker of the Royal Victoria Hospital in Montreal[31]: 'In Montreal betamethasone administration to patients at risk of premature delivery quickly gained acceptance by both physicians and patients. We now rarely deliver a baby prior to 36 weeks gestation or weight less than 2500 g without administration of two or more injections of betamethasone'. Their dosage schedule was 12 mg every 12 hours for four doses, then every seven days thereafter; sometimes these patients were on steroids for months because they were started relatively early in pregnancy due to concern about preterm labor.

Possible benefits

There are considerations in defense of corticosteroid therapy in pregnancy. One of these is financial. If steroids reduce RDS by one-third, that means potentially that around 3000 cases of RDS per year could be prevented. The cost of care in a neonatal intensive care unit for these 300 infants with RDS over a span of 14 days with a very conservative cost estimate of $1000 per day could mean a saving of about $42 million yearly through the use of steroids. Alleviating parental trauma associated with RDS is of inestimable value. It is important to point out, however, that prematurely born infants in whom RDS has been prevented remain, nevertheless, prematures with all the problems associated with prematurity. Furthermore, studies do not establish clearly that mortality is decreased by treatment with corticosteroids. Mortality of premature infants is actually a crude estimate and related more to competency of a neonatal intensive care unit than to a particular therapeutic regimen.

Limitations and possible dangers

In evaluating the good and bad effects of steroids in developing organisms, we may first ask how the steroids act. The steroid is not a brilliant thinking substance; instead it goes to any cell that has a protein receptor site. This means that it will act upon not only lung cells, but also liver cells, brain cells, kidney cells, gut cells, muscle cells, and any cell that is dividing rapidly in the fetus[8]. The steroid is picked up by the receptor at the cell membrane, then transported to the nucleus; it seeks out a configuration of the rapidly dividing DNA and attaches itself to the acid protein, whereupon DNA synthesis stops.

Thymidine kinase, an enzyme associated with DNA synthesis, is inhibited, with the resultant stimulation of transcription and production of messenger RNA. This enters the cytoplasm, stimulating protein synthesis by the endoplasmic reticulum. Hopefully this will be new enzyme protein to produce more surfactant.

Steroids go to cells throughout the body, decreasing the cell numbers by inhibiting DNA synthesis, thus resulting in lower than normal body weight. Steroids affect myelinization of nerve fibres[17]; the lung weight is smaller at term[19]; immune responses may be altered dramatically[9] (in fact there is evidence of long-term thymic inhibition); and most importantly, perhaps, steroids affect DNA synthesis in brain[3]. Additionally steroids are known to have behavioural effects[18,30].

In the fetal rat, glycogen normally increases in the liver until term;

after term there is a rapid drop in glycogen as glucose is mobilized. Normally phosphorylases are induced prior to delivery to break down glycogen. A series of enzymes appear before birth to metabolize glycogen and glucose in the newborn, when enzymes for absorption and metabolism of milk appear and those needed to wean at 23 days of life develop. If steroids are given to the fetus 3–5 days before birth, all this changes[16]. The high levels of glycogen are not stored in the liver. Neonatal animals are hypoglycemic and undergrown and they literally become metabolic cripples throughout life, because of inadequate development of neonatal digestive and weaning enzymes.

More importantly, perhaps, DNA levels in the cerebrum and cerebellum are markedly diminished after administration of steroids[12]. Steroids decrease brain growth and therefore head size and cause gliosis and a reduction in numbers of brain cells in rhesus monkeys[13]. Steroids produce effects even at a very low dosage, despite assertions that effects are seen only after large doses. A study by Loeb[25] showed that heart, skeletal muscle and kidney are particularly susceptible to steroid action in low doses, similar to doses given to the human. Even other so-called 'resistant' tissues, including the brain, show some effect from steroids. Steroids elevate cholesterol levels in human infants[2], particularly the very low density lipoprotein associated with coronary disease in the human; this remains elevated for long periods of time after these drugs are stopped. Steroid treatment also increases maternal infections, particularly with ruptured membranes[32].

In one study, hydrocortisone was given to preterm infants during the first 24 hours of life to prevent or ameliorate RDS[6]. The rationale was that if it could be given to the fetus to prevent RDS, why not give it to the preterm infants with RDS after birth. The steroid was ineffective in this role, but the development of these babies was followed. At the end of one year the investigators reported that of the eight deaths, six had had intraventricular hemorrhage, only one of whom had been among the untreated group. Also at the age of one year, motor development and EEG abnormalities were increased in the group treated with hydrocortisone, but numbers were too small for statistical significance[14].

The question is asked frequently about steroid effects on fetuses in mothers receiving prednisone and other steroid compounds chronically for asthma and other conditions. Such resultant babies are significantly undergrown compared to the untreated ones, according to a study published in *Science*[29]. Steroids thus seem to affect human fetal body growth adversely, even though low doses are given chronically to mothers who presumably metabolize these drugs very well.

Very bothersome is the data from Ballard[5] who, in evaluating various reported clinical studies, reduced the doses to cortisol equivalents, remembering that cortisol is the active component. Compounds like betamethasone and dexamethasone are artificial, not natural, compounds so that it is useful to reduce the dosage to cortisol equivalents. Using Liggins' and Howie's study[22] as a standard at 5 cortisol equivalents per kilo per 24 hours, some investigators have given considerably more hydrocortisone. Morrison[26] gave the equivalent of 16.7 cortisol equivalents per kilogram per 24 hours, which is in the range of some animal experiments showing effects on brain. Zuspan[34], using 1000 mg doses of hydrocortisone, administered 67 cortisol equivalents and was in a range even higher than several experimental studies.

Conclusion

In their 'zeal to heal' physicians often disregard the potential hazards of their therapy. Corticosteroids may well produce adverse effects in humans, especially where large doses are administered, but also perhaps with any level of therapy. Furthermore, from the study by Quirk *et al.*[28] we learn '. . . the present study demonstrates that careful attention to the management of the labor and delivery of the low birth weight infant so reduces the incidence of RDS that the pulmonary maturational effects of glucocorticosteroid therapy are not clinically demonstrated.' Thus, with a large potential for doing harm and with decreasing evidence[28] that steroids are really as efficacious as was initially believed, great caution must be exercised in their use. If steroids are to be given, there are at least some considerations to guide us.

First, since there is little effectiveness of corticosteroids given after 32 weeks gestation, steroids would be given only if the patient is going to deliver earlier than 32 weeks gestation. Second, there must be some determination of fetal lung maturity. If the fetal lung is immature in the patient threatening to deliver, then there is some rationale for administering steroids. Third, doses of steroids should be spaced so that delivery occurs more than 24 hours after the second dose. Fourth, the mother must be accorded the right of refusal through informed consent telling her that corticosteroids for this purpose are experimental, pointing out both benefits and potential hazards. Fifth, the resultant infant should be committed to a long-term follow-up study evaluating development.

In following these precepts, even should adverse effects be revealed later, at least our consciences can be clear that we exercised the best available judgment in treating a fetus susceptible to a potentially damaging condition, that informed consent was exercised and that, in following the infant, we have the opportunity to encourage or stop such studies in the future according to the outcomes of the infant.

References

1 AMIEL-TISON, C., BARBIANI, M., HORNYTH, H., TCHONBROUTSKY, C. and HENRION, R. Changes in incidence of IRDS and deaths due to IRDS during the last 10 years in the Port-Royal Maternity Hospital, without prenatal glucocorticoid treatment. In *Proceedings of 6th European Congress of Perinatal Medicine*, edited by O. Thalhammer and A. Pollack. Vienna, Norographic (1978)

2 ANDERSON, G. E. and FRIIS-HANSEN, B. Hypercholesterolemia in the newborn: occurrence after antepartum treatment with betamethasone-phenobarbital-ritodrine for the prevention of RDS. *Pediatrics*, **62,** 8 (1978)

3 BALASZ, R. and COTTERRELL, M. Effect of hormonal state on cell numbers and functional and maturation of the brain. *Nature*, **236,** 348 (1972)

4 BALLARD, P. L. and BALLARD, R. A. Glucocorticoid receptors and the role of glucocorticoids in fetal lung development. *Proceedings of the National Academy of Sciences of the United States of America*, **69,** 2668 (1972)

5 BALLARD, P. L. In *Mead Johnson Symposium on Perinatal and Developmental Medicine*. (Marco Island, Florida) Evansville, Mead Johnson (1978)

6 BADEN, M., BAUER, C. R., COLLE, E., KLEIN, G., TAEUSCH, H. W. and STERN, L. A controlled trial of hydrocortisone therapy in infants with respiratory distress syndrome. Pediatrics, **50,** 526 (1972)

7 BUCKINGHAM, S., MCNARY, W. F., SOMMERS, S. C. and ROTHSCHILD, J. Is lung an analogue of Moog's developing intestine? I. Phosphatases and pulmonary alveolar differentiations in fetal rabbits. *Federation Proceedings*, **27,** 328 (1968)

8 BUTLER, R. E. and O'MALLEY, B. W. Steroid hormone action–1976. In *Perinatal Endocrinology, Mead Johnson Symposium on Perinatal and Developmental Medicine No. 8* edited by R. S. Bloom, J. B. Warshaw, J. C. Sinclair, 3. Evansville, Mead Johnson (1976)

9 CLARMAN, H. N. Corticosteroids and lymphoid cells. *New England Journal of Medicine*, **287,** 388 (1972)

10 DELEMOS, R., SHERMATA, D. W., KNELSON, J. K., KOTAS, R. and AVERY, M. E. Acceleration of appearance of pulmonary surfactant on the fetal lamb by administration of corticosteroids. *American Review of Respiratory Diseases*, **102,** 459 (1970)

11 DELEMOS, R. and MCLAUGHLIN, G. W. Induction of the pulmonary surfactant in the fetal primate by the intrauterine administration of corticosteroids. *Pediatric Research*, **7,** 425 (1973)

12 DELEMOS, R. A. Glucocorticoid effect: organ development in monkeys. In *Lung Maturation and the Prevention of Hyaline Membrane Disease* (Report of the 70th Ross Conferences on Pediatric Research), edited by T. D. Moore, 771. Colmbus, Ohio, Ross Laboratories (1976)

13 EPSTEIN, M. F., FARRELL, P. M., SPARKS, J. W., PEPE, G., DRISCOLL, S. G. and CHEZ, R. A. Maternal betamethasone and fetal growth and development in the monkey. *American Journal of Obstetrics and Gynecology*, **127,** 261–263 (1977)

14 FITZHARDINGE, P. M., EISEN, A., LEITENYI, C., METRAKOS, K. and RAMSEY, M. Sequelae of early steroid administration to the newborn infant. *Pediatrics*, **53,** (1974)

15 GIANNOPOULOUS, G., MILLAY, S. and SOLOMON, S. Cortisol receptors in rabbit fetal lung, *Biochemical and Biophysical Research Communications*, **47,** 411 (1972)

16 GREENGAARD, O. Enzymic differentiation in mammalian tissues. *Essays in Biochemistry*, **7,** 159 (1971)

17 GUMBRIAS, M., ODA, M. and HUTTENLOCHER, P. The effects of corticosteroids on myelination of the developing rat brain. *Biology of the Neonate*, **22,** 355 (1973)

18 HOWARD, E. and GRANOFF, D. M. Increased voluntary running and decreased motorcoordination in mice after neonatal corticosterone implantation. *Experimental Neurology*, **26,** 651 (1968)

19 KOTAS, R. V., MIMS, L. C. and HART, L. K. Reversible inhibitions of lung cell number after glucocorticoid injection into fetal rabbits to enhance surfactant appearance. *Pediatrics*, **52,** 358 (1974)

20 KUBLI, F. Discussion. In *Pre-term Labour*, (Proceedings of the 5th Study Group of the Royal College of Obstetricians and Gynaecologists, London), edited by A. B. M. Anderson, R. Beard, J. M. Brudenell, P. M. Dunn. London, Royal College of Obstetricians and Gynaecologists (1977)

21 LIGGINS, G. C., Premature delivery of fetal lambs infused with glucocorticoids. *Journal of Endocrinology*, **45,** 515 (1969)

22 LIGGINS, G. C. and HOWIE, R. N. A controlled trial of antepartum glucocorticoid treatment for prevention of the respiratory distress syndrome in premature infants. *Pediatrics*, **50,** 515 (1972)

23 LIGGINS, G. C. and HOWIE, R. N. The prevention of RDS by maternal steroid therapy. In *Modern Perinatal Medicine*, edited by L. Gluck, 415. Chicago, Year Book Medical Publishers, Inc. (1974)

24 LIGGINS, G. C. Prenatal glucocorticoid treatment: Prevention of respiratory distress syndrome. In *Lung Maturation and the Prevention of Hyaline Membrane Disease* (Report of the 70th Ross Conference on Pediatric Research), edited by R. D. Moore, 97. Columbus, Ohio, Ross Laboratories (1976)

25 LOEB, J. N. Corticosteroids and growth. *New England Journal of Medicine* **295,** 547 (1975)

26 MORRISON, J. C., WHYBREW, W. D., BUCOVAZ, E. T. and SCHNEIDER, J. M. Injection of corticosteroids into mother to prevent neonatal respiratory distress syndrome. *American Journal of Obstetrics and Gynecology*, **131,** 358 (1978)

27 MOTOYAMA, E. K., ORZALEZI, M. M., KIKKAWA, Y., KAIBARA, M., LOW, B., ZIGAS, C. J. and COOK, C. D. Effect of cortisol on the maturation of fetal rabbit lungs. *Pediatrics*, **48,** 547 (1971)

28 QUIRK, J. G., ROKER, R. K., PETRIE, R. H. and WILLIAMS, A. M. The role of glucocorticoids, unstressful labor and atraumatic delivery in the prevention of RDS. *American Journal of Obstetrics and Gynecology*, **134,** 768 (1979)

29 REINISCH, M. J. and SIMON, N. G. Prenatal exposure to prednisone in humans and animals retards intrauterine growth. *Science*, **202,** 436 (1978)

30 SHAPIRO, S. Some physiological, biochemical and behavioural consequences of neonatal hormone administration: cortisol and thyroxine. *General and Comparative Endocrinology*, **10,** 214 (1958)

31 STOCKER, J. Prenatal glucocorticoid treatment: Reduction in neonatal deaths. In *Lung Maturation and the Prevention of Hyaline Membrane Disease*, (Report of the 70th Ross Conference on Pediatric Research), edited by T. D. Moore, 97. Columbus, Ohio, Ross Laboratories (1976)

32 TAEUSCH, H. W., FRIGOLETTO, F., KITZMILLER, J. and AVERY, M. E. Risk of respiratory distress syndrome after prenatal dexamethasone treatment. *Pediatrics*, **63,** 64 (1969)

33 TAEUSCH, W. Glucocorticoids and respiratory distress syndrome: Clinical questions. In *Report of the 78th Ross Conference on Pediatric Research*, edited by L. Gluck. Columbus, Ohio, Ross Laboratories (1980)

34 ZUSPAN, F. P., CORDERO, L. and SENCHYSEHYN, S. Effects of hydrocortisone on lecithin/sphingomyelin ratio. *American Journal of Obstetrics and Gynecology*, **128,** 571 (1977)

12
Induction of preterm labour – why, when and how?

M. C. Macnaughton

Introduction

Labour is induced most commonly at term, with the object of reducing perinatal mortality and morbidity due to postmaturity or placental insufficiency. Much has been written in recent years on this subject and there has been and still is controversy about the indications for induction of labour at this time.

Discussion of induction of labour at term is not the object of this chapter. Rather the question of induction of labour before 37 completed weeks of pregnancy, namely preterm labour, will be discussed. The reasons for, and the appropriate timing of, preterm induction are evaluated. In addition, and most importantly, the methods of induction at this earlier stage of pregnancy will be described since this may be one of the main problems confronting the obstetrician who decides that it is time the pregnancy was ended.

Induction of preterm labour or caesarean section?

Whenever a decision is made to intervene to deliver the baby, thought must be given as to how this may best be accomplished – by induction of labour or by elective caesarean section. Where preterm delivery is called for this choice is often a particularly difficult one because of the relative risks of mortality and morbidity to both mother and child.

In general, caesarean section serves the interests of the baby best but increases both the immediate and long-term risks to the mother. While caesarean section continues to increase in safety there may be special risk factors deriving from the medical or obstetric complication which is necessitating early delivery. Added to this is the occasional discovery, more common at early gestation, of a lower segment so poorly formed that the classical type of operation has to be performed. Even a vertical lower segment procedure is more risky for the mother in future pregnancies.

Caesarean section cannot then be undertaken lightly and the choice must be for induction of labour if either caesarean section appears to offer the baby little or no material advantage over vaginal delivery, or the prospects of intact survival of the baby are not good enough to justify the maternal morbidity risk of caesarean section. A neonatal death after a first pregnancy in a patient who is left to face her obstetric future with a classical uterine scar is the worst of all worlds.

The crux of the matter lies in assessing the baby's chances of survival and this is one of the most difficult problems in modern obstetric practice. The main factors which determine the neonatal mortality rate are gestational age and birth weight but clearly this may be further influenced by the occurrence of ante-, intra- or postpartum hypoxia or neonatal hypothermia and by the quality of the facilities and expertise available for care of the neonate. Within any paediatric department the approximate survival rates at a given gestational age and birth weight should be known[24]. It may, however, be necessary to modify this equation where there is evidence of fetal compromise due, for instance, to hypoxia.

Figure 12.1 shows the minimal gestational age at which caesarean section was performed for a fetal indication in 71 European departments[14], plotted as a cumulative frequency curve. The median value indicated is around 33 weeks although there is a large scatter starting at 29 weeks of pregnancy presumably reflecting a spectrum of neonatal care facilities and results. It is likely that a re-survey of these departments in 1981 would reveal that the minimal gestational age had become even earlier.

The problem lies principally with babies who weigh under 1500 g since, apart possibly from the complications of breech delivery or fetal hypoxia, the intact survival rate over this weight group is high.

Stewart[27] has produced good evidence that the mortality of neonates under 1500 g is considerably less following caesarean section than following vaginal delivery either spontaneous, by forceps or by breech with forceps for the after coming head (*Tables 12.1 and 12.2*) All the data from University College Hospital[27] support the view that intact survival of the very premature baby i.e. under 1500 g is more likely when abdominal delivery is undertaken than when vaginal delivery is

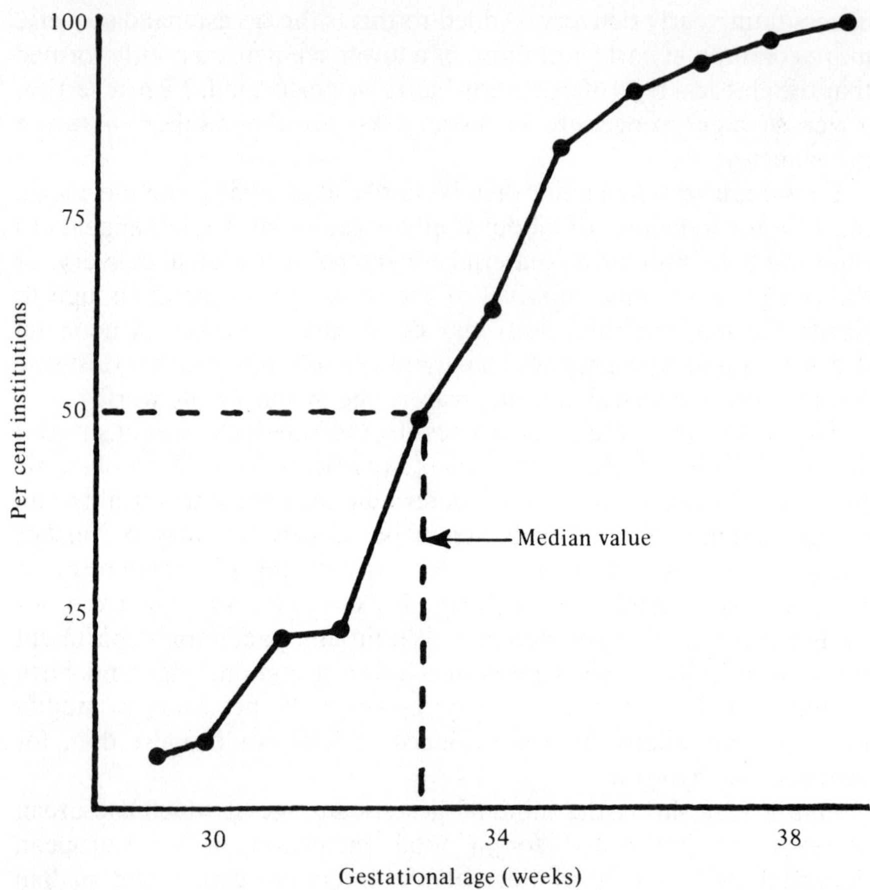

Figure 12.1 Minimal gestational age at which caesarean section is performed on fetal indication (From Kubli[14], courtesy of the author and the Royal College of Obstetricians and Gynaecologists)

allowed. Bowes[2] reported that when the birth weight was between 500 and 1000 g the mortality was 73 per cent from vaginal delivery and 36 per cent from caesarean section.

Although there is a widely held impression that the preterm breech is better delivered by the abdominal rather than the vaginal route, concrete evidence does not exist. A recent study, however, by Giersson[13] in Glasgow Royal Maternity Hospital lends further support to this view and suggests that intracranial haemorrhage, a common cause of death among premature breech deliveries, may be prevented by caesarean section. A failing common to all these studies, however,

Table 12.1 Mortality according to the method of delivery in 589 infants of birth weight < 1500 g born 1966–76 (From Stewart[27], courtesy of the author and the RCOG)

Method of delivery		*% Mortality*	
500–1500 g	Spontaneous vertex	45	
	Forceps	39	
	Breech	52	
	Caesarean section	18	$P < 0.001$

is that the groups delivered vaginally and abdominally may not be strictly comparable and Cruickshank and Pitkin[7] have pointed out that the only way to answer this question is by a carefully designed prospective investigation with randomised assignment to different treatment groups. This would allow comparison of a policy of universal caesarean section with a policy which involved modern methods of intensive intrapartum management which would include caesarean section on indication and vaginal delivery for the remainder.

Rush *et al.*[25] reported 109 cases of elective preterm delivery. Among the 57 delivered by elective caesarean section after 28 weeks gestation there were 2 perinatal deaths. In the induced group of 52 patients there was only one neonatal death. In this case, the mother had acute renal failure at 29 weeks and the infant died of hyaline membrane disease. However, in this series, only 15 out of the 109 babies weighed under 1500 g and 39 weighed over 2500 g. It is not possible from the paper to decide which babies in the low birth weight group were

Table 12.2 Mortality according to the method of delivery in infants of birth weight < 1500 g during 1966–70 and 1971–76 (From Stewart[27], courtesy of the author and the RCOG)

Method of delivery	*% Mortality*		
	1966–70	1971–76	
Spontaneous vertex	47	47	
Forceps	36	40	
Breech ± forceps for the after coming head	53	51	
Caesarean section	31	14	$P < 0.05$

delivered by caesarean section and which by induced labour. However, where preterm labour was elective, Rush, Davey and Segall[26] found that the perinatal mortality was about half that which occurred when preterm labour was spontaneous and without obvious maternal or fetal disease.

In most groups, Rush, Davey and Segall[26] found that survival was the rule after 31 weeks or if the infant had a birth weight of at least 1500 g and he considered that postponing delivery until 32 weeks of gestation would considerably reduce early neonatal mortality except where fetal growth retardation was present.

The present conclusion would therefore seem to be that caesarean section should be considered when the baby is alive and estimated to weigh under 1500 g or where there is an abnormal presentation. Above this weight preterm induction is justified with proper intrapartum monitoring and expert neonatal facilities. The critically important point is that the child should be delivered in as good a condition as possible. While survival is not uncommon among infants of less than 1500 g born with Apgar scores of 3 or less at 5 minutes, high Apgar scores are associated with an improved chance of survival[2].

Reasons for induction of preterm labour

There are two basic reasons for induction of preterm labour. The first is when, in the maternal interest, continuation of the pregnancy would present such hazards to the life or health of the mother that the pregnancy must be ended. The second and more common reason is when the intrauterine environment of the fetus is deteriorating to such an extent that it will either die or suffer damage unless it is removed from the uterus. At present, it is much more likely in this country to be performed in the fetal interest. There are, however, some indications where the interests of both mother and fetus are at stake. Such an example is severe renal disease of the mother where it may be desirable to terminate the pregnancy as soon as the child is of reasonable viability in order to prevent damage to the mother from further deterioration in renal function associated with the pregnancy. At the same time the fetus may also be at considerable hazard from poor growth and nutrition and may face the possibility of intrauterine death. It is therefore also in the best interests of the fetus that the pregnancy should be terminated as soon as the dangers of prematurity have been passed.

It will be evident, therefore, that the reasons for induction of preterm labour may be complex and that the interests of mother and child both in the index pregnancy and in subsequent pregnancies have to be taken into account when induction of preterm labour is indicated.

Maternal disease and induction of labour

Rarely, induction of preterm labour may have to be performed if either serious disease in the mother has developed or pre-existing disease has deteriorated. Such conditions include heart disease, various types of renal disease which are not responding to treatment, late vomiting in pregnancy, hypertensive disease which could lead to eclampsia, and malignant conditions. Induction of labour is usually best avoided in a patient with cardiac disease but if required, this will more often be for obstetric reasons and not for cardiac reasons. Antepartal fetal monitoring helps the clinician to identify when the fetus is at risk. This can be done by biochemical methods such as oestriol and human placental lactogen measurements (reviewed by Chard[6]) and biophysical methods of assessing the fetal heart either by stressed or unstressed methods. In a good review of this by Linzey and Freeman[17], they conclude that the oxytocin challenge test (OCT) is very useful in that a negative OCT reassures the clinician and prevents unnecessary premature intervention. They suggest that the combination of both OCT, oestriol values and L/S ratio are the appropriate tests for timing intervention in those conditions.

Not everyone subscribes to this view and many prefer a non-stress test (Flynn and Kelly[10]). It has also been reported by Egley and Suzuki[8] that there are a number of cases of deaths which follow negative OCT. It is evident that further work is required on the antenatal electronic monitoring of the fetal heart as a method of detecting antenatal fetal problems.

The reasons for elective preterm labour are well set out in two papers by Rush *et al.*[25] and Rush, Davey and Segall[26]. The first of these papers is from Oxford and the second from Capetown. Since the populations are very different, they are not directly comparable but what is apparent is that in both areas the commonest indication for elective preterm delivery is hypertension. In both studies, especially the one from South Africa, this was also the commonest cause of perinatal death.

Table 12.3 Indications for elective preterm delivery (excluding lethal deformity (After Rush *et al.*[25])

	Per cent of Cases
Hypertension	40.3
Antepartum haemorrhage	13.7
Diabetes	10.0
Fetal growth retardation	7.3
Rhesus isoimmunisation	7.3
Miscellaneous maternal conditions	17.4
Miscellaneous fetal conditions	3.6

Table 12.3 shows the different conditions for which elective preterm delivery was performed in Oxford in cases without lethal deformity.

In the Scottish Perinatal Survey[20] the commonest medical condition of the mother associated with perinatal death was essential hypertension. It is therefore understandable that hypertension, whether pregnancy-associated or pre-existing is the most common reason for induction of preterm labour.

Induction of preterm labour in hypertension

This is necessary when deterioration of the maternal condition is signified by a rise in blood pressure, the appearance of proteinuria, symptoms suggestive of developing eclampsia or low abdominal pain which might suggest abruption of the placenta. A sudden increase in weight even in the absence of proteinuria and hypertension should be noted since this may herald the rapid development of these conditions. Evidence of fetal growth retardation may be found by serial ultrasonographic measurements either by biparietal or thoracic diameters. It may be anticipated in cases of proteinuria and deteriorating renal function[12], and low or falling oestriol measurements. Frequent measurement of the serum uric acid and fetal heart rate may also be helpful in choosing the time for induction.

Elective preterm delivery in antepartum haemorrhage

Antepartum haemorrhage is still a major cause of perinatal death. In Scotland in 1977 the perinatal death rate from this cause was 2 per 1000[20]. The type of antepartum haemorrhage most commonly causing death was abruption of the placenta. This accounted for 70 per cent of the haemorrhage related deaths. It was interesting to note that two-thirds of the babies weighed more than 1500 g; 58 per cent of these were dead before the onset of labour so that it is doubtful if induction of labour would have saved any of these infants.

Placenta praevia is a less common cause of perinatal death in the Scottish Survey (0.2 per 1000), less in fact than that due to undiagnosed antepartal haemorrhage (0.5 per 1000).

In cases of abruptio placentae where the fetus is alive, the safest mode of delivery is caesarean section. Induction of labour before 37 weeks is only indicated if the baby is already dead or if caesarean section is contraindicated by the development of a blood coagulopathy in the mother.

Lunan[18] considered that a number of babies could have been saved in his series of abruptio placentae if delivery had been undertaken more expeditiously by caesarean section.

Caesarean section is indicated if the haemorrhage is due to a major degree of placenta praevia. Indications for induction of labour in other types of antepartum haemorrhage before 37 weeks are where the haemorrhage is continuing and there is danger to the mother. However, if a premature baby has been compromised, caesarean section may be the better method of delivery.

Elective preterm delivery in diabetes

In diabetes the decision whether to deliver vaginally or by caesarean section is primarily taken on obstetric rather than medical grounds. The timing of the delivery will depend on a number of factors, the most important being the degree of diabetic control of the mother, the presence and severity of pre-eclampsia, the degree of polyhydramnios, the size and maturity of the baby, the previous obstetric history and other clinical factors which infer special risk.

The main risk to the fetus is intrauterine death which is greatest in the last 4 weeks of pregnancy and increases as term approaches, especially when there is imperfect control of the diabetes. However, the earlier the fetus is delivered the greater is the danger of death from prematurity and respiratory distress syndrome (RDS). The estimation of the L/S has greatly reduced the risk of RDS and there is only a small risk of the baby developing RDS if the value is 2.0 or greater.

One difficulty with the L/S ratio was reported by Whitfield, Sproule and Brudenell[33] who found that nearly one-third of diabetic women failed to show the terminal rise in the ratio which occurs in the latter weeks of pregnancy in the non-diabetic woman. The reason for this difference is not known but the presence of a satisfactory L/S ratio in a diabetic woman greatly increases the likelihood of a successful outcome of pregnancy.

It is frequently difficult to know when to deliver the fetus. After 38 weeks, the danger of prematurity is usually overcome and although it used to be common practice to deliver the fetus before this time, with modern methods of blood sugar monitoring it has become quite usual, if there are no other complications to allow the patient to go to 38 weeks before labour is induced[19]. Nowadays, delivery before 38 weeks is not commonly required and should be avoided unless there are the most cogent reasons.

With good diabetic control, 70 per cent of patients are now delivered after 37 weeks[22]. The mode of delivery is of less importance than the timing. Until recently, many diabetic women were delivered by caesarean section but the increased risk of RDS among babies delivered abdominally compared with those delivered by the vaginal route, combined with improvements in the techniques of induction, especially in women with initially unripe cervices, has caused a swing away from caesarean section. These techniques of induction will be discussed later in the chapter.

Induction of preterm labour for fetal growth retardation

Fetal growth retardation is an important reason for preterm induction of labour. Here again assessment of the degree of compromise which the fetus has sustained may determine whether delivery is best accomplished by the abdominal or vaginal route. The prime consideration is that it should be made available to the paediatrician in the best possible condition.

In the Scottish Perinatal Mortality Survey[20] there were 302 perinatal deaths of babies of low birth weight. In 34 per cent of these (103 deaths) the mother had no obvious obstetric complication and the cause of the low birth weight was growth retardation. Of these 103 babies, 63 (61 per cent) were delivered before 37 weeks and the majority (73 per cent) died in the antenatal period.

If these babies had been recognised, carefully monitored by the many methods available and delivered either by induction of preterm labour or by caesarean section, many might have survived.

Growth retardation is very difficult to diagnose and much work is currently being directed towards improving the methods of detection. It is not the place in this chapter to evaluate the different methods of measuring fetal growth *in utero* and each department will have its own way of doing this.

If the diagnosis of fetal growth retardation is made, then careful monitoring is required. Before delivery is decided upon, an L/S ratio may be helpful and if possible delivery should be postponed until the ratio is more than two. Labour may then be induced or the patient delivered by caesarean section. If it is thought that retardation is severe or the baby is less than 32 weeks gestation, caesarean section may be the best method of delivery. Careful monitoring in labour preferably by electronic methods and fetal scalp blood sampling, if necessary, is essential if vaginal delivery is decided upon.

Fetal growth retardation may occur without any other signs of obstetric disease or may be associated with pre-eclampsia, essential hypertension and renal disease. The obstetrician has to be on the lookout for this abnormality in patients with these conditions and must be continually assessing the fetal condition so that he can choose the optimal time for delivery.

Rhesus isoimmunisation and induction of preterm labour

The numbers of cases of rhesus disease causing perinatal death has been greatly reduced in recent years but occasional cases persist. In the Scottish Survey rhesus disease accounted for 0.3 deaths per 1000 total births. The disease should be almost totally preventable now by routine use of anti-D immunoglobulin but a few women are escaping detection and some have been sensitized prior to the introduction of anti-D immunoglobulin.

Here again the timing of preterm induction will depend on the state of the fetus. This is assessed by measurement of the titre of antibodies in the blood and the level of bilirubin in the liquor. As babies can now be kept alive *in utero* by intrauterine transfusion until they are of reasonable viability, the judgment as to when to deliver depends on the individual case. Probably the earliest safe time to deliver the child is about 32–33 weeks and the risks of delivery must be weighed against those of intrauterine transfusion.

The prediction chart devised by Liley[15] and the refinement introduced by Whitfield[32] are helpful in this respect. The action line described by Whitfield is a guide as to when the obstetrician should intervene. Around 32–33 weeks the obstetrician has to decide whether to deliver the baby or to perform intrauterine transfusion and delay the delivery until the fetus is more mature. Palmer and Gordon[23] found that the neonatal mortality at 32 weeks in infants treated by intrauterine transfusion was 52.4 per cent and suggested that transfusion at this stage was less efficacious than premature induction of labour. Measurement of amniotic fluid phospholipids may provide a useful guide to timing induction of labour and clearly a number of factors, including the standard of neonatal care facilities available need to be considered. The exact timing of delivery of each case has then to be considered on its own merits.

Preterm delivery in fetal death and when lethal fetal abnormality is detected

When either of these conditions is detected labour should be induced and this has to be done in such a way as to minimize the danger to the mother. The most important aspect of this is the method of induction which will now be discussed.

Method of induction of preterm labour

The various conditions for which preterm labour has to be induced have been discussed – the why and the when. Perhaps the most important aspects of the induction of preterm labour is 'how'. The object of the induction of preterm labour is to deliver the baby in as good a state as possible and the method of induction is one of the most important aspects of this.

Human labour is not really the sudden event it usually appears to be. Its physiological control mechanisms evolve gradually over several weeks in the latter part of pregnancy. It therefore follows that the further these have evolved and the more imminent is spontaneous labour the more likely is induction to be easy and successful. This is borne out in clinical practice. Amniotomy, together with intravenous oxytocin infusion, is an admirable method of inducing term labour but its efficacy declines the further one moves into the preterm period. At these earlier gestations the myometrium is generally less sensitive to oxytocin and the cervix much less ripe so that it is harder to generate uterine contractions and much more uterine work is required to overcome cervical resistance. Induction of labour may then be much more akin to induction of second trimester abortion, a procedure for which prostaglandins have proved particularly valuable. For these reasons the use of prostaglandins has greatly improved our ability to induce preterm labour safely and effectively.

The responsiveness of the uterus and the state of the cervix when induction is performed is crucial to the method of induction and to the outcome of the labour. Bishop[1] was the first to evolve a pelvic score which takes into account dilatation, effacement, consistency and the

Table 12.4 Modification of the Bishop Score to assess cervical ripeness (From Calder, Embrey and Hillier[3], courtesy of the author and the RCOG)

	0	*1*	*2*	*3*
Dilation (cm)	<1	1–2	2–4	>4
Length (cm)	>4	2–4	1–2	<1
Consistency	firm	average	soft	
Position	posterior	mid-anterior		
Level	0–3	0–2	0–1;0	+

position of the cervix together with the level of head in the pelvis. This has more recently been modified by Calder, Embrey and Hillier[3] who measured the length of the cervix in centimetres rather than the percentage effacement which is more difficult to assess (*see Table 12.4*).

The unripe cervix at term is considered to be abnormal but for many of the complications requiring preterm delivery, the cervix can be expected to be unripe unless there has been some episode of spontaneous preterm labour or perhaps abruption of the placenta. The earlier that preterm labour has to be induced, the more unripe is the cervix likely to be but it should be remembered that ripening of the cervix occurs throughout the third trimester of pregnancy[5] so that by 36 weeks the cervix is usually fairly ripe. It follows, therefore, that the degree of ripeness of the cervix can help to determine the technique used to induce preterm labour.

If the cervix is found to be ripe this implies that the uterus is likely to respond to oxytocin although this is not always the case. When the cervix is found to be unripe near term it may be possible to defer delivery until cervical ripening occurs but if there is primary need to deliver the child preterm then methods are required which will overcome this problem. The method of induction will also be determined to some extent by whether the baby is alive or dead.

Preterm induction of labour can be a complicated procedure due to the unripe cervix, non-engagement of the presenting part, poor inducibility features and to the relative fetal immaturity as well as the presence of adverse fetal or maternal factors which are the reason for the induction. The combination of the unripe cervix leading to a long labour, and the poor fetal state which is frequently the reason for the induction may be hazardous to the fetus and delivery may therefore be more safely accomplished by the abdominal route. When induction of labour is performed it is essential that both the fetus and the mother are closely monitored and if there is any doubt about the fetal condition then caesarean section is indicated.

Probably the best method of inducing labour when the cervix is favourable is by amniotomy followed by intravenous oxytocin in increasing doses as first described by Turnbull and Anderson[31]. This method has been used in many centres over the last decade and has been found to be very satisfactory.

This method would not be satisfactory when fetal death or severe malformation is present because there is a possibility of introducing infection at amniotomy and a method should be used where the membranes can be preserved intact.

In these cases, Thiery[30] has suggested that prostaglandins E_2 or $F_{2\alpha}$ given by the intravenous or the extra-amniotic route have proved to be effective in cases of severe malformation or intrauterine death. When the fetus has been dead for a week or more disseminated intravascular coagulation must be excluded or treated before labour is induced.

When the cervix is unripe, therapy is necessary to ripen it before induction of labour. It has been the practice over many years to induce labour in these cases by prolonged intravenous oxytocin but this has been found to be fairly unsatisfactory[16]. Since the uterus at the preterm stage of gestation is less sensitive to oxytocin, resort to caesarean section was frequently necessary in these cases when induction failed. Oral prostaglandins have also been unsatisfactory for this purpose[11]. Another technique used was that of Embrey and Mollison[9] who introduced a Foley catheter through the cervix so that the inflated balloon lay just inside the internal cervical os. The time taken to effect cervical changes may be several days with this method but it is effective in some cases.

The most recent method advocated for cervical ripening is that developed by Calder, Embrey and Tait[4]. This method involves the use of prostaglandin E_2 in 'Tylose' gel injected via a catheter into the extra-amniotic space. A single dose of prostaglandin E_2 400 μg is suspended in 5 ml of 5 per cent methyl hydroxyethyl cellulose (Tylose) and delivered via a trans-cervical Foley catheter (20 ml balloon) into the extra-amniotic space. Uterine contractions result and after about three to six hours the catheter is extruded because the cervix is dilated and effaced. The membranes can then be ruptured and intravenous oxytocin started as is usually done in those cases where the cervix is already ripe.

This technique has proved to be safe, effective and acceptable by patients. Considerable experience has been obtained in several centres[29] and there have been no reports of serious maternal or fetal complications. Fears about the possibility of infection have not been realised in practice.

More recently Mackenzie and Embrey[21] have used a larger dose of prostaglandin in a sodium carboxymethyl cellulose gel given high into the posterior vaginal fornix 16–18 hours before induction of labour and achieved similar results to those obtained with the extra-amniotic group.

These methods are pre-requisites to the successful induction of preterm labour where the cervix is found to be unripe. In cases where induction is being performed for maternal pathology the use of prostaglandins, intravenously if the cervix is ripe, may be more efficacious and safer for the mother and will avoid the possibility of water intoxication which is one of the problems with oxytocin. This subject has been well reviewed by Thiery and Amy[28]. With the development of more sophisticated delivery systems for the prostaglandins and the possibility that particular analogues may show enhanced efficacy both for cervical ripening and uterine stimulation, the role of these agents for induction of preterm labour is likely to increase.

Acknowledgements

I should like to thank my colleague, Dr Andrew Calder, for his most helpful advice in the preparation of this chapter.

References

1 BISHOP, F. H. Pelvic scoring for elective induction. *Obstetrics and Gynecology*, **24,** 266–268 (1964)

2 BOWES, W. A. Results of the intensive perinatal management of very low birth weight infants. In *Pre-term Labour* edited by A. Anderson, R. Beard, J. M. Brundenell and P. M. Dunn. (Proceedings of the 5th Study Group of the Royal College of Obstetricians and Gynaecologists) 331–355. London, Royal College of Obstetricians and Gynaecologists (1977)

3 CALDER, A. A., EMBREY, M. P. and HILLIER, K. Extra-amniotic prostaglandin E_2 for the induction of labour at term. *Journal of Obstetrics and Gynaecology of the British Commonwealth*, **81,** 39–46 (1974)

4 CALDER, A. A., EMBREY, M. P. and TAIT, T. Ripening of the cervix with extra-amniotic prostaglandin E_2 in viscous gel before induction of labour. *British Journal of Obstetrics and Gynaecology*, **84,** 264–268 (1977)

5 CALDER, A. A. The management of the unripe cervix. In *Human Parturition* (Boerhaave Series Vol 15), edited by M. J. N. C. Keirse, A. B. M. Anderson, J. Bennebroek Gravenhorst, 201–217. The Hague, Martinus Nijhoff (1979)

6 CHARD, T. The hormonal assessment of fetal and placental function in fetal medicine. *Clinics in Obstetrics and Gynaecology*, edited by R. W. Beard, 85–102. London, W. B. Saunders Co. Ltd. (1974)

7 CRUICKSHANK, D. P. and PITKIN, R. M. Delivery of the premature breech. *Obstetrics and Gynecology*, **50,** 367–369 (1977)

8 EGLEY, C. C. and SUZUKI, K. Intra-uterine fetal demise after negative oxytocin challenge tests. *Obstetrics and Gynecology*, **50,** (Supplement) 54–57 (1977)

9 EMBREY, M. P. and MOLLISON, B. G. The unfavourable cervix and induction of labour using a cervical balloon. *Journal of Obstetrics and Gynaecology of the British Commonwealth*, **74,** 44–48 (1967)

10 FLYNN, A. M. and KELLY, J. Evaluation of fetal well-being by ante-partum fetal heart monitoring. *British Medical Journal*, **1,** 936–939 (1977)

11 FRIEDMAN, E. A. and SACHTLEBEN, M. R. Preinduction priming with oral prostaglandin E_2. *American Journal of Obstetrics and Gynecology*, **121,** 521–523 (1975)

12 GANT, N. F. and WORLEY, R. J. Differential diagnosis of hypertension in pregnancy. In *Hypertensive States in Pregnancy*, edited by E. M. Symonds, 613–633. London, W. B. Saunders Co. Ltd. (1977)

13 GIERSSON, R. Premature breech delivery (unpublished observations)

14 KUBLI, F. In *Pre-term Labour* (Proceedings of the 5th Study Group of the Royal College of Obstetricians and Gynaecologists), edited by A. Anderson, R, Beard, J. M. Brudenell, P. M. Dunn, 360. London, Royal College of Obstetricians and Gynaecologists (1977)

15 LILEY, A. W. Intrauterine transfusion of the fetus in haemolytic disease. *British Medical Journal*, **2,** 1107 (1963)

16 LILLIENTHAL, C. M. and WARD, J. B. Medical induction of labour. *Journal of Obstetrics and Gynaecology of the British Commonwealth*, **78,** 317–321 (1971)

17 LINZEY, E. M. and FREEMAN, R. K. Fetal monitoring. In *Year Book of Obstetrics and Gynecology* edited by R. M. Pitkin, J. R. Scott, 85–110. Chicago, Year Book Medical Publishers Inc., (1978)

18 LUNAN, C. B. The role of caesarean section in management of abruptio placentae. *Journal of Obstetrics and Gynaecology of the British Commonwealth*, **80,** 120–124 (1973)

19 MCCUISH, A. C. and LUNAN, C. B. Personal communication (1980)

20 MCILWAINE, G. M., HOWAT, R. C. L., DUNN, F. and MACNAUGHTON, M. C. The Scottish Perinatal Mortality Survey. *British Medical Journal*, **2,** 1103–1106 (1979)

21 MACKENZIE, I. Z. and EMBREY, M. P. Cervical ripening with intra-vaginal PGE_2 gel. *British Medical Journal*, **2,** 1381–1384 (1977)

22 MONTGOMERY, D. A. D. and HARLEY, J. M. G. Diabetes mellitus and pregnancy. In *Medical Disorders in Pregnancy*, edited by C. R. Whitfield, 356–370 London, W. B. Saunders Co. (1977)

23 PALMAR, A. and GORDON, R. R. A critical review of intrauterine fetal transfusion. *British Journal of Obstetrics and Gynaecology*, **83,** 688–693 (1976)

24 ROBERTON, N. R. C. Personal communication. (1979)

25 RUSH, R. W., KEIRSE, M. J. N. C., HOWAT, P., BAUM, J. D., ANDERSON, A. B. M. and TURNBULL, A. C. Contribution of pre-term delivery to perinatal mortality. *British Medical Journal*, **2,** 965–968 (1976)

26 RUSH, R. W., DAVEY, D. A. and SEGALL, M. L. The effect of pre-term delivery on perinatal mortality. *British Journal of Obstetrics and Gynaecology*, **85,** 806–811 (1978)

27 STEWART, A. Follow-up of pre-term infants. In *Pre-term Labour*, (Proceedings of the 5th Study Group of the Royal College of Obstetricians and Gynaecologists) edited by A. Anderson, R. Beard, J. M. Brundell, P. M. Dunn 372–384. London, Royal College of Obstetricians and Gynaecologists (1977)

28 THIERY, M. and AMY, J. J. Spontaneous and induced labor: two roles for the prostaglandins. In *Obstetrics and Gynecology*, edited by R. M. Wynn 127–171. New York, Appleton-Century Crofts (1977)

29 THIERY, M., DEFOORT, P., BENIJTS, G., VAN EYCK, J., HENNAY, T., VAN KETS, H. and MARTENS, G. Effectiveness of extra-ovular injection of prostaglandin E_2 in Tylose gel to ripen the cervix prior to elective induction of labour at term. *Prostaglandins*, **14,** 381–388 (1977)

30 THIERY, M. Induction of labour with prostaglandins. In *Human Parturition* (Boerhaave Series Vol. 15), edited by M. J. N. C., Keirse, A. B. M. Anderson, J. Bennebroek Gravenhorst, 155–164. The Hague, Martinus Nijhoff (1979)

31 TURNBULL, A. C. and ANDERSON, A. B. M. Uterine cntractility and oxytocin sensitivity during human pregnancy in relation to the onset of labour. *Journal of Obstetrics and Gynaecology of the British Commonwealth*, **75,** 278–288 (1968)

32 WHITFIELD, C. R. A three year assessment of an action line method of timing intervention in rhesus iso-immunisation. *American Journal of Obstetrics and Gynecology*, **108,** 1239–1244 (1970)

33 WHITFIELD, C. R., SPROULE, W. B. and BRUDENELL, J. The amniotic fluid lecithin/sphyngomyelin ratio (L.S.A.R.) in pregnancies complicated by diabetes. *Journal of Obstetrics and Gynaecology of the British Commonwealth*, **80,** 918–922 (1974)

13

Where should preterm labour be conducted?

Jack M. Schneider

Introduction

The preterm delivery of the normally-developed fetus continues to outweigh all other causes of neonatal mortality with particular vulnerability noted for the very low birth weight infant weighing less than 1500 g. Success in dramatically lowering the neonatal mortality rate followed the introduction of intensive care capabilities for the newborn. In an attempt to further reduce perinatal mortality, emphasis is now shifting to the *in utero* management of the fetus–fetal intensive care.

This presentation sets forth the background regarding what has been termed regionalization of perinatal health care, the demonstrated and implied advantages of fetal and neonatal intensive care provided in selective settings and some of the problems or shortcomings with the proffered approaches. The issue is whether or not a systematic approach to the organization of perinatal health care delivery can have a favorable impact on the outcome of pregnancy by influencing where preterm labor is conducted.

Background

Regionalization of perinatal health care delivery

Several models of regional perinatal service organization have demonstrated a positive effect on perinatal outcome[15, 30, 45, 46, 57]. Even in Sweden, the recurrent international leader of low infant mortality rates[59], a regionalization effort in one of the counties based on communication, education and appropriate transfer reduced perinatal mortality essentially to the same extent as demonstrated earlier in Wisconsin[46].

The development of perinatal regional systems has been influenced in the past decade by professional organizations[2, 34, 53, 57]. Of special note, an interprofessional and multidisciplinary task force defined guidelines for a regional perinatal care system which have been adopted in fact or with non-conceptual modification by the US federal government and over 50 percent of the states[7]. The document developed by this task force characterizes responsibilities, specialized services and personnel requirements of each of the perinatal units in a three-tiered system of care[57]. Common to all facilities providing perinatal services is the need to respond to the emergency complicating the maternal, fetal and/or neonatal status with timely evaluation and initial definitive care. Implicit is the transfer of the patient(s) when long-term needs exceed the capabilities of the unit providing the emergency care. As far as possible, prenatal assessment for risk factors is to be utilized to select those women who might benefit from care by another practitioner and/or at another institution directed to prevention of the emergency situation[4, 21].

Successful regional perinatal care programs have emphasized communication and education, comtemporary consultation and professional competence in the management of maternal, fetal and neonatal complications.

The where, what, and why of it

Personal experience with the antagonism engendered at least initially by 'where' of perinatal health care delivery has led the author to think in terms of the 'what' and 'why' of the various requisites for appropriate care. Indeed, only the 'who' of perinatal health care delivery fosters a more negative reaction.

The content of any list of requirements bearing relevance to a problem is generally not unique regardless of author. Others are more often able to embrace the concepts proffered if the reasoning for each can be set forth. The author's view of the requisites to conduct premature labor anywhere are as follows.

(1) Personnel (immediately available, appropriate expertise).
(2) Definition of management plan.

(3) Commitment of *all* personnel to management plan.
(4) Ultrasonography and radiography availability.
(5) Amniocentesis capability.
(6) Laboratory – special studies availability.
(7) Familiarity with use of tocolytic drugs and corticosteroids (if used).
(8) Expertise in management complications due to drug interventions.
(9) Equipment for continuous fetal assessments during labor.
(10) Rapid response time for emergency cesarean section.
(11) Equipment for resuscitation and stabilization of newborn.
(12) Continuous re-assessment of all exigencies of defined management plan.
(13) Defined provision for consultation and referral-transport.

Wherever possible, the 'why' of the list is defined later in this chapter. The 'how' of the conduct of premature labor is covered elsewhere in this book (Chapters 14 and 15).

Preterm labor constitutes an obstetric emergency. Timeliness is next to holiness regarding definition and execution of an appropriate plan of management to prevent, forestall or qualitatively optimize the process of preterm delivery. Unnecessary delays or procrastination impart a remarkable risk to both mother and baby.

Early assessment is more likely to permit the time necessary for the appropriate interventions to work, thereby lowering the complication rate. If the use of a tocolytic agent and/or steroid is contemplated, the former is more effective the earlier it is initiated and the latter requires 48–72 hours for maximal effectiveness. The later in labor a tocolytic agent is employed, the higher the complication rate associated with the higher required dosage.

Many of the cases of preterm labor have associated rupture of the membranes. Early evaluation of the woman, favors the collection of amniotic fluid per vagina for measurement of L/S ratio[47], determination of the presenting part, and discovery of the prolapsed cord.

The determination of the L/S ratio takes approximately three hours. It is not appropriate to await reopening of the laboratory in hours or even days while the risk of respiratory distress syndrome (RDS) due to delay in administering steroids, the risk of complication from a tocolytic agent or the risk of infection increase. About 30 percent of the patients considered to be in preterm labor have lung maturity indicated by L/S ratio assessment which negates delay of delivery[47]. Indeed, in many of these instances, intrauterine growth retardation is unexpectedly present[43, 48, 61]. Whereas the majority of cases of suspected intrauterine infection do not portend serious infection for the neonate, mortality and serious morbidity are more common when the neonate is infected, and sepsis is more common the longer the membranes have been ruptured. Furthermore, the results of cervical or transabdominal uterine cultures correlate well with the pathogens recovered from the septic newborn.

Ultrasonography is useful in defining the presenting part; estimating fetal size; diagnosing abruptio placentae; defining multiple gestation; suggesting fetal abnormality; and facilitating safe amniocentesis, particularly when the membranes are ruptured.

At 28 weeks' gestation, approximately 25 percent of fetal presentations are breech[44]. While the route of delivery for the fetus weighing less than 1500 g and presenting cephalically remains controversial, cesarean section for the breech presentation is accepted by most. Data also suggest an improved neonatal survival with cesarean section for the under 1000 g birth weight fetus presenting as the vertex[18, 51, 52]. Management is commonly altered by the finding of more than one fetus and/or fetal abnormality–both conditions being significantly associated with preterm labor. Radiographic evaluation may play an important role in identifying the abnormal fetus.

Assessment of fetal size by ultrasonography is not perfect, but precision is greatest in the highest risk period (26–32 weeks' gestation) for perinatal mortality and morbidity. Ultrasonography provides a more critical assessment of fetal weight than can be attained by transabdominal palpation. There is a clinical tendency to underestimate the weight of the very low birth weight fetus supported by this author's experience[38]. The importance of this is demonstrated by the fact that when estimated fetal weight and birth weight correlated (65 percent of cases), the perinatal mortality rate was approximately 20 percent; while in cases where birth weight was significantly underestimated (35 percent of cases), the perinatal mortality rate was close to 50 percent[38].

The intrauterine growth retarded fetus is a more common finding with the presumptive diagnosis of preterm labor than at term[43, 48]. While a single ultrasonogram will define only about half of these cases, the finding of a low weight fetus with an unexpectedly high L/S ratio is very suggestive of intrauterine growth retardation. Such fetal lung maturity assessment results not only preclude the need for a tocolytic agent or corticosteroid but avoid temporizing in the intrauterine growth retarded fetus–a high risk group for both distress during labor and neonatal complications.

Amniotic fluid, obtained as soon as possible by either vaginal collection[47] or amniocentesis, should be assessed for fetal lung maturity and/or intra-amniotic infection in either those cases where a tocolytic agent has been effective in abating labor and the use of steroids is contemplated or those cases when a growth retarded fetus is suggested by history and/or ultrasound. Amniotic fluid evaluation for bacteria by Gram stain may indicate preterm labor associated with infection even though the membranes are intact[8]. Temporizing in the face of amnionitis is not advocated. A continuous laboratory capability is essential for these assessments and others such as blood gas determinations.

While there is some evidence for improved outcome for the very low birth weight when delivery is delayed by tocolytic agents long enough for steroids to play a role in decreasing the occurrence or severity of RDS, this is neither a panacea nor the ultimate solution for preterm delivery. The randomized controlled trial to prove efficacy of the various tocolytic agents has yet to be published. Even if the physician and patient, by virtue of informed consent, are willing to accept responsibility for the use of a tocolytic agent and/or steroids, as many as 50 percent of the associated maternal–fetal conditions preclude drug use[62]. In addition, the differentiation between preterm and false labor is precise only when assessed retrospectively. Furthermore timely maternal–fetal transport must be done if the requirements for fetal and neonatal intensive care cannot be met. Inevitably, unnecessary maternal–fetal transports will occur, further demonstrating the imprecision of the diagnosis of preterm labor.

The practitioner electing to use tocolytic agents must assure the availability of personnel expert in neonatal and maternal resuscitation. A particular requirement with the β-mimetic agents is expertise in adult cardiopulmonary support.

Intrapartum management of the fetus has been shown to have a positive effect on the initial and follow-up status of the neonate[5,10,11,19,31,37,38,40,41]. The optimal management of preterm labor requires an intensive-care setting to ensure the availability of personnel who are attentive to details directed to the prevention or early detection and appropriate intervention of intrapartum fetal distress associated with hypoxia or acidosis or both. The required personnel-to-patient ratio is generally not available at an institution with a low annual delivery rate nor can it be reasonably expected in small medical partnerships. Even when the necessary individual expertise is available, the practitioner must ensure that colleagues who provide coverage have the same expertise and commitment to the prescribed management plan. The outcome for the infant delivered prematurely will not be influenced by the doctor who is not in attendance regardless of his or her capabilities.

Both RDS[10,22,31] and intraventricular hemorrhage[35] have been shown to be correlated with the condition of the preterm fetus during labor. These two complications account for the majority of mortality and long-term morbidity of the less than 1500 g birth weight newborn[36].

Low Apgar scores[14,55], abnormal fetal heart rate patterns[22,28], decreased fetal heart rate baseline variability[28] and fetal acidosis[22] are associated with an increased risk of RDS in the neonate. Fetal acidosis has a particularly adverse effect on pulmonary surfactant production and pulmonary perfusion in the very low birth weight infant. Borkowf, Grausz and Delfs[10], in reviewing trends in perinatal mortality over a 12-year period of evolution of a perinatal center, cite a remarkable decrease in the percentage of neonatal deaths due to RDS in infants weighing 1000–1999 g. They attribute the decrease to be due in part to the prevention of fetal asphyxia. Similarly, Milligan and Sheenan[31] in making a case for an equal partnership between obstetric and neonatal perinatologists, ascribe the lowered RDS incidence and corrected survival of 100 percent of babies weighing between 1000 and 2000 g in large part to the avoidance of fetal hypoxia and trauma. Other factors, such as the use in steroids and tocolytic agents, may also have contributed to the improvement.

Bowes, Halgrimson and Simmons[11], obstetricians associated with one of the early neonatal intensive care units in the USA, have presented the best case for the important influence of intrapartum care of patients in preterm labor. *No* β-mimetic tocolytic or corticosteroid drugs were used during the two year study period to assess the effect of maternal–fetal intensive care on the perinatal outcome of patients in premature labor. Comparison of the neonatal mortality of infants weighing 501–1500 g for the study and earlier care periods showed the significant effect of maternal–fetal intensive care. While the techniques of intrapartum fetal assessment, e.g. fetal heart rate monitoring, and newborn resuscitation were in place in the five years preceding the study, they were not routinely applied because of the obstetricians' bias that since the anticipated very low birth weight infant generally could not be expected to survive intact, the risks to the mother were not warranted. This bias in obstetrical practice has been documented by Paul, Koh and Monfared[38].

Bowes, Halgrimson and Simmons[11], and Paul, Koh and Monfared[38] noted another obstetrical bias which negatively influenced neonatal outcome – namely the use of a low Apgar[3] score to prohibit resuscitation immediately after birth. The original work of Apgar[5] included few infants of very low birth weight. Contemporary experience has demonstrated that low Apgar scores in very low birth weight infants are common, while Thomson, Searle and Russell[56] have shown the lack of predictability of the Apgar score for long-term follow-up status in this group of infants.

While debate continues as to the value of continuous fetal heart rate monitoring, the literature supports its value in the low birth weight fetus[20]. The fetal heart rate patterns recorded with electronic monitoring in the premature fetus have been shown to be of the same configuration and to have the same implications including relationship to pH determinations as defined for the term fetus[60]. For all its shortcomings, the fetal monitor is the single assessment tool available to raise a suspicion of fetal distress during labor. To be helpful, this instrument must be available and utilized and personnel expert in interpretation of the continuous data and carrying out the appropriate interventions must be available.

Zanini, Paul and Huey[60] have suggested that ominous fetal heart rhythm patterns become worse more quickly in the preterm fetus than is the case at term. This consideration, as well as the more frequent association of prolapsed cord and abruptio placentae with preterm labor, and the higher risk of RDS and intraventricular hemorrhage with hypoxia in the preterm fetus mandate a rapid response time for delivery by cesarean section. Cesarean delivery of the very low birth weight baby has been stated to be associated with both decreased neonatal mortality and lower long-term morbidity[51, 52].

Moore[33] states that more deaths occur in the first 5 min of life than the next 50 years. It is generally accepted that initial neonatal resuscitation and stabilization have the greatest impact on neonatal outcome. The lower weight-specific mortality rates for inborn babies compared to transfer babies adds credence to this opinion. The major effect on neonatal mortality of a regional perinatal care program care has been shown to be in the first four hours of life, suggesting a positive result from timely, appropriate intervention for the neonate[46]. These and other data[50] make the availability of expert resuscitation at birth an essential consideration.

Continuous assessment of the status of the mother and fetus will facilitate timely alterations in the management plan and appropriate interventions including consultation and referral-transport if exigency exceeds capability. When maternal–fetal or neonatal transport is elected, final outcome regarding mortality and morbidity is directly related to the status of the patient when received at the accepting facility. While the quality of transport plays a role, the timeliness of the decision to transfer may be the more important consideration.

Neonatal care and transport

Intensive care has significantly reduced neonatal mortality. Lee *et al.*[26] have probably presented the most cogent, yet unbiased, case for the dramatic decrease in neonatal mortality being due to changes in practice patterns coincident with establishment of neonatal intensive care units. In contrast, before the advent of such special care for newborns (1950–1960: USA) *no* improvement was noted in weight-specific neonatal mortality in any category under 2500 g[26].

Before the establishment of neonatal intensive care units, neither the size of the hospital, the number of deliveries per year nor the availability of specialists in obstetrics and pediatrics seemed to influence perinatal outcome[46]. The recent decline in very low birth weight mortality in the USA has been evident in hospitals delivering 2000 or more infants annually[15] and/or those with designated newborn intensive care centers[13]. Bakketeig, Hoffman and Sternthal[5] compared perinatal mortality between country groups in Norway with differing obstetric services. They demonstrated that the level of obstetric care at the time of delivery affected early neonatal mortality more than fetal mortality. The decrease in neonatal mortality occurred simultaneously with the introduction of contemporary perinatal care practices. Similarly, workers in Sweden showed a higher perinatal mortality for progeny of mothers living in the vicinity of less specialized hospital facilities contrasted to that of mothers living in the same county but within the vicinity of a more highly specialized hospital[26].

Important to the consideration of the conduct of preterm labor, the reduction in neonatal mortality rate due to intensive care has been most notable in the very low birth weight infant. Reports now show survival of the neonatal period (28 day) of the order of 90 percent for infants weighing between 1000 and 1500 g and 50 percent for infants weighing between 500 and 1000 g. Indeed, the low perinatal death rate in the under 1500 g birthweight group in the US is significantly less than that reported in Sweden[42].

Not only has neonatal intensive care reduced mortality but the benefits for the transported neonate requiring such care have been shown to outweigh the risks of transport when contrasted with outcome for the infants kept at facilities without a neonatal intensive care unit[29, 30, 54, 58]. On the other hand, comparative analysis of inborn infant neonatal mortality with that of the transferred neonate in the same weight group has consistently favored the inborn birth when a difference was demonstrated[19, 25, 29, 32, 58].

The findings that babies born in a facility with neonatal intensive care fared better than those that were transported, as well as the fact that maternal transport is less demanding and less costly than neonatal transport, has led to a shift in emphasis from neonatal transport to the transport in utero of the baby at risk[24].

Maternal–fetal transport

Maternal transport is not new but the emphasis on transport of a healthy woman for the sake of her fetus/neonate is a fairly recent development[9, 11, 12, 16, 17, 19, 29, 32, 49]. With the successful lowering of neonatal mortality following development of neonatal transport, it was a natural evolution that maternal–fetal transport should gain emphasis for conditions such as preterm labor at high probability of requiring professional expertise and specialized equipment for the baby.

Specific approaches to maternal–fetal transport are largely based on geography. While the issues pertinent to air transport have been well described[17] and ground transport by ambulance is usually recommended, early transport before labor is well-established can in many instances be safely done in the family conveyance at much less cost than transfer of the premature neonate. Brown[12] advocates attempts to delay labor progression and attendance of a physician during transport of the woman who is in active labor.

The implied advantages of maternal–fetal transport for the conduct of preterm labor are as follows.

(1) Earlier, less costly, safer than neonatal transport.
(2) Maternal–fetal in-hospital care less costly than neonatal intensive care.
(3) Timely availability of appropriate personnel.
(4) Immediately available equipment for fetal and neonatal intensive care.

(5) Decreased expected neonatal mortality.
(6) Decreased neonatal morbidity.
(7) Maternal–neonatal bonding facilitated.
(8) Positive alterations in traditional patterns of care unrelated to preterm labor.

Transport of a healthy fetus inside a mother who is generally well is simpler, less costly and safer than transport of an ill infant. Pomerance *et al*[39], Anderson *et al*[1], and others have found the cost for maternal–fetal hospitalization during periods requiring intensive care to be far less than either the short or long term expense of neonatal intensive care. Additionally, *in utero* transport facilitates subsequent maternal–neonatal bonding and attachment which may play an important role in infant development[23].

Both direct and indirect evidence support the premise that maternal–fetal transport is beneficial. The reason for transport is usually preterm labor, with or without ruptured membranes. The good results cited by Bowes *et al.*[11] included more than 50 percent maternal–fetal transports. Harris, Isaman and Giles[19], and Souma[49] using the Lubchenco predictive perinatal risk score[27] to demonstrate the advantage of maternal–fetal transport over transport of the newborn, showed a remarkably lower than *expected* neonatal death rate (60 percent and 68 percent respectively). Knuppel *et al.*[24], correcting perinatal deaths for congenital anomalies and irrevocable fetal hypoxia at the time of admission, have reported a perinatal survival rate of 100 percent for infants transferred *in utero* and born after 27 weeks gestation (n = 76 at 28–34 weeks). The largest reported experience with maternal–fetal transport is that of Harris, Isaman and Giles [19]. In an attempt to make a valid comparison between maternal–fetal and neonatal transport, these workers compared the neonatal outcome of infants from both transport approaches who required neonatal intensive care. Their analysis excluded approximately 50 percent of the progeny of maternal–fetal transport because they did not require such care. Even with their large experience approaching 500 transports, only 20 percent of the infants had a birth weight of less than 1500 g. Although the overall mortality difference between the maternal–fetal and neonatal transfers was not statistically significant, a lower absolute neonatal mortality in the maternal–fetal transport category was demonstrated in spite of significantly lower mean birth weight, shorter mean gestational age and a higher mean projected mortality risk utilizing the Colorado classification of Lubchenco, Searls and Brazie[27].

In particular, neonatal mortality risk in the maternal–fetal transport group was significantly reduced in infants of birth weights of 500–1500 gm and gestational ages of 24–34 weeks. These findings suggest strongly that the quality of obstetric care acted either to decrease the early neonatal death rate at the outlying perinatal units and/or to increase the quality of the newborn at the moment of birth at the regional center.

As previously noted, inborn births benefit from a lower rate of RDS, and this benefit is conveyed to babies born following maternal–fetal transport[31]. In addition, neonatal morbidity has also been decreased in these very low birth weight infants transferred before birth[11,29,31,32]. A decreased length of hospital stay has been noted for the neonate born after maternal–fetal transport as compared with that of the baby transported after birth[1,29].

Modanlou *et al*[32] matched 50 maternal–fetal transports with 50 neonatal transfers for birth weight, gestational age and outcome. While these authors were unable to show a decrease in neonatal mortality when matched-pair comparative analysis was performed, they did demonstrate a significant decrease in neonatal morbidity for the babies born following maternal–fetal transport. Perhaps the short transport distances, on average 18 miles, and the high referral rate from hospitals participating in a formal perinatal education program had a positive influence on perinatal outcome.

Finer delineation of the issues related to maternal–fetal transport requires additional data. Although the case for transport seems to be evolving positively, it is difficult to control for biases in data comparing maternal–fetal and neonatal transport. Selection of patients occurs in both transport groups. For example, in cases of preterm labor, comparison cannot include patients for whom labor progresses too rapidly to permit transport. Perhaps the delay of delivery in the transport group,as suggested by worsened perinatal outcome related to length of ruptured membranes, is important. Likewise, it is usually not possible to assess critically those neonatal deaths which occur before transfer can be effected. In addition, of the surviving infants, only those who are sick are transferred, thereby excluding the well baby from comparative weight-group analyses. A randomized study of the respective impact of maternal–fetal and neonatal transport within a single care system is highly desirable but seemingly impossible.

Subtle positive alterations in traditional patterns of care related to clinical situations other than preterm labor are a benefit of maternal–fetal transport. It is an experience common to all transport programs that while consultation about the case at hand is occurring, other, similar cases are discussed.

Problem areas

The antepartal risk assessment for preterm labor is rewarding only as an epidemiological exercise. Coupled with the difficulty of making a prospective diagnosis of preterm labor, timely interventions may defy the best intentions.

Ego considerations operate at both ends of the referral line. In many settings the experienced obstetrician is asked to transfer the care of his patient to an institution where the delivery may be by a housestaff-trainee making it difficult for the obstetrician to understand any direct benefit to the patient. An impact on fetal mortality, the traditional focal point for the obstetrician, has not yet been – and may never be – conclusively shown in any of the regionalization–transport schemes. Maintenance of enthusiasm by the obstetrician at the receiving unit who, as Souma[49] so well states, 'is most frequently asked to accept a healthy patient in order subsequently to provide a sick patient to another physician' may be understandably difficult.

The intensive care of the fetus and/or neonate must be viewed as complementary, not competitive, with the obstetrician and pediatrician in a balanced partnership. While a laudable goal, training programs in years past have not provided the opportunities to facilitate such a relationship. Some pediatricians have sensed an obstructionist pattern in their obstetric colleagues with neither a realization of the difficulties inherent in assessing a patient (fetus) not yet born nor a willingness to get involved in the decision-making process of maternal–fetal transport. Just as the pediatricians needed convincing before becoming fully committed to a regional system of neonatal transport[46], so obstetricians have the same need before committing to fetal transport.

The assumption of liability for maternal–fetal transports is not well defined although it is generally stated that the transferring institution has responsibility until the patient arrives at the receiving institution.

An increasing number of maternal–fetal transports must be denied because of unavailability of a bed in the neonatal intensive care unit. When one calculates the potential need for such transport for preterm labor in a service region of 12 000–15 000 births per year – allowing for over-referral because of the difficulty in precise diagnosis – the scope of the problem becomes obvious. In 10–20 percent of instances of maternal–fetal transport, the patient is discharged from the hospital undelivered, most commonly because of successful intervention[12, 24, 49].

The expense of a regional perinatal care program is high. Differential payment schedules for maternal–fetal intensive care have not kept pace with the increased funding for neonatal intensive care. Furthermore, payment for the more costly neonatal transport is more available than for the less expensive maternal–fetal transport. Fetal intensive care in the very low birth weight groupings does not necessarily contribute unfavorably to neonatal intensive care costs. Bowes *et al.*[11], for example, noted that when neonatal death occurred in the very low birth weight baby, the infant perished by 12 days of age in 87 percent of the cases. The cost of neonatal intensive care for the very low birth weight infant has been estimated as high as $100 000[39]. Maternal–fetal care that effects a decrease in the number or an increase in the gestational age of infants delivering prematurely should reduce these costs. Women of low socio-economic status, whose care is often under-funded and who commonly enter late into the care system are at increased risk for preterm labor. Such patients are often not given care soon enough commensurate with their increased risk.

Consumer considerations other than financial play a role in the conduct of preterm labor. Dislocation from family and community, transference of trust to new care providers and intolerance of long-term side-effects of the tocolytic agents are notable. That consumers and providers are increasingly endorsing a systematic approach to the problem of preterm labor, however, is evidenced by the burgeoning number of maternal–fetal transports[9, 11, 19, 24, 49], often with an associated significant decrease in neonatal transports[24].

Conclusion

While the frequency of the preterm delivery of the very low birth weight infant has not changed favorably in the past 25 years[26], alterations in perinatal medical care have significantly lowered the mortality of these infants. An increasing data base supports the concept that the chances of quality survival for the baby whose birth weight is less than 1500 g relates to the availability of high-quality fetal–neonatal intensive care.

Until preterm labor can be prevented, practitioners will have the responsibility of assuring timely, appropriate interventions when preterm labor does occur in order to achieve optimal potential for the newly born.

References

1 ANDERSON, C. L., ALADJEM, S., AYUSTE, O., *et al.* An analysis of maternal transport within a suburban metropolitan region. *American Journal of Obstetrics and Gynecology*, in press (1980)

2 AMERICAN MEDICAL ASSOCIATION HOUSE OF DELEGATES. *Centralized Community or Regionalized Perinatal Intensive Care*. Chicago, American Medical Association (1971)

3 APGAR, V. A proposal for new method of evaluation of the newborn infant. *Current Researches in Anesthesia and Analgesia*, 260–267 (1953)

4 AUBRY, R. Identification of the high-risk perinatal patient. In *Perinatal Intensive Care*, edited by S. Aladjem, A. K. Brown, 63–76. St. Louis, Mosby (1976)

5 BAKKETEIG, L. S., HOFFMAN, H. J. and STERNTHAL, P. M. Obstetric service and perinatal mortality in Norway. *Acta Obstetricia et Gynecologica Scandinavica*, **57,** (Supplement 77), 1–19 (1978)

6 BEARD, R. W. and RIVERS, R. P. A. Fetal asphyxia in labour. *Lancet*, **2,** 1117–1119 (1979)

7 BERGER, G. S., GILLINGS, D. B. and SIEGEL, E. The evaluation of regionalized perinatal health care programs. *American Journal of Obstetrics and Gynecology*, **125,** 924–932 (1976)

8 BOBITT, J. R. and LEDGER, W. J. Unrecognized amnionitis and prematurity. *Journal of Reproductive Medicine*, **19,** 8–12 (1977)

9 BOEHM, F. H. and HAIRE, M. F. One-way maternal transport: an evolving concept. *American Journal of Obstetrics and Gynecology*, **134,** 484–492 (1979)

10 BORKOWF, H. I., GRAUSZ, J. P. and DELFS, E. The effect of a perinatal center on perinatal mortality. *Obstetrics and Gynecology*, **53,** 633–640 (1979)

11 BOWES, W. A., HALGRIMSON, M. and SIMMONS, M. A. Results of the intensive perinatal management of very low-birth-weight infants (501 to 1500 grams). *Journal of Reproductive Medicine*, **23,** 245–250 (1979)

12 BROWN, F. B. The management of high-risk obstetric transfer patients. *Obstetrics and Gynecology*, **51,** 674–676 (1978)

13 DAY, R. L. What evidence exists that intensive care has changed survival? *Problems of Neonatal Intensive Care Units*. (Report of the 59th Ross Conference on Pediatric Research) Columbus, OH, Ross Laboratories, (1969)

14 DONALD, I. R., FREEMAN, R. K., GOEBELSMANN, U., NAKAMURA, R. M. Clinical experience with the amniotic fluid lecithin/sphingomyelin ratio. I. Antenatal prediction of pulmonary maturity. *American Journal of Obstetrics and Gynecology,* **115,** 547–552 (1973)

15 FINAL REPORT of Massachusetts Maternity and Newborn Regionalization Project. Massachusetts Department of Public Health (1976)

16 GILES, H. R., ISAMAN, J., MOORE, W. J. and CHRISTIAN, C. D. The Arizona high-risk maternal transport system: An initial view. *American Journal of Obstetrics and Gynecology,* **128,** 400–407 (1977)

17 GRAVEN, S. N. and SOMMERS, J. G., Editors. *Proceedings Maternal Air Transport Conference,* (Denver, Colorado, March 1979.) Evansville, Mead Johnson (1980)

18 HAESSLEIN, H. C. and GOODLIN, R. C. Delivery of the tiny newborn. *American Journal of Obstetrics and Gynecology,* **134,** 192–200 (1979)

19 HARRIS, T. R., ISAMAN, J. and GILES, H. R. Improved neonatal survival through maternal transport. *Obstetrics and Gynecology,* **52,** 294–300 (1978)

20 HOBBINS, J. C., FREEMAN R. and QUEENAN, J. T. The fetal monitoring debate. *Obstetrics and Gynecology,* **54**(1), 103–109 (1979)

21 HOBEL, C. J., HYVARINEN, M. A., OKADA, D. M. and OH, W. Prenatal and intrapartum high risk screening. *American Journal of Obstetrics and Gynecology,* **117,** 1–9 (1973)

22 HOBEL, C. J., HYVARINEN, M. A. and OH, W. Abnormal fetal heart rate patterns and fetal acid-base balance in low birth weight infants in relation to respiratory distress syndrome. *Obstetrics and Gynecology,* **39,** 83–88 (1972)

23 KLAUS, M., JERAULD K., KREGER, N., MCALPINE, W., STEFFA, M. and KENNELL, J. W. Maternal attachment: importance of the first postpartum days. *New England Journal of Medicine,* **286,** 460–463 (1972)

24 KNUPPEL, R. A., CETRULO, C. L., INGARDIA, C. J., KAPPY, K. A., KENNEDY, J. L., HERSCHEL, M. J., AUMANN, G., LAKE, M. and SBARRA, A. Experience of a Massachusetts perinatal center. *New England Journal of Medicine,* **300,** 560–562 (1979)

25 KORONES, S. B. Mortality of inborn and transferred neonates, (1976–1979). (unpublished data)

26 LEE, K., PANETH, N., GARTNER, L. M., PEARLMAN, M. A. and GRUSS, L. Neonatal mortality: an analysis of the recent improvement in the United States. *American Journal of Public Health,* **70,** 15–21 (1980)

27 LUBCHENCO, L. O., SEARLS, D. T. and BRAZIE, J. V. Neonatal mortality rate: Relationship to birth weight and gestational age. *Journal of Pediatrics,* **81,** 814–822 (1972)

28 MARTIN, C. M., SIASSI, B. and HON, E. H. Fetal heart rate patterns and neonatal death in low birth weight infants. *Obstetrics and Gynecology,* **44,** 503–510 (1974)

29 MERENSTEIN, G. B., PETTETT, G., WOODALL, J. and HILL, J. M. An analysis of air transport results in the sick newborn: II. Antenatal and neonatal referrals. *American Journal of Obstetrics and Gynecology,* **128,** 520–525 (1977)

30 MEYER, H. B. P. Transport of high-risk infants in Arizona. In *Regionalization of Perinatal Care,* (Report of the Sixty-sixth Ross Conference on Pediatric Research), edited by P. Sunshine, 65–67 Columbus, OH, Ross Laboratories (1974)

31 MILLIGAN, J. E. and SHEENAN, A. T. Perinatal management and outcome in the infant weighing 1000 to 2000 grams, *American Journal of Obstetrics and Gynecology,* **163,** 269–272 (1980)

32 MODANLOU, H. D., DORCHESTER, W. L., THOROSIAN, A. and FREEMAN, R. K. Antenatal versus neonatal transport to a regional perinatal center: a comparison between matched pairs. *Obstetrics and Gynecology,* **53,** 725–729 (1979)

33 MOORE, W. M. O. Antenatal care and the choice of place of birth. In *The Place of Birth,* edited by S. Kitzinger and J. A. Davis. II. Oxford, University Press, (1978)

34 NATIONAL STUDY OF MATERNITY CARE. Chicago, American College of Obstetrics and Gynecology (1970)

35 PAPE, K. and WIGGLESWORTH, J. S. Haemorrhage. In *Ischaemia and the Perinatal Brain.* Edited by K. Copeland, chapter 7, London, Spastics International Publications, (1979)

36 PAPILE, L., BURSTEIN, J., BURSTEIN, R. and KOFFLER, H. Incidence and evolution of subependymal and intraventricular hemorrhage. *Journal of Pediatrics,* **92,** 529–534 (1978)

37 PARER, J. T. Fetal heart rate monitoring. *Lancet,* **2,** 632–633 (1979)

38 PAUL, R. H., KOH, K. and MONFARED, A. H. Obstetric factors influencing outcome in infants weighing from 1001 to 1500 grams. *American Journal of Obstetrics and Gynecology,* **133,** 503–508 (1979)

39 POMERANCE, J. J., UKRAINSKI, C. T., UKRA, T., HENDERSON, D. H., NASH, A. H. and MEREDITH, J. Cost of living for infants weighing 1000 grams or less at birth. *Pediatrics,* **61,** 908–910 (1978)

40 QUILLIGAN, E. J., PAUL, R. H. and SACKS, D. A. Results of fetal and neonatal intensive care. In *Modern Perinatal Medicine,* edited by L. Gluck. 425–430. Chicago, Year Book Medical Publishers (1974)

41 REY, H. R., BOWE, E. T. and JAMES, L. S. Impact of fetal heart rate monitoring and fetal blood sampling on infant mortality and morbidity. *Pediatric Research,* **8,** 176–183 (1974)

42 ROOTH, G. Socio-economic aspects of perinatal medicine. In *Perinatal Medicine,* edited by G. Rooth and L. E. Bratteby, 11. Stockholm, Almquist and Wiksell International, (1976)

43 RUSH, R. W., DAVEY, D. A. and SEGALL, M. L. The effect of preterm delivery on perinatal mortality. *British Journal of Obstetrics and Gynaecology,* **85,** 806–811 (1978)

44 SCHEER, K. and NUBAR, J. Variation of fetal presentation with gestational age. *American Journal of Obstetrics and Gynecology,* **125,** 269–270 (1976)

45 SCHNEIDER, J. M. and RYAN, G. M. Regionalization of Perinatal Health Care. In *Gynecology and Obstetrics* Vol. 3, edited by J. J. Sciarra, Chapter 108, Hagertown, MD, Harper and Row Publishers, Inc. (1979)

46 SCHNEIDER, J. M. Development and educational aspects of a regionalized program. In *Regionalization of Perinatal Care,* (Report of the Sixty-sixth Ross Conference on Pediatric Research), edited by P. Sunshine, 14–19. Ross Laboratories, Columbus, OH (1974)

47 SCHNEIDER, J. M., MORRISON, J. C., SIBAI, B. M., LIPSHITZ, J. and ANDERSON, G. D. Prediction of neonatal RDS based on vaginal-amniotic fluid pulmonary maturity studies. Unpublished data (1980)

48 SCOTT, K. and USHER, R. Fetal malnutrition: its incidence causes and effects. *American Journal of Obstetrics and Gynecology,* **94,** 951–963 (1966)

49 SOUMA, M. L. Maternal transport: behind the drama. *American Journal of Obstetrics and Gynecology,* **134,** 904–908 (1979)

50 STANLEY, F. J. and ALBERMAN, E. D. Infants of very low birthweight I. Perinatal factors affecting survival. *Developmental Medical Child Neurology,* **20,** 300–312 (1978)

51 STEWART, A., TURCAN, D., RAWLINGS, G. and REYNOLDS, E. R. Prognosis for infants weighing 1000 g or less. *Archives Diseases of Childhood,* **52,** 97–104 (1977)

52 STEWART, A. L. Follow-up of pre-term infants. In *Pre-term Labour* (Proceedings of the Fifth Study Group of the Royal College of Obstetricians and Gynaecologists,) edited by A. B. M. Anderson, R. Beard, J. M. Brundenell, P. M. Dunn, 372–384. London, Royal College of Obstetricians and Gynaecologists (1977)

53 SWYER, P. R., GOODWIN, J. W. (Editors) *Regional Services in Reproductive Medicine.* Joint Committee of the Society of Obstetricians and Gynaecologists of Canada and the Canadian Pediatric Society, Sherbrooke, Quebec, (1971)

54 SWYER, P. R., HARDIE, M. J. Reproductive medicine in Toronto with particular reference to neonatal care in the Hospital for Sick Children. In *Current Concepts of Neonatal Intensive Care.* Edited by Swyer, P. R., Stetson, J. B. St. Louis, Warren H. Green, 591 (1972)

55 THIBEAULT, D. W. and HOBEL C. J. The interrelationship of the foam stability test, immaturity, and intrapartum complications in the respiratory distress syndrome. *American Journal of Obstetrics and Gynecology,* **118,** 56–61 (1974)

56 THOMSON, A. L., SEARLE, M. and RUSSELL, G. Quality of survival after severe birth asphyxia. *Archives Diseases of Childhood* **52,** 620–626 (1977)

57 *Toward Improving the Outcome of Pregnancy: Recommendations for the Regional Development of Maternal and Perinatal Health Services.* Committee on Perinatal Health. White Plains, NY, The National Foundation—March of Dimes, (1976)

58 USHER, R. Changing mortality rates with perinatal intensive care and regionalization. *Seminars in Perinatology* **1,** 309–319 (1977)

59 WALLACE, H. M. and GOLDSTEIN H. The status on infant mortality in Sweden and the United States. *Journal of Pediatrics,* **87,** 995–1000 (1975)

60 ZANINI, B., PAUL, R. H. and HUEY, J. R. Intrapartum fetal heart rate: correlation with scalp pH in the preterm fetus. *American Journal of Obstetrics and Gynecology,* **136** (1), 43–47 (1980)

61 ZLATNIK, F. Premature labor: its management and therapy. *Journal of Reproductive Medicine,* **9,** 93–118 (1972)

62 ZLATNIK, F. The applicability of labor inhibition to the problem of prematurity. *American Journal of Obstetrics and Gynecology,* **113,** 704–706 (1972)

14
The management of preterm labour

David T. Y. Liu and Denys V. I. Fairweather

Introduction

Substantial improvement in perinatal and infant mortality and morbidity following preterm delivery has been recorded during the past 10 years[2,15,18] especially in those infants weighing 1500 g or less[78]. This success followed changes in paediatric attitudes toward management of the preterm infant, including a more energetic approach to resuscitation, ventilation and intensive care. In the light of these changes, many obstetricians have re-examined their management of the patient in preterm labour or in whom premature delivery was contemplated and concluded that the conservative or 'hands-off' approach with its high perinatal mortality and morbidity is no longer justified. On the other hand active obstetric management routines will vary depending on the particular circumstances of each case. Paediatric results are naturally influenced by the quality and state of the infants at delivery and if appropriate obstetric intervention can avert factors such as trauma or anoxia which affect the infants' condition at birth, a valuable partnership can be envisaged between obstetricians and paediatricians to enable better management of preterm labour and delivery with even further improvement in infant survival and prognosis.

A recent *British Medical Journal* leader[12] suggesting that drugs to inhibit threatened preterm labour particularly before the thirty-second week of pregnancy are of relatively limited value concluded that improvement in perinatal mortality and morbidity is more likely to come from concentrating efforts on the identification of high-risk pregnancies, on their early admission when labour supervenes, and on measures to ensure that infants at risk are delivered in optimum condition in centres of perinatal skill.

This chapter reviews relevant information related to the management of preterm labour and attempts to formulate constructive guidelines for a balanced approach to the problem.

Factors affecting development of management routines and assessment of their value

Definition of preterm

The World Health Organisation Consultation on Methodology of Reporting and Analysis of Perinatal and Maternal Morbidity and Mortality, Bristol, 1972, recommended that infants delivered at less than 36 complete weeks (less than 259 days from last menstrual period) should be defined as preterm. The American Academy of Pediatrics Committee on The Fetus and Newborn (1976) extended the gestation time a further week to include 37 weeks (less than 266 from LMP). Differences in definition obviously alter the concept of incidence of preterm labour and confuse the issue when success in treatment is discussed.

Infant survival rates and duration of pregnancy

Figure 14.1 illustrates diagrammatically the relationships between body weight, gestation and likelihood of survival. After 36 weeks when the fetus weighs 2500 g any further gestation will not appreciably alter fetal prognosis. Survival rates are similar for infants between 32 weeks (1500 g) and 36 weeks (2500 g). Furthermore, there appears to be little (two to three per cent) difference in survival rates between infants born after 36 weeks and those of 32–36 weeks[35].

The legal definition of viability is still set at 28 weeks of gestation. However since few infants of less than 26 weeks gestation or 750 g survive it may be prudent to suggest those criteria for the lower limit for active intervention to achieve delivery in the interest of the infant as opposed to that of the mother. Individual neonatal centres must determine their own capability for safe handling of these very low birth weight immature infants.

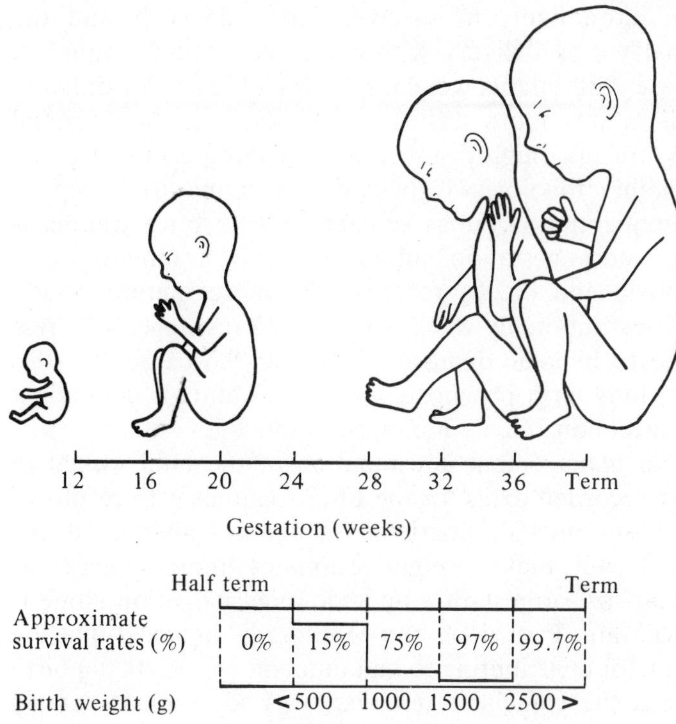

Figure 14.1 Diagrammatic representation of fetal growth with the current survival rates of infants of different birth weights. The birth weight histograms only approximate to the average body weight for the aligned gestation. (After Hull[35])

Fetal weight

After 36 weeks gestation the fetus normally weighs at least 2500 g. Because gestational age may be difficult to establish, it is understandable why less than 2500 g was first suggested as an alternative definition of preterm. This, however, is an unsatisfactory alternative because low fetal weight may be due to retarded fetal growth and not fetal immaturity. Usher, McLean and Scott[85] and Alberman[2] have shown that in infants weighing 2500 g or less, the gestational age in nearly 40 per cent may be 38 weeks or more. Although it is important to distinguish between these two groups of low birth weight infants because neonatal complications differ, any infants weighing more than 1500 g are more likely to survive. They can withstand the process of normal vertex delivery without undue adverse sequelae. This is not the case with infants weighing 1500 g or less. Not only are these very small infants more difficult to manage in the neonatal period, but they are also highly susceptible to intrapartum hypoxia and trauma. Whether this low weight is due to immaturity or poor growth is inconsequential as far as susceptibility to birth trauma is concerned. The short gestation infant is easily traumatized, is sensitive to hypoxia and bleeds readily. The more mature poorly grown infant is constitutionally weak with limited resistance to stress and is also prone to hypoxic damage. Whatever the causes for this low fetal weight, long-term prognosis for these infants is dependent on delivery being conducted to minimize trauma[22].

One problem in management is estimation of the fetal weight *in utero*. Accurately recorded dates for the LMP together with results of several sonar measurements (biparietal diameter – abdominal circumference, etc.) will make weight estimates more precise as assessment of fetal size or gestation by abdominal palpation alone is difficult and inaccurate. Paul, Koh and Monfared[59] believed that the most important factor contributing to bad outcome in the 1000 g birth weight infants was the clinician's tendency to underestimate actual fetal size. In their series when they attempted to estimate weights as under or over 1000 g, underestimation occurred in 35 per cent compared with only eight per cent with overestimation.

Definition of preterm labour

One of the most difficult yet most urgent problems in the management of preterm labour is knowing when labour has actually commenced. Misdiagnosis of the onset of labour confuses the concept of therapeutic success and accounts for the large placebo effect [36, 94], which has led many obstetricians to question the value of treating preterm labour. A major difficulty in diagnosis occurs because the onset of labour is insidious. Uterine activity gradually increases throughout pregnancy. There is a progression from inherent basal activity[17] to Braxton Hicks contractions, to more regular and persistent activity in the latent phase of labour, followed by the strong contractions of the active phase. Cervical dilatation may mimic this progression, changing from little dilatation at the beginning of pregnancy to the recognisably ripe cervix which is soft, opened 2–3 cm, and which readily dilates with the onset of regular uterine contractions. Recurrent painful uterine activity which persists is universally accepted as suggestive of the onset of labour. The level of activity which the patient or obstetrician considers as diagnostic of labour is both subjective and variable. At term, when labour is expected, 10 per cent[57] of patients who considered themselves in labour were mistaken. Before term, when labour is not expected, or alternatively the patient is overtly anxious in case labour occurs, it is not surprising to find a high incidence of false labours. The experience from the John Radcliffe Hospital, Oxford, suggests that up to 50 per cent of patients who present with preterm labour could be mistaken[4].

Careful assessment of patients admitted in suspected labour should eliminate those who are in fact in false labour, but in one survey in New York[43] obstetricians were mistaken in their diagnosis in over 30 per cent of patients. The diagnosis may be suggested by the following.

(1) Signs and symptoms reported by the patient.
(2) Signs observed by the attending obstetric staff.
(3) Physiological changes observed following examination of the patient.

Errors in diagnosis by obstetric attendants can be reduced by closer attention to the physiological changes associated with the onset of preterm labour, especially the uterine contractions and cervical dilatation. The three components in a contraction are its duration, frequency, and strength. Although the strength of a contraction is undoubtedly an important feature in cervical dilatation, its accurate measurement in preterm labour is difficult. External tocography at best only indicates the presence of a contraction. Since the cervix may dilate in response to a wide range of intrauterine pressures, it is not useful and can be misleading, to define labour by an arbitrary level of intrauterine pressure. This, however, does not mean that some knowledge of intensity of contractions is unimportant. An indication of intensity may be reflected in the duration of the contraction. Although Steer *et al.*[75] and Pontonnier *et al.*[61] found little correlation between intrauterine pressure and duration of contractions, it is suggested that a sustained pressure is more effective than a short period of high pressure for dilating any viscoelastic tissue. Normally it takes 40–60 s before the whole uterus participates in a contraction. A contraction of shorter duration may mean that all myometrial tissue has not participated in the contraction, or that the contraction, whatever the intensity, is necessarily less effective.

The frequency of uterine contractions is important. Observing normal term labour in the active phase we know that uterine contractions recur at least once every five minutes, which suggests that repeated pressure at this interval (two contractions or more in 10 minutes) is sufficient to ensure dilatation of the cervix. It could be argued that these conditions need not apply to preterm labour, but if contractions lasting at least 40 seconds recur every five minutes and persist for an hour or more, then it is not unreasonable to assume that dilatation of the cervix may result and that treatment to check these contractions should be instituted. Cervical dilatation measured at the internal os, reflects uterine activity and has frequently been used as an indicator of progress in labour. The cervix dilates progressively throughout pregnancy and by 32 weeks a dilatation of 2–3 cm is present in nearly one-third of all parous and multiparous patients[70, 92]. In his classical study Bishop[8] showed that for any given cervical dilatation the length of time till labour supervenes varies greatly from one patient to another. This emphasised the point made by Brooks[14] and Wood *et al.*[92] that cervical dilatation on its own need not suggest preterm labour.

Active labour commences at a cervical dilatation of 4 cm[60, 79]. This is the case for both primigravidae[24] or multigravidae[25] and for induced or spontaneous labour[7, 49]. Continuing uterine contractions and a cervical dilatation of 4 cm indicates the need for urgent therapy if preterm delivery is to be avoided.

Cervical effacement follows regular uterine contractions or in the incompetent cervix, the more subtle process of increasing intrauterine pressure as the uterus enlarges. Significant cervical effacement (more than 50 per cent) reflects the result of increased uterine activity and indicates there is little residual resistance to rapid dilatation if increased uterine pressure is allowed to continue. Uterine contractions and an effaced cervix necessitate urgent treatment to prevent irrevocable dilatation. If the cervix is dilated beyond 5 cm, attempts to stop labour are usually unsuccessful.

It becomes apparent from the above discussion that various gradations of uterine activity can be defined when the state of the cervix is known. Merely defining preterm labour as the presence of regular painful uterine contractions which bring about progressive dilatation of the cervix is not enough. The following clinical definitions/observations can be easily made and used to indicate possible treatment.

(1) Cervical effacement (75–100 per cent) without uterine contractions but with dilatation of more than 3 cm requires consideration of cerclage to prevent further dilatation which will initiate further uterine activity.
(2) Uterine contractions recurring at least once every five minutes, lasting 40 seconds and continuing for an hour or more associated with less than 3 cm dilatation and no effacement. One can safely wait and reassess this patient over an hour or two. If uterine activity persists, it can usually be abolished by treatment with tocolytic drugs and further cervical dilatation thus prevented.
(3) Uterine activity as in (2) with effaced cervix and 3 cm or more dilatation necessitates immediate therapy to prevent preterm delivery. There is no justification in this category of patients for a wait-and-see policy. The choice of treatment should also be aimed at rapid control of uterine activity. Administration of drugs in increments is not advisable since thereby time is lost[50].
(4) Uterine contractions with cervical dilatation beyond 6 cm have a poor prognosis for prevention of preterm delivery. At most the contractions may be controlled temporarily to allow preparations to be made for delivery or transfer of the patient to a unit better suited to the delivery and care of a very low birth weight infant.

Grading preterm labour

There is no established measure which delineates the grade or stage to which preterm labour has progressed when patients first present. This increases the difficulty in determining the significance or comparison of results from any form of therapy, and thus the criticism by Hemminki and Starfield[32] that few therapeutic trials to date are meaningful, is valid. The presence of ruptured fetal membranes, cervical dilatation, mucoid show, and regular uterine contractions all influence the likelihood of success in inhibiting preterm labour. The influence of each variable described above has not been determined but is known to vary widely. Labour need not follow the presence of a show. Even with ruptured membranes, four weeks may elapse before uterine contractions supervene[54]. Attempts have been made to use Bishop's pelvic score, a tocolytic index[6, 65] and degrees of uterine activity with or without associated bleeding[47, 48, 63, 73] to stage the degree of progression in labour. Because most of these attempts relied on arbitrary scores their predictive value tends to be equally non-discriminating. There is clearly a need to examine statistically as reported by Liu and Blackwell[50] the contribution towards outcome by each component of any proposed score so that correct weighting for each component can be determined to allow construction of a realistic composite preterm labour score or index.

Liu and Blackwell found that uterine contractions *per se* gave little guide towards the eventual outcome of preterm labour and cannot, as frequently assumed, be used as the baseline from which to measure the need for or success of therapy. Whatever the mode of therapy or the drug used, a third of these patients are likely to delivery within the first 24 hours, less than half will continue pregnancy for 48 hours and only about a quarter are not delivered at the end of a week. As expected, the lower the allocated preterm labour score, the more likely it is for pregnancy to continue. A score of seven or more forewarns of imminent preterm delivery.

Aims in management

A clear idea of expected achievement is important. Ideally the aim should be to deliver a baby in good condition with the mother's future health unimpaired and the baby developing normally. There are times when obstetricians are forced to compromise by preserving a healthy mother at the expense of her baby. Rarely, as in maternal death, or imminent maternal death, the welfare of the preterm fetus will be considered as having priority over that of the mother.

Although the prognosis for preterm infants has improved in the last two decades, mere delivery of a live infant is not a complete criterion for obstetric success. Fetal death is relatively cheap in terms of emotional and financial expense. A damaged infant is costly in all aspects for the family involved, and the society upon which it will depend. Obstetricians must learn to be more critical of reports which define perinatal and neonatal success only in conventional statistical terms. With improved design in life support systems and nursing expertise many small preterm infants can be kept alive for more than seven days. Perinatal or neonatal mortality rates may have little meaning in preterm studies and survival beyond 28 days, the ability to be discharged from hospital without morbidity, outcome after two years[1], or performance in adolescence may be more realistic guides of successful treatment. These topics are further discussed in Chapter 17.

Current therapeutic measures for management of preterm labour can also affect the mother in terms of mortality and morbidity. Cervical cerclage requires an anaesthetic with the associated risks, and the suture itself may predispose to local or intrauterine infections. Prolonged usage of β-sympathomimetic drugs can stress the myocardium and interfere with electrolyte balance[82]. Maternal fatalities have been reported[41] when β-mimetics were used in conjunction with corticoids. For obtaining best results for fetal salvage of the very low birth weight infants liberal use of caesarean section delivery is required. This is a major operation carrying its own morbidity and a fairly constant mortality rate of 0.8 per 1000 operations (Report on Confidential Inquiries into Maternal Deaths in England and Wales, 1973–1975).

Theoretically the aims of preterm management for mother and fetus are clear. This may not be true in practice when frequently the mother may have associated obstetric or medical complications and the degree of fetal compromise is difficult to ascertain. As the patient and her husband, or family, will eventually bear the brunt of the consequence of therapy, the authors strongly advise adequate counselling and involvement of the patient and her family in discussions concerning management so that they are well-informed of the problems.

Attitudes in management

Correct diagnosis and appropriate treatment are important but all too often the vital initial assessment is delegated to a junior member of the obstetric team. This casual attitude must be changed if fetal prognosis is to be improved. An experienced obstetrician should assess the patient when preterm labour is suspected. Differential diagnoses should be considered. If preterm labour is present, the category of uterine activity as defined earlier is ascertained so that appropriate management can be organised.

The merits of treatment in specialist centres have been discussed in a previous chapter. Suffice it to stress that this active approach was initiated mainly by paediatricians[27, 34, 62, 64, 72, 87]. More constructive steps by obstetricians will further enhance achievement by our paediatric colleagues. One such step is the willingness to transfer patients with preterm labour to regionalized specialist centres once it is determined that the infants are too small to be managed by the staff and facilities available in their own departments. Efficient transfer requires close liaison between referral hospitals and the specialist centres. Adequate facilities for transport of the mother and fetus or newborn should be available. Whenever possible, transfer of the fetus *in utero* is preferred[53, 67]. Patients, however, frequently present too late in preterm labour to allow transfer and in these cases preparation for preterm delivery should be initiated and transport organized to transfer the neonate (in a transfer incubator[9]) as soon as initial resuscitation has been completed.

Roberton[66] from Cambridge, England, has shown that proper care in the first hour is most important for preterm infants, especially those whose birth weight is 1500 g or less. He advocated early intubation and ventilation with 60–80 per cent oxygen, umbilical catherization, correction of hypotension and maintenance of the neonate's temperature. In their survey, Stanley and Alberman[74] showed that the temperature of infants arriving at neonatal units was a major determinant of mortality in hyaline membrane disease.

Keeping the neonate warm, early intubation and ventilation and transferring in a warm (36°C) incubator are simple procedures with far reaching consequences for the preterm infant. Because delivery may occur before transfer can be arranged, an important part of management of preterm labour, especially in peripheral hospitals, is to ensure that all attending obstetricians and nursing staff are aware of the above simple procedures and capable of carrying them out.

If the attitude for *in utero* transfer of the small preterm fetus is encouraged, then invariably one must consider the question of predicting preterm labour. Certain patients such as those with multiple gestation, low maternal weight (below 50.8 kg) and smokers are at increased risk[23]. Previous midtrimester deliveries, bleeding in early pregnancy[68, 86] which may be responsible for raised maternal plasma α-fetoprotein[13, 88] and maternal stress[55, 58] may contribute. Early engagement of the fetal head[89] and cervical shortening[3, 92] are other suggested indicators, but as discussed in Chapter four these are only general and indiscriminate indicators. Even if a group of at-risk patients are identified the problem of preventing preterm labour still remains.

Recent attempts at prevention of preterm labour either by prophylactic cervical cerclage[40, 90] or long-term oral tocolytic agents[52, 56] have met with little success. If prevention is not easy, then the emphasis must be on better management when the condition arises.

Management of special problems in preterm labour

Congenital abnormalities

With advances in antenatal diagnosis the number of patients with a congenital abnormality of the fetus presenting in preterm labour should be somewhat reduced. If major fetal abnormality is suspected vaginal delivery should be allowed and caesarean section avoided. The value of careful assessment of the patient in preterm labour by an experienced obstetrician is again stressed.

Bleeding and preterm labour

When there is only slight bleeding associated with uterine contractions and placenta praevia, inhibition of uterine activity may prevent further placental separation and may be worth considering. Bleeding due to placenta praevia, unlike that in abruptio is usually obvious and can be used to monitor the safety of continuing preventive therapy. It should be emphasised that therapy is only considered where bleeding is minimal: heavy bleeding suggests significant placental separation and the need to effect delivery.

Ruptured membranes

As indicated in Chapter 6 a high proportion (30–50 per cent) of preterm labour is associated with ruptured fetal membranes[46, 48, 54, 57, 83]. Most obstetricians would agree with Embrey[21] that once the membranes have ruptured the majority (75 per cent) of patients will proceed to labour within 24 hours. The earlier in pregnancy the membranes rupture the longer is the interval before the onset of labour[28]. When the emphasis of individual factors influencing the likelihood of controlling preterm labour was studied, Liu and Blackwell[50] found the presence of ruptured membranes to be the most significant factor which predicted a poor prognosis. One should, however, distinguish between the two types of patients with ruptured membranes: those with and those without concurrent uterine activity. Treatment with tocolytic drugs, particularly when uterine contractions are not present, can in a proportion (less than one third) of patients, prolong pregnancy for a week or more[26, 38, 42, 91]. The prime concern if pregnancy is allowed to continue is the risk of cord prolapse and intrauterine infection. The dangers of preterm birth must be balanced against these risks. Contrary to the low incidence of infection reported by some[38, 80] a retrospective study (Liu, unpublished) at University College Hospital, London of 55 consecutive patients who delivered infants of less than 1500 g after membranes had been ruptured for more than 48 hours, showed a substantial infection rate in both mother and the newborn. Fourteen out of 55 neonates (25.5 per cent) showed evidence of infection ranging from mild umbilical sepsis to septicaemia as verified by blood cultures and over half (32 of 55) of the mothers had signs of early puerperal infection such as a pyrexia of 38°C, and vaginal pathogens identified by cultures.

For patients with ruptured membranes and contractions, attempts should be made to defer preterm birth if the gestational age is less than 32 weeks, whereas delivery is probably safer for fetuses of more than this age. The conservative approach for patients with ruptured membranes but without uterine contractions is to await the spontaneous onset of labour. A vaginal examination under aseptic conditions is carried out to ensure that the umbilical cord has not prolapsed; to obtain specimens for bacteriology, surfactant content and possibly zinc–protein estimation[44]. A high phosphate/zinc ratio in liquor indicates that there is little defence against infection[71] and delivery should be considered.

Preterm labour in the second trimester

Few infants born at less than 26 weeks gestation will survive. Control of preterm labour in these patients is undoubtedly important but this must not be at the expense of the mother or her future reproductive capability. We would therefore avoid operative obstetric intervention in these patients.

Besides cervical incompetence, we may see an increasing number of patients in this gestation range now presenting with a history of having had an amniocentesis or fetoscopy examination for suspected genetic abnormalities. The latter group of patients often also have poor obstetric histories so there are additional reasons why preterm delivery must be avoided.

Caesarean section or vaginal delivery?

It is difficult to lay down hard and fast rules to answer this question as there are so many variables to be considered in the management of the individual case. Some of these have already been mentioned at the beginning of this chapter. The following guidelines are suggested on the basis of our experience at University College Hospital, London. We tend to be guided more by the estimated fetal weight than by the gestational age in deciding the method of delivery as the former – e.g. in the small-for-dates situation – seems more relevant. We have therefore set out the guidelines by fetal weights, making reference where necessary to equivalent gestation periods when the fetus is normally grown.

Infants 500–1500 g (24–31 weeks)

In the past only a minority of obstetricians have been prepared to perform a caesarean section for fetal reasons before 30 weeks gestation. A more conservative approach to delivery was chosen on the basis of the poor prognosis for survival and the high rate of reported handicap in the very low birth weight (less than 1500 g) survivors[19, 33, 51]. The influence of the method of delivery on survival and outcome of these very low birth weight infants was emphasised by Stewart and Reynolds[76], higher survival rates being associated with delivery by caesarean section. This was shown to be especially important for infants of 1000 g or less where 64 per cent survived after vaginal delivery. Other workers have confirmed the beneficial effect of abdominal delivery of low birth weight or severely premature infants[27, 45]. In addition more recent follow-up studies of these very low birth weight survivors have indicated a much improved long-term prognosis[34, 76, 78].

Since caesarean section is not without risk for the mother it is useful to know when this active approach should be undertaken and the recent study by Fairweather and Stewart[22] provides guidelines. They analysed the outcome of 490 live born infants with birth weights between 500 and 1500 g admitted to the Neonatal Unit at University College Hospital, London during the seven years 1971–1977. Three hundred and eighty seven babies (79 per cent) were from singleton and 103 from multiple pregnancies. Of these 490 infants, 30.6 per cent weighed 500–1000 g; the rest were between 1001 and 1500 g inclusive. Spontaneous onset of preterm labour occurred in 80 per cent of these deliveries. Ten per cent of those patients had the added complication of maternal hypertension and about 40 per cent antepartum haemorrhage. The remaining 20 per cent of patients were delivered preterm following induction of labour or elective caesarean section for maternal hypertension (73 per cent); history of bleeding (14 per cent) and fetal growth retardation (12 per cent). The remaining patients (one per cent) were delivered by caesarean section because of diabetes (three patients) and Rhesus disease (two patients). Among booked cases and those transferred *in utero* (299) attempts were made using drugs, including isoxuprine and salbutamol, to stop preterm labour when the membranes were intact and fetal or maternal conditions were favourable. Steroids were not used routinely to enhance lung maturation.

Table 14.1 Liveborn infants 500–1500 g, University College Hospital, 1971–1977. Twenty-eight day mortality × birth weight

Birth weight (g)	*Number*	*% 28 Day mortality*	*Significance*
500–750	32	75	n/s
751–1000	118	55	$P<0.001$
1001–1250	176	35	$P<0.0005$
1251–1500	164	20	
500–1500	490	37	

Fifty-two per cent (255) of the 490 infants were born vaginally with the vertex presenting, 21 per cent (103) vaginally by the breech while 26 per cent were delivered by caesarean section. In addition five infants (one per cent) were delivered vaginally as brow/face. The mortality rate at 28 days (37 per cent) was clearly influenced by birth weight (*Table 14.1*), being significantly improved by every 250 g increase in weight from 750 g onwards. The effect of gestational age (*Table 14.2*) was also noted, showing that from 27 weeks of gestation each additional week of maturity conferred significant benefit until gestational age of 29 weeks though thereafter further increase in gestation did not significantly alter the mortality rate.

The influence by mode of delivery on the 28 day mortality rate is shown in *Table 14.3*, for the weight ranges 500–1000 and 1001–1500 g as well as for the whole group. There was no significant increase in mortality between spontaneous vertex and forceps deliveries nor

Table 14.2 Liveborn infants 500–1500 g, University College Hospital, 1971–1977. Twenty-eight day mortality × gestation

Gestation (weeks)	*Number*	*% 28 Day mortality*	*Significance*
22–23	3	100	–
24	7	86	–
25	10	90	n/s
26	45	62	n/s
27	59	64	$P<0.02$
28	90	43	$P<0.05$
29	76	26	n/s
30	76	28	n/s
31	40	15	
32	40	18	
33+	44	11	
All	490	37	

Table 14.3 Liveborn infants 500–1500 g. University College Hospital, 1971–1977. Twenty-eight day mortality × method of delivery × birth weight

Method of delivery	*% 28 Day mortality (n)*					
	500–1000 g		*1001–1500 g*		*500–1500 g*	
Vertex spontaneous	71	(58)	21	(102)	39	(160)
Vertex forceps	64	(25)	33	(69)	41	(94)
Vertex ventouse	–	(–)	0	(1)	0	(1)
Breech spontaneous	76	(33)	40	(49)	55	(82)
Breech with forceps for the after coming head	67	(6)	33	(15)	43	(21)
All breech	74	(39)	39	(64)	52	(103)
Brow/face spontaneous	100	(2)	67	(3)	80	(5)
Caesarean section in labour	50	(10)	12	(43)	19	(53)
Caesarean section elective	24	(17)	16	(57)	17.5	(74)
All caesarean section	33	(27)	14	(100)	18	(127)
Total	64	(151)	25	(339)	37	(490)

n = Total number of cases in each group

between forceps and breech deliveries or between elective and emergency caesarean sections. However mortalities among caesarean section deliveries were significantly lower than vertex ($P<0.001$), forceps ($P<0.001$) and all breech deliveries ($P<0.001$). The mortality for spontaneous vertex compared with all breech deliveries was also significant ($P<0.05$). For each method of delivery Fairweather and Stewart[22] found that the mortality of infants weighing 1000 g or less was significantly higher than that of those weighing more than 1000 g. In each weight group mortality from breech delivery was significantly higher than that for vertex and very significantly higher than that for caesarean section. In the 1001–1500 g group forceps delivery was also significantly ($P<0.01$) more hazardous than caesarean section. Even in infants weighing 500–750 g those delivered by caesarean section had a lower mortality than breech deliveries. Indeed breech delivery was the only method for which the 28 day mortality did not fall progressively as birth weight increased. Similarly, after 26 weeks, for every two week period until 34 weeks gestation the mortality for infants delivered by caesarean section was lower than that for breech delivery.

Birth by caesarean section is associated with a lower mortality rate than spontaneous or assisted vaginal delivery especially where presentation is by the breech and these findings concur with other reports[11, 20, 37]. Indeed Goldenberg and Nelson[29] suggested that serious consideration should be given to prophylactic caesarean section for all preterm breeches when delivery is anticipated. They found that the preterm breech fetus was 16 times more likely to die during labour than was the preterm fetus presenting cephalically and that the increased mortality and morbidity was greater than that attributable to low birth weight alone. Hasslein and Goodlin[31] suggest that with infants weighting 800–1350 g (26–31 weeks) it is preferable, in the absence of a well-developed lower uterine segment, to perform a classical caesarean section. However we feel that in the majority of cases the lower segment approach is quite feasible. The series at University College Hospital did not support the view that the lower segment incision 'frequently' needed to be extended to a T and there is no doubt that classical incision scars are more vulnerable to rupture in future pregnancies.

Fairweather and Stewart's data also suggested that there was no significant effect on the mortality rate in different delivery categories when the infant was either of low or appropriate weight for gestation. In singleton infants the mortality rate was significantly higher when the onset of labour was spontaneous and the membranes remained intact to within an hour of delivery compared with those where the membranes had ruptured earlier in labour. Additionally they found no evidence to support the belief that the application of forceps was advantageous in the delivery of these very low birth weight infants.

Based on the University College Hospital findings we support the following guidelines for safe delivery of infants weighing 1500 g or less when preterm labour cannot be stopped or when delivery has to be undertaken for either maternal or fetal reasons.

When labour has commenced spontaneously and the estimated fetal weight is 750 g or more or gestational age is more than 26 weeks, delivery by caesarean section should be considered when:

(1) other than the vertex is presenting,
(2) there is associated antepartum haemorrhage,
(3) labour is not progressing, and
(4) fetal distress develops.

Karp *et al.*[39] from their study of premature breech delivery concluded that vaginal delivery could be undertaken safely when the presentation was either a full or frank breech. However they found that with the footling breech, especially those weighing 1000–1500 g, caesarean section was indicated because of the risks of prolapse of the cord and entrapment of the after coming head. Our experience leads us to advise caesarean section for all breech presentations where the fetus weighs less than 1500 g.

Vaginal delivery should be anticipated when:

(1) the vertex is presenting,
(2) there is steady progress of cervical dilatation,
(3) there is no fetal distress (presence of meconium staining, alternation from normal fetal heart rate patterns, or evidence of hypoxia), and
(4) the maternal condition is satisfactory.

The membranes should be ruptured once labour is definitely established and cervical dilatation is proceeding beyond 3 cm. Delivery should be spontaneous with the aid of an episiotomy and controlled delivery of the head unless there is obvious delay in the second stage when forceps should be applied.

Infants 1500–2500 g (31–36 weeks)

In this group management policy clearly varies depending on which end of the scale it is estimated that the fetal weight falls. In the lower half management would be very much along the lines suggested above for the smaller infants, whilst as gestation advances and the fetal weight increases the policy should be closer to that suggested for infants in the next weight group. In general terms vaginal delivery should be allowed if the presentation is vertex and there are no obstetric complications. Low birth weight, preterm infants presenting by the breech are highly susceptible to trauma if delivered vaginally[11, 29] and will benefit if birth is by caesarean section[10, 40, 77]. There may be a case in this weight range for considering the argument, already referred to above, put forward by Karp *et al.*[39] in favour of vaginal delivery for certain cases. Woods[93] also advances the view that caesarean section is not justified on a routine basis for infants weighing between 1500 and 2500 g presenting by the breech. We suggest that each case must be assessed by an experienced obstetrician to decide on the management in light of the particular circumstances, the stage and progress of labour and the presentation at the time of admission. If other than easy vaginal delivery is anticipated, when an episiotomy and controlled delivery of the after coming head may be all that is necessary, caesarean section should be considered.

Infants over 2500 g (over 36 weeks)

In this weight group and at this stage of gestation we consider that there is no need to elaborate any routine differing from that for the management of labour normally applicable to mature infants.

General comments

Monitoring in labour

Although the value of electronic fetal monitoring during labour has not been specifically shown to be of value in these low birth weight infants, Guilliams and Held[30] advised its use and in practice although sometimes there may be technical difficulties, and the time available for recording may be short, it is agreed that in all cases of preterm labour intrapartum monitoring may serve to alert the clinician to otherwise unsuspected poor fetal condition. If progress in labour is poor or there is evidence of fetal distress or deterioration in maternal condition emergency caesarean section should clearly be considered.

Episiotomy

If progress in labour is satisfactory we feel that delivery should be aided by an episiotomy and controlled delivery of the head. The role of episiotomy in the delivery of the preterm infant is difficult to justify on the basis of statistical data and we are not aware of any studies which have been addressed particularly to this aspect. On general principles, however, because episiotomy is known to reduce the length of second stage and because the fetus is at risk of hypoxia during the second stage we feel that routine episiotomy is a reasonable suggestion. Fairweather and Stewart[22] found no evidence to support the belief that prophylactic application of forceps was advantageous in the delivery of the very low birth weight infants and we suggest that routine policies advising the use of forceps in these cases be reviewed, and where continued that it be made quite clear that their use is concerned primarily with achieving controlled delivery of the head and preventing tentorial tears.

Analgesia–anaesthesia

Choice of analgesia in labour and anaesthesia for delivery of the preterm infant has received relatively scant attention in the literature. We doubt whether in the past our practice for pain relief in preterm labour differed greatly from that normally used for term labours. However in recent years we detect some changes, mainly a reduction in the use of pethidine with self-administered nitrous oxide and oxygen by inhalation at the end of labour, and an increase in the use of epidural anaesthesia for management of these cases. There is no doubt that even though epidurals may lead to some increase in the number of forceps deliveries they allow for much better controlled delivery. Crawford[16] claimed that vaginal delivery of the premature breech with epidural anaesthesia was as good as, if not better than, caesarean section but his series can be criticised because of the heterogenous grouping of cases and the failure to investigate the incidence of long-term sequelae. If there is not time to administer epidural anaesthesia we advocate the use of local anaesthesia to the perineum or pudendal nerve block for episiotomy and forceps delivery. For caesarean section we usually recommend general anaesthesia as in the situation of preterm labour the mothers tend to be more anxious and not so relaxed as to allow use of epidural or local anaesthetic. Some authors[81] have proposed the routine use of local anaesthesia for caesarean sections in high risk cases – including prematurity – and the value of epidurals in these cases has also been advocated on the basis that the infant's condition at birth is improved and breathing established more rapidly. Obviously the smaller amounts of analgesic or general anaesthetic agents used during labour and delivery the better will be the infant's response at birth.

Cord-clamping

The time of cord-clamping in the preterm infant may be critical as placental blood may amount to almost 50 per cent of the normal newborn blood volume[69]. Avery[5] indicates the problems associated with total transfusion of all placental blood but Usher[86] reported that premature infants with red blood cell volume of 35–42 ml/kg had the best survival from respiratory distress syndrome. Such levels correlate to those found when the cord is clamped 45–60 s after delivery with the infant held at a lower level than the uterus.

Conclusions

Provided that they received skilled management throughout the perinatal period preterm infants are potentially viable even when their birth weights are as low as 750 g and the gestational age is only 26 weeks. At all birth weights in the range 500–1500 g and at gestational age of between 26 and 34 weeks, the 28 day mortality is significantly lower for infants presenting by the breech and delivered by caesarean section compared with those delivered vaginally. This is true irrespective of whether the infant is presenting by the vertex or the breech at the time of operation. Further, infants delivered vaginally by the breech are in a worse condition at birth, possibly having suffered more hypoxia, than infants delivered by other routes.

They also have a higher incidence of serious mental and neurological handicap at follow-up. We therefore suggest that when preterm labour cannot be stopped or when delivery of a very low birth weight infant (less than 1500 g) has to be undertaken for either maternal or fetal reasons, preferably the mother should be transferred to a special unit where there are facilities for both expert obstetric care and a neonatal intensive care unit staffed and equipped to deal with high risk infants. If this is impossible, and also where dealing with heavier infants (1500–2500 g), the delivery should be conducted along the lines outlined above providing adequate facilities for resuscitation of the infant, including the presence of an experienced neonatalogist, and arrangements made where indicated for immediate transfer of the infant to a neonatal intensive care unit.

The obstetric care of preterm labour greatly influences both the short and long-term prognosis for the infant and close collaboration between obstetrician and paediatrician in the active management of these cases is essential if further improvement in infant survival and prognosis is to be achieved.

References

1 AGERHOLM, M. Handicap and the handicapped: a nomenclature and classification of intrinsic handicaps. *Royal Society of Health Journal*, **95,** 3–8 (1975)

2 ALBERMAN, E. Stillbirths and neonatal mortality in England and Wales by birthweight. *Health Trends*, **6,** 14–17 (1974)

3 ANDERSON, A. B. M. and TURNBULL, A. C. Relationship between length of gestation and cervical dilatation, uterine contractability, and other factors during pregnancy. *American Journal of Obstetrics and Gynecology*, **105,** 1207–1214 (1969)

4 ANDERSON, A. B. M. In *Pre-term Labour* (Proceedings of the Fifth Study Group of the Royal College of Obstetricians and Gynaecologists) edited by A. B. M. Anderson, R. Beard, J. M. Brudenell, P. M. Dunn, 4. London, Royal College of Obstetricians and Gynaecologists (1977)

5 AVERY, G. B. In *Neonatology: pathophysiology and management of the newborn*. Edited by G. B. Avery, Philadelphia, J. B. Lippincott Co. (1975)

6 BAUMGARTEN, K. and GRUBER, W. Tokolyseindex. *Perinatale Medicine*, Bd. **5.** Edited by J. W. Dudenhausen and E. Saling, 58–59 (1974)

7 BEASLEY, J. M. and KURJAK, A. Influence of a partograph on the active management of labour. *Lancet*, **2,** 348–51 (1972)

8 BISHOP, E. H. Pelvic scoring for elective induction. *Obstetrics and Gynaecology*, **24,** 266–268 (1964)

9 BLAKE, A. M., McINTOSH, N., REYNOLDS, E. O. R. and ST. ANDREW, D. Transport of newborn infants for intensive care. *British Medical Journal*, **4,** 13–19 (1975)

10 BOWES, W. Results of the intensive perinatal management of very low birth weight infants (501–1500 g). In *Pre-term Labour*. (Proceedings of the Fifth Study Group of the Royal College of Obstetricians and Gynaecologists), edited by A. B. M. Anderson, R. Beard, J. M. Brudenell, P. M. Dunn, 331–335. London, Royal College of Obstetricians and Gynaecologists (1977)

11 BRENNER, W. E., BRUCE, R. D. and HENDRICKS, C. H. The characteristics and perils of breech presentation. *American Journal of Obstetrics and Gynecology*, **118,** 700–712 (1974)

12 BRITISH MEDICAL JOURNAL LEADER Drugs in threatened preterm labour. *British Medical Journal*, **1,** 71 (1979)

13 BROCK, D. J. H., BARRON, L., JELEN, P., MATT, M. and SCRIMGEOUR, J. B. Maternal serum-alpha-fetoprotein measurements as an early indicator of low birthweight. *Lancet*, **2,** 267–268 (1977)

14 BROOKS, R. Congenital cervical incompetence in primigravidae. *American Journal of Obstetrics and Gynecology*, **86,** 52–65 (1963)

15 CASSADY, G. In *Clinical Perinatology*. Edited by S. Aladjem Campus, and A. K. Brown, 422. St. Louis, C. V. Mosby (1974)

16 CRAWFORD, J. S. Lumbar epidural analgesia for the singleton breech presentation. *Anaesthesia*, **30,** 119–120 (1975)

17 CSAPO, A. I. In *Uterine contraction: side effects of steroidal contraceptives*. Edited by J. B. Josimovich, 223. New York, John Wiley (1973)

18 DAVIES, P. A. Outlook for the low birthweight baby – then and now. *Archives of Diseases in Childhood*, **51,** 817–819 (1976)

19 DRILLIEN, C. M. Incidence of mental and physical handicaps in school age children of very low birthweight. *Pediatrics* (Springfield), **27,** 452–464 (1961)

20 DUENHOELTER, J. H., WELLS, C. E., REISCH, J. S., SANTOS-RAMOS, R. and JIMENEZ, J. M. A paired controlled study of vaginal and abdominal delivery of the low birthweight breech fetus. *Obstetrics and Gynaecology*, **54,** 310–313 (1979)

21 EMBREY, M. P. Premature rupture of the membranes. *Journal of Obstetrics and Gynaecology of the British Empire*, **60,** 37–43 (1953)

22 FAIRWEATHER, D. V. I. and STEWART, A. L. How to deliver the under 1500 g infant. *Reid's Controversy in Obstetrics and Gynaecology* 3rd Edn, Eastbourne, Holt-Saunders (in press)

23 FEDRICK, J. and ANDERSON A. B. M. Factors associated with spontaneous preterm birth. *British Journal of Obstetrics and Gynaecology*, **83,** 342–350 (1976)

24 FRIEDMAN, E. A. Primigravid labour, graphicostatistical analysis. *Obstetrics and Gynaecology*, **6,** 567–589 (1955)

25 FRIEDMAN, E. A. Cervimetry: objective method for study of cervical dilatation in labour. *American Journal of Obstetrics and Gynecology*, **71,** 1189–1193 (1956)

26 FROLICH, H., BAUMGARTEN, K., GRUBER, W., KLEARCHON, N., SEIDL, A. and URBAN, G. In *Premature Labour* (Proceedings of the International Symposium on the Treatment of Fetal Risks), edited by K. Baumgarten and A. Wesselius de Casparis, 11. Vienna, University of Vienna Medical School (1972)

27 FULLER, W. E. Management of premature labour. *Clinical Obstetrics and Gynaecology*, **21,** 542 (1972)

28 GILLIBRAND, P. N. Premature rupture of the membranes and prematurity. *Journal of Obstetrics and Gynaecology of the British Commonwealth*, **74,** 678–682 (1967)

29 GOLDENBERG, R. L. and NELSON, L. G. The premature breech. *American Journal of Obstetrics and Gynecology*, **127,** 240–244 (1977)

30 GUILLIAMS, S. and HELD, B. Contemporary management and conduct of preterm labour and delivery: a review. *Obstetrical and Gynaecological Survey*, **34,** 248–255 (1979)

31 HASSLEIN, H. C. and GOODLIN, R. C. Delivery of the tiny newborn. *American Journal of Obstetrics and Gynecology*, **134,** 192–200 (1979)

32 HEMMINKI, E. and STARFIELD, B. Prevention and treatment of premature labour by drugs: review of controlled clinical trials. *British Journal of Obstetrics and Gynaecology*, **85,** 404–417 (1978)

33 HOLT, K. S. The quality of survival. In *Occasional Papers 2, 3* and *4.* Institute of Research into Mental Retardation, London, Butterworths (1972)

34 HOMMERS, M. and KENDALL, A. C. The prognosis of the very low birthweight infant. *Developmental Medicine and Child Neurology*, **18,** 745–752 (1976)

35 HULL, D. Contributions of preterm birth to perinatal mortality. In *Preterm Labour* (Proceedings of the Fifth Study Group of the Royal College of Obstetricians and Gynaecologists), edited by A. B. M. Anderson, R. Beard, J. M. Brudenell, P. M. Dunn, 5–16. London, Royal College of Obstetricians and Gynaecologists (1977)

36 INGEMARSSON, I. Effect of terbutaline on premature labour: a double-blind placebo-controlled study. *American Journal of Obstetrics and Gynecology*, **125,** 520–524 (1976)

37 INGEMARSSON, I., WESTGREN, M. and SVENNINGSEN, N. W. Long term follow up of preterm infants in breech presentation delivered by caesarean section – a prospective study. *Lancet*, **2,** 172–175 (1978)

38 KAPPY, K. A., CETRULO, C. L., KNUPPEL, R. A., INGARDIA, C. J., SBARRA, A. J., SCERBO, J. C. and MITCHELL, G. W. Premature rupture of the membranes: a conservative approach. *American Journal of Obstetrics and Gynecology*, **134,** 655–661 (1979)

39 KARP, L. E., DONEY, J. R., McCARTHY, J., MEIS, P. J. and HALL, M. The premature breech. Trial of labour or caesarean section. *Obstetrics and Gynaecology*, **53,** 88–92 (1979)

40 KEIRSE, M. J. N. C., RUSH, R. W., ANDERSON, A. B. M. and TURNBULL, A. C. Risk of preterm delivery in patients with previous preterm delivery and or abortion. *British Journal of Obstetrics and Gynaecology*, **85,** 81–85 (1978)

41 KUBLI, F. In *Pre-term Labour* (Proceedings of the Fifth Study Group of the Royal College of Obstetricians and Gynaecologists) edited by A. B. M. Anderson, R. Beard, J. M. Brudenell, P. M. Dunn, 218. London, Royal College of Obstetricians and Gynaecologists (1977)

42 KVIST-CHRISTENSEN, K., CHRISTENSEN, P., INGEMARSSON, I. A study of complications in preterm delivery after prolonged premature rupture of the membranes. *Obstetrics and Gynaecology* 670–677 (1976)

43 LANDSMAN, R. In *Pre-term Labour* (Proceedings of the Fifth Study Group of the Royal College of Obstetricians and Gynaecologists) edited by A. B. M. Anderson, R. Beard, J. M. Brudenell, P. M. Dunn, 371. London, Royal College of Obstetricians and Gynaecologists (1977)

44 LEDGER, W. J. Bacterial infections complicating pregnancy. *Clinical Obstetrics and Gynaecology*, **21,** 445–475 (1978)

45 LEHMANN, W. D., JONATHA, W. and FORSTNER, H. A. Progress in diagnosis and treatment of pregnancies with low birthweight infants. *Geburtshilfe und Frauenheilkunde*, **38,** 606–618 (1978)

46 LIGGINS, G. C. and HOWIE, R. N. A controlled trial of antepartum glucocorticoid treatment for prevention of respiratory distress syndrome in premature infants. *Pediatrics*, **50,** 515–525 (1972)

47 LIGGINS, G. C. and VAUGHAN, G. S. Intravenous infusion of salbutamol in the management of premature labour. *Journal of Obstetrics and Gynaecology of the British Commonwealth*, **80,** 29–35 (1973)

48 LIU, D. T. Y., MELVILLE, H. A. H. and MEASDAY, B. Premature labour – parameters for comparison employing methylxanthine therapy. *Australian and New Zealand Journal of Obstetrics and Gynaecology*, **15,** 145–149 (1975)

49 LIU, D. T. Y. and KERR-WILSON, R. Cervical dilatation in spontaneous and induced labours. *British Journal of Clinical Practice*, **31,** 177–179 (1977)

50 LIU, D. T. Y. and BLACKWELL, R. J. The value of a scoring system in predicting outcome of preterm labour and comparing the efficacy of treatment with aminophylline and salbutamol. *British Journal of Obstetrics and Gynaecology*, **85,** 418–424 (1978)

51 LUBCHENCO, L. O., HORNER, F. A., REED, L. H., HIX, I. E., METCALF, D., COHIG, R., ELLIOTT, H. C. and BOURG, M. Sequelae of premature birth. *American Journal of Diseases in Childhood*, **106,** 101–115 (1963)

52 MARIVATE, M., DE VILLIERS, K. Q., FAIRBROTHER, P. Effect of prophylactic outpatient administration of fenoterol on the time of onset of spontaneous labour and fetal growth rate in twin pregnancy. *American Journal of Obstetrics and Gynecology*, **128,** 707–708 (1977)

53 MERENSTEIN, G. B., PETTET, G. B., WOODALL, J. and HILL, J. M. An analysis of our transport results in the newborn. II. Antenatal and neonatal referrals. *American Journal of Obstetrics and Gynecology*, **128,** 520–525 (1977)

54 MILLER, J. M., PUPKIN, M. J. and CRENSHAW, JR., C. Premature labour and premature rupture of the membranes. *American Journal of Obstetrics and Gynecology*, **132,** 1–6 (1978)

55 NEWTON, R. W., WEBSTER, P. A. C., BINU, P. S., MASKREY, N. and PHILLIPS, A. B. Psychosocial stress in pregnancy and its reaction to the onset of premature labour. *British Medical Journal*, **1,** 411–413 (1979)

56 O'CONNER, M. C., MURPHY, H. and DALRYMPLE, I. J. Double blind trial of ritodrine and placebo in twin pregnancy. *British Journal of Obstetrics and Gynaecology*, **86,** 706–709 (1979)

57 O'DRISCOLL, M. In *Pre-term Labour* (Proceedings of the Fifth Study Group of the Royal College of Obstetricians and Gynaecologists) edited by A. B. M. Anderson, R. Beard, J. M. Brudenell, P. M. Dunn, 369. London, Royal College of Obstetricians and Gynaecologists (1977)

58 PAPIERNIK, E. and KAMINSKI, M. Multifactorial study of the risk of prematurity at 32 weeks of gestation. *Journal of Perinatal Medicine*, **2,** 30–36 (1974)

59 PAUL, R. H., KOH, K. S. and MONFARED, A. H. Obstetric factors influencing outcome in infants weighing from 1001–1500 grams. *American Journal of Obstetrics and Gynecology*, **133,** 503–508 (1979)

60 PHILPOTT, R. H. Graphic records in labour. *British Medical Journal,* **4,** 163–165 (1972)

61 PONTONNIER, G., PUECH, F., GRANDJERN, H. and ROLLAND, M. Some physical and biochemical parameters during normal labour. *Biology of Neonate*, **26,** 159–173 (1975)

62 RAWLINGS, G., REYNOLDS, E. O. R., STEWART, A. L. and STRANG, L. B. Changing prognosis for infants of very low birthweight. *Lancet*, **1,** 516–519 (1971)

63 RENAUD, R., IRRMAN, M., GANDAR, R. and FLYNN, M. J. The use of ritodrine in the treatment of premature labour. *Journal of Obstetrics and Gynaecology of the British Commonwealth*, **81,** 182–186 (1974)

64 REYNOLDS, E. O. R. Effects of alterations in mechanical ventilation settings on pulmonary gas exchange in hyaline membrane disease. *Archives of Disease in Childhood*, **46,** 152–159 (1971)

65 RICHTER, R. and HINSELMANN, M. Treatment of threatened premature labour by betamimetic drugs: comparison of fenoterol and ritodrine. *Obstetrics and Gynaecology*, **1,** 81–87 (1979)

66 ROBERTON, N. R. C. Birth asphyxia, early and late effects. In *The Management of Labour* (Proceedings of the 3rd Study Group of the Royal College of Obstetricians and Gynaecologists) edited by R. Beard, J. M. Brudenell, P. M. Dunn, D. Fairweather, 220. London, Royal College of Obstetricians and Gynaecologists (1975)

67 ROBERTON, N. R. C. and TIZARD, J. P. M. Prognosis for infants with idiopathic respiratory distress syndrome. *British Medical Journal*, **2,** 271–274 (1975)

68 ROBERTS, G. Unclassified antepartum haemorrhage – incidence and perinatal mortality in a community. *Journal of Obstetrics and Gynaecology of the British Commonwealth*, **77,** 492–495 (1970)

69 SAIGAL, S., O'NEILL, A. and SURAINDER, Y. Placental transfusion and hyperbilirubinaemia in the premature. *Pediatrics*, **49,** 406 (1972)

70 SCHAFFNER, F. and SCHANZER, S. N. Cervical dilatation in the early third trimester. *Obstetrics and Gynaecology*, **27,** 130–133 (1966)

71 SCHLIEVERT, P., JOHNSON, W. and GALASK, R. P. Bacterial inhibition by amniotic fluid. *American Journal of Obstetrics and Gynecology*, **125,** 899–905 (1976)

72 SHAW, J. C. L. Parenteral nutrition in the management of sick low birthweight infants. *Pediatric Clinics of North America*, **20,** 333–358 (1973)

73 SIVASAMBOO, R. In *Premature Labour* (Proceedings of the International Symposium on the Treatment of Fetal Risks), edited by K. Baumgarten and A. Wesselius de Casparis, 16. Vienna, University of Vienna Medical School (1972)

74 STANLEY, F. J. and ALBERMAN, E. D. Infants of very low birthweight. I. Perinatal factors affecting survival. *Developmental Medicine and Child Neurology*, **20,** 313–322 (1977)

75 STEER, P. J., LITTLE, D. J., LEWIS, N. L., KELLY, M. C. M. and BEARD, R. W. Uterine activity in induced labour. *British Journal of Obstetrics and Gynaecology*, **82,** 433–441 (1975)

76 STEWART, A. L. and REYNOLDS, E. O. R. Improved prognosis for infants of very low birthweight, *Pediatrics* (Springfield) **54,** 724–735 (1974)

77 STEWART, A. L. In *Pre-term Labour* (Proceedings of the Fifth Study Group of the Royal College of Obstetricians and Gynaecologists), edited by A. B. M. Anderson, R. Beard, J. M. Brudenell, P. M. Dunn, 372–384. London, Royal College of Obstetricians and Gynaecologists (1977)

78 STEWART, A. L., TURCAN, D. M., RAWLINGS, G. and REYNOLDS, E. O. R. Prognosis for infants weighing 1000 grams or less at birth. *Archives of Disease in Childhood*, **52,** 97–104 (1977)

79 STUDD, J. J. W. and DUIAGAN, N. Graphic records in labour. *British Medical Journal*, **4,** 426 (1972)

80 TAYLOR, E. S., MORGAN, R. L., BRUNS, P. D. and DROSE, V. E. Spontaneous premature rupture of the fetal membranes. *American Journal of Obstetrics and Gynecology*, **82,** 1341–1348 (1961)

81 TERAMO, K., KIVALO, I., TARKKANEN, U. and TIMONEN, S. Caesarean section under local anaesthesia for high-risk fetuses. *Lancet*, **1,** 646 (1971)

82 THOMAS, D. J. B., DOVE, A. F. and ALBERTI, K. G. M. M. Metabolic effects of salbutamol infusion during premature labour. *British Journal of Obstetrics and Gynaecology*, **84,** 497–499 (1977)

83 TURNBULL, A. C. In *Pre-term Labour* (Proceedings of the Fifth Study Group of the Royal College fof Obstetricians and Gynaecologists) edited by A. B. M. Anderson, R. Beard, J. M. Brudenell, P. M. Dunn, 127. London, Royal College of Obstetricians and Gynaecologists (1977)

84 TURNBULL, E. P. N. and WALKER, J. Outcome of pregnancy complicated by threatened abortion. *Journal of Obstetrics and Gynaecology of the British Empire*, **63,** 553–559 (1956)

85 USHER, R. H., McLEAN, F. and SCOTT, K. E. Judgement of fetal age. II. Clinical significance of gestational age and an objective method for its assessment. *Pediatric Clinics of North America*, **13,** 835–862 (1966)

86 USHER, R. H. The special problems of the premature infant. In *Neonatology: pathophysiology and management of the newborn.* Edited by G. B. Avery, Philadelphia, J. P. Lippincott (1975)

87 USHER, R. H. Changing mortality rates with perinatal intensive care and regionalisation. *Seminars in Perinatology*, **1,** 309–319, (1977)

88 WALD, N., CUCKLE, H., STIRRAT, G. M., BENNETT, M. J. and TURNBULL, A. C. Maternal serum alpha-fetoprotein and low birthweight *Lancet*, **2,** 268–270 (1977)

89 WEEKES, A. R. L. and FLYNN, M. S. Engagement of the fetal head in primigravida and its relationship to duration of gestation and time of onset of labour. *British Journal of Obstetrics and Gynaecology*, **82,** 7–11 (1975)

90 WEEKES, A. R. L., MENZIES, D. N. and DE BOER, C. H. The relative efficacy of bed rest, cervical suture, and no treatment in the management of twin pregnancy. *British Journal of Obstetrics and Gynaecology*, **84,** 161–164 (1977)

91 WESSELIUS DE CASPARIS, A., THIERY, M., YOLESIAN, A., BAUMGARTEN, K. BROSENS, I., GAMISSANS, O., STOLK, J. G. and VIVIER, W. Results of a double blind, multicentre study with ritodrine in premature labour. *British Medical Journal*, **3,** 144–147, (1971)

92 WOOD, C., BANNERMAN, R. H. O., BOOTH, R. T. and PINKERTON, J. H. M. The prediction of premature labour by observation of the cervix and external tocography. *American Journal of Obstetrics and Gynecology*, **91,** 396–402 (1965)

93 WOODS, J. M. Effects of low birth weight breech delivery on neonatal mortality. *Obstetrics and Gynaecology*, **53,** 735–740 (1979)

94 ZLATNIK, F. and FUCHS, F. A controlled study of ethanol in threatened premature labour. *American Journal of Obstetrics and Gynecology*, **112,** 610–612 (1972)

15
Treatment of the prematurely born infant

Ernest N. Kraybill

Introduction

The medical, psychosocial and economic consequences of preterm births are in striking disproportion to their numbers. In North Carolina Memorial Hospital (a regional perinatal center) during a recent seven year period, low birth weight infants accounted for 92 percent of neonatal deaths, yet constituted only 15 percent of live births. Although the quality of surviving preterm infants has improved during recent years, the incidence of neurologic handicap is still high, especially among smaller prematures who required mechanical ventilation[8]. The average medical cost for 30 surviving infants weighing 1000 g or less at birth was \$40 287 in one regional center[21]. Several studies have shown that the risk of abuse and neglect is higher for preterm than for full term infants[7,10,14].

Two contrasting hypotheses could be formulated to explain the increased rates of death and disability among preterm infants (*Figure 15.1*). First, there could be an intrinsic defect in the fetus which accounts for both the preterm birth and the subsequent risk of abnormality or death. Alternatively, the fetus could be intrinsically normal, but have suffered the unfortunate 'accident' of preterm birth, with risk of subsequent handicap or death resulting from perinatal and postnatal events.

For certain premature infants who have birth anomalies, congenital infection, or fetal growth disturbances, the first hypothesis may be correct. For most preterm infants, however, there is little evidence to support the former hypothesis and much to support the latter one. If the higher mortality and handicap risks of preterm infants are indeed related to perinatal and postnatal events they are, at least theoretically,

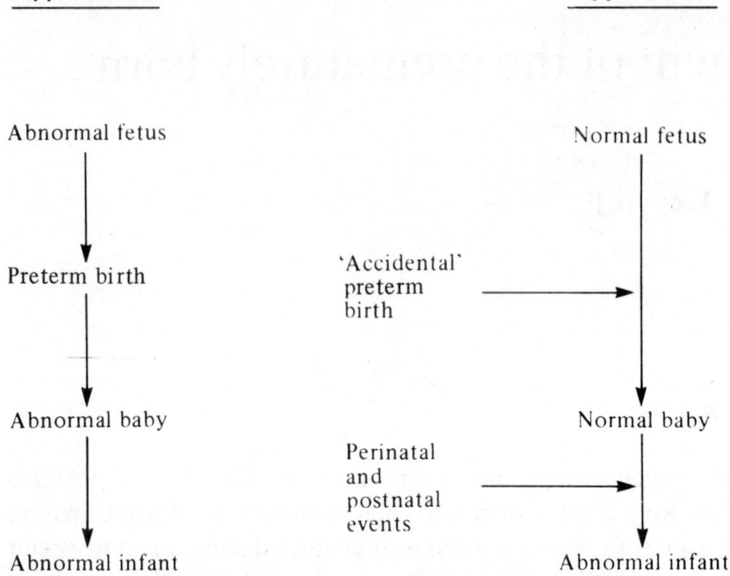

Figure 15.1 Pathogenesis of childhood handicap related to preterm birth

preventable. Present knowledge and practice has permitted a reduction in these risks, but has not eliminated them.

The previous chapter has been devoted to management of preterm labor in such a way as to minimize the hazards to the fetus. The present chapter will summarize certain aspects of the care of preterm infants which may affect the risk of handicap or death (*see Table 15.1*).

Preventive measures

Cold stress

The classic studies of Silverman, Fertig and Berger[23], demonstrated that low birth weight infants who were cared for at suboptimal environmental temperatures had a higher mortality rate than comparable infants nursed in a warmer environment. This phenomenon can be related to the increased oxygen cost of metabolizing brown fat, (non-shivering thermogenesis), coming as it often does at a time when the amount of oxygen available to neonatal organs is already marginal due to respiratory insufficiency.

Attention to thermal needs of preterm infants properly begins in the delivery room. The delivery room temperature, often cooled for the comfort of the obstetrician and mother, affects the infant most during the brief interval immediately following birth. A warmer setting is in the best interests of the premature. Prompt drying can reduce evaporative heat loss. Radiant heat exchange may be reversed by used of an overhead radiant heater which permits easy access for resuscitation. Warmed blankets are nearly as effective[6], but do limit access.

In the nursery, the preterm infant's large surface area relative to body mass allows extra heat loss by radiation and convection. If relative humidity of the environment is low, evaporative heat loss may also be substantial. Thermoneutrality (the body temperature at which the oxygen consumption is lowest) can be maintained by a wide variety of warming devices which utilize radiating or convecting heat sources. Either type device can be controlled to maintain a constant desired skin temperature through feedback from a thermistor applied to the infant's skin. Oxygen administered for treatment of respiratory distress is warmed and humidified to prevent excessive heat loss from the respiratory tract.

Table 15.1 Preventive medicine for premature infants

(Sometimes) preventable cause	*Pathophysiology*	*(Possible) unfavorable outcome*
Cold stress	Increased O_2 consumption	Increased mortality risk
Asphyxia	Cortical necrosis Periventricular-intraventricular hemorrhage; hydrocephalus Periventricular leukomalacia	Learning disability Mental retardation Seizure disorder Cerebral palsy
Hyperbilirubinemia	Kernicterus	
Malnutrition	Reduced brain growth (?)	
Infection	Cerebritis, ventriculitis, meningitis	
Hyperoxia	Retrolental fibroplasia	Myopia, blindness
Separation, communication failure	Failure of 'bonding' psychosocial family disorder	Neglect, abuse

Asphyxia and other causes of central nervous system injury

Although adverse events affecting preterm infants seldom occur singly, asphyxia is considered the most important factor associated with neurologic handicap or death. This devastating event commonly occurs in one or more of three settings – during or immediately following birth, during respiratory distress sydrome, or during apnea of prematurity.

Delivery room care

The promptness with which the preterm infant accomplishes onset of respiration, alveolar gas exchange and transition from fetal to neonatal circulatory pathways is influenced by many factors, some of which cannot be altered postnatally. Those factors already determined at birth include the degree of maturity of the lungs and central nervous system and the degree to which circulation and oxygenation have been maintained during labor and birth.

Several avenues of intervention in the delivery room may prevent or mitigate asphyxia, and thereby reduce the risk of respiratory distress syndrome. Thermal control, discussed earlier, is of prime importance. The infant's circulating blood volume, largely determined by the timing of cord clamping, may influence cardiorespiratory adaptation but its role is incompletely understood. The physiologic consequences of early versus late cord clamping, though extensively studied in the full-term infant, have not been similarly investigated in the preterm infant. Immediate cord clamping may cause hypovolemia and hypotension. Late cord clamping, which probably occurs only rarely in preterm infants, may result in decreased lung compliance, as occurs in full-term infants[19]. With present knowledge it seems prudent to avoid both very early and very late cord clamping.

Establishment of adequate ventilation and oxygenation is essential. The basic procedures, i.e., suctioning of the airway, drying of the skin and assignment of the one minute Apgar score, can usually be accomplished before clamping of the cord. If spontaneous respiration has not occurred during the first minute, manual ventilation must be started promptly. Infants who show evidence of intrapartum asphyxia, manifest by hypotonia and low or falling heart rate, require earlier ventilation.

Endotracheal intubation, though associated with certain risks, is the most efficient method of establishing a route for manual ventilation in the very small, severely depressed preterm. A decision to employ this technique should take into consideration the skill and experience of the physician as well as the condition of the infant. Even if such skill is lacking, it is possible to resuscitate the depressed infant via a properly applied face mask.

Emphasis is given to adequacy of ventilation, before administration of alkali or blood volume expanders. Those few infants who fail to respond to adequate ventilation may have suffered progressive asphyxia and acidosis during labor, may have an inadequate circulating blood volume or may have depression of the respiratory center due to maternal drugs. Each of these is evaluated independently. Alkali may be given safely to an infant whose 5 min Apgar score is less than seven. Blood volume expansion is reserved for those infants who have not responded to ventilation and correction of acidosis and who show evidence of poor skin perfusion. Placental blood, if collected in a sterile fashion, heparinized and filtered, may be used effectively for rapid volume expansion in cases of severe hypovolemia. Respiratory depression due to maternal narcotics is effectively treated with a narcotic antagonist.

Respiratory distress syndrome

An impressive body of research spanning three decades has elucidated the pathogenesis of respiratory distress syndrome (RDS), provided the rationale for therapy and resulted in a significant reduction in mortality. With current techniques including continuous positive airway pressure, mechanical ventilation, parenteral nutrition, cardiorespiratory monitoring and other aspects of critical neonatal care, death due to acute respiratory failure has become rare. If death occurs during the acute illness it is almost always associated with intraventricular hemorrhage.

Unfortunately, increased survival rates from RDS appear to have been achieved at the cost of chronic pulmonary sequellae. Bronchopulmonary dysplasia, described by Northway, Rosan and Porter[18] in 1967, may affect 20 percent of survivors of severe RDS in some centers. The spectrum of disease appears to be broad. In mild form, requirement for supplemental oxygen may be prolonged a few weeks beyond that expected of babies with uncomplicated RDS. In severe form, there may be pulmonary insufficiency requiring prolonged mechanical ventilation; the requirement for supplemental oxygen may extend into the second year of life. Whether such infants will ultimately develop completely normal pulmonary function is not known.

The etiologic factors associated with bronchopulmonary dysplasia remain poorly understood. Prolonged exposure of the respiratory tract to high concentrations of oxygen and to high pressure mechanical ventilation have been implicated. Large volumes of intravenous fluids and left-to-right shunting of blood through the ductus arteriosus may also be involved. The contribution of the primary disease (RDS) is, of course, impossible to distinguish from that due to therapeutic measures. Current efforts to prevent or mitigate this complication are directed toward limiting inspired oxygen concentration and peak airway pressures to the minimum necessary for adequate oxygenation. In many centers, fluid intake is being restricted because of its apparent relationship to patency of the ductus arteriosus[3], and possibly to bronchopulmonary dysplasia.

Apnea of prematurity

Otherwise 'normal' preterm infants are frequently observed to have periodic breathing which merges with apnea (usually defined as a respiratory pause of 20 s or greater, associated with bradycardia). This unique behavior of premature infants may be due to failure to sustain hyperventilation in response to hypoxia and a decreased ventilatory response to hypercarbia, in the presence of hypoxia[22]; both may be evidence of immaturity of neural respiratory control. Apnea of prematurity is diagnosed by excluding known environmental or pathologic causes of apnea such as cold stress, hyperthermia, intracranial hemorrhage, infection, metabolic disturbances and airway obstruction.

If properly monitored and treated, this phenomenon is self-limiting and compatible with normal survival. Obviously if undetected or inadequately treated, death or hypoxic brain injury may result. Electronic cardiorespiratory monitoring is effective in alerting care personnel to the occurrence of apnea. Mild apnea requires only stimulation or occasional manual ventilation. In severe cases, theophylline, caffeine, and continuous positive airway pressure have all been shown to be effective. Mechanical ventilation is rarely required.

The possible relationship between apnea of prematurity and risk for sudden infant death syndrome has led to continuing anxiety on the part of physicians as well as parents, after discharge of a preterm infant who had apnea. The use of electronic cardiorespiratory monitoring at home places a heavy burden on parents, but may be advisable in certain situations.

Although asphyxia is properly considered the major factor resulting in neurological handicap, two other disorders, often associated with asphyxia, may occur as independent events and result in severe neurologic injury.

Kernicterus. Kernicterus has long been recognized as a consequence of the toxic effects of bilirubin on the immature brain. The syndrome of lethargy, hypotonia and high-pitched cry, progressing to opisthotonus, seizures and finally choreoathetosis, spasticity and mental retardation was first associated with bilirubin concentrations in excess of 20 mg/dl in full-term infants with erythroblastosis fetalis[1].

More recent evidence has modified our understanding of this disorder. Bilirubin encephalopathy is now known to represent a spectrum of severity, of which kernicterus is only the extreme. Moreover, the risk of central nervous system effects is related to other factors in addition to the absolute serum concentration of bilirubin. Those factors include the amount of serum albumin available for bilirubin binding, the presence of competitive inhibitors and serum pH. Gestational age appears to be a factor but whether this is through the above-mentioned factors is not clear.

Exchange transfusion, once the sole method of preventing bilirubin encephalopathy, remains an important technique but is now used less frequently because of phototherapy. Light in the wavelengths around 45 nm (450 Å) causes bilirubin in the skin to be broken down into smaller, water soluble molecules which are non-toxic and are excreted in the urine.

Two major questions about phototherapy remain unanswered. The criteria for instituting phototherapy are imprecise because of uncertainty about when the premature brain is at risk of bilirubin damage. More important, though, is the continuing uncertainty about whether phototherapy is completely safe. The lack of confirmed reports of serious side-effects after two decades of use is reassuring, but the possibility of subtle, long-term side-effects cannot be ruled out.

Intraventricular hemorrhage. Once thought to be a rare, fatal event in prematures, intraventricular hemorrhage has been shown by computerized tomography to occur in about 40 percent of infants weighing less than 1500 g at birth[20]. In another prospective study[15], nearly half of the hemorrhages shown by computerized tomography were not predicted by clinical findings. Bleeding occurs first in the subependymal germinal matrix, adjacent to the ventricular system. In many cases the resulting hematoma ruptures into the lateral ventricle and may result in obstructive hydrocephalus.

Unlike subdural hemorrhage, which is usually due to trauma, intraventricular hemorrhage is most strongly associated with asphyxia. A recent study[16] has suggested that low cerebral blood flow may be a predisposing factor in the preterm infant with respiratory distress syndrome.

Experience to date indicates that severe intraventricular hemorrhage causing hydrocephalus carries an unfavorable though not hopeless prognosis. Insufficient follow-up data are available to predict the neurologic outcome of infants with mild to moderate hemorrhage. However, it is apparent that some such infants can have completely normal development.

Until the pathogenesis of intraventricular hemorrhage is more clearly understood preventive efforts are centered on prevention of asphyxia. Other possible etiologic factors including administration of sodium bicarbonate and variations in intravascular volume await further investigation.

Malnutrition

The rapid growth, characteristic of the human fetus during the third trimester of gestation, is rarely matched after preterm birth. The immature gastrointestinal tract is incapable of accepting, digesting and absorbing enough food to provide energy needs for growth, after basal and activity requirements are met. Conventional intravenous feedings provide only a fraction of full caloric requirements and contain no protein or fat. Hence, preterm infants who are nourished by conventional methods, either oral or parenteral, suffer some degree of malnutrition.

Experiments with animals suggest that the effect on various organs, including brain, of malnutrition during early infancy is dependent upon timing of the malnutrition[25]. It is difficult to extrapolate this information to human infants, mainly because of the large number of other variables affecting neurologic development. Nevertheless, there is legitimate concern that poor nutrition may contribute to neurologic handicap in very immature infants.

Human milk has certain features, such as low osmolality, low renal solute load, easy digestability and immunological properties which would be advantageous to premature infants. However, certain nutritional characteristics, particularly its protein, calcium and phosphorus content, may not be adequate to support needed growth in very low birth weight infants[9]. The finding that milk from mothers of prematures has a higher nitrogen concentration than that from mothers of term infants[2] suggests that some nutritional adaptation occurs. Nevertheless, nutritional supplementation is advisable if human milk is fed to very low birth weight infants.

There are significant risks associated with any method of feeding the very small preterm infant. Current nutritional practice includes various modifications of the technique of parenteral nutrition developed by Wilmore and Dudrick[24] for surgical patients. Parenteral solutions of protein hydrolysate or amino acids with carbohydrate, minerals and vitamins are used, often in conjunction with a parenteral lipid solution. Such parenteral feedings may be provided simultaneously with small enteric feedings. With these combined techniques it is possible to provide balanced nutrition and often to permit some growth to occur during the acute phase of respiratory illness. Such techniques have generally resulted in more rapid growth and shorter hospital stays; effects on mortality are uncertain. There are significant risks, of infectious, mechanical and metabolic nature, associated with parenteral nutrition and the long-term consequences have not been adequately studied.

The special problem of necrotizing enterocolitis may seriously jeopardize nutrition in certain preterm infants. This disease occurs almost exclusively in preterm infants and is frequently preceded by asphyxia which may damage bowel mucosa in such a way as to permit bacterial invasion. Although no single organism has been implicated, there is evidence to suggest that the disease may occur as an epidemic within a newborn intensive care unit[4]. Mild cases, without bowel perforation or necrosis, are treated with antibiotics and bowel rest. During this period parenteral fluids provide the only source of nutrition. If the disease is more severe, bowel resection may be required. Extensive resection of small bowel may leave the infant with marginal absorptive surface and thus jeopardize nutrition for many months. There is a significant mortality.

Infection

The special vulnerability of the preterm infant to infection is explained in part by developmental immaturity of the host's defense system and in part by unique avenues of exposure. While still *in utero*, infection may be acquired transplacentally or via the amniotic fluid; in some instances amnionitis may precede preterm labor. A number of organisms which infect the birth canal, including herpes simplex, group B streptococcus, chlamydia, gonococcus, and coliform bacteria, may contaminate the fetus during vaginal delivery and cause life-threatening neonatal infections. In the nursery, infection may be transmitted by hospital personnel, by tubes and instruments, by blood transfusions and even by mothers' milk.

Recent advances in understanding the pathogenesis of infection in neonates have generally not been matched by a reduction in morbidity and mortality due to infection. One notable exception to this is congenital rubella, which has become rare as a result of widespread immunization. The incidence of many other neonatal infections, including those due to group B streptococcus and herpes simplex, remains unchanged or may be increasing.

Fatal perinatal infection is more frequent in fetuses of mothers who had low weight gain during pregnancy[17]. It remains to be shown whether special nutritional counselling during pregnancy can reduce such risk; however, such programs seem warranted, especially among low socio-economic groups. Other preventive measures which may be applied include avoidance of exposure of the pregnant mother to known infections and prompt treatment of bacterial infections during pregnancy. The special problem of premature rupture of the fetal membranes is discussed in Chapter 6.

There is general agreement that maternal genital herpes simplex infection with intact membranes is a contraindication to vaginal delivery. There is no such certainty about how to protect the fetus in up to 30 percent of mothers whose birth canals harbour group B streptococci. The problem of treating the infant is compounded by the clinical and radiographic similarity between respiratory distress syndrome and congenital pneumonia due to group B streptococcus. This problem has led some physicians to treat with antibiotics all preterm infants who have respiratory distress of early onset, until infection is ruled out by appropriate cultures. It has not been demonstrated, however, whether this practice reduces morbidity or mortality.

Important preventive measures which may be applied in the newborn nursery include the provision of adequate space and personnel and careful attention to techniques for preventing cross-infection, particularly handwashing. During epidemics of respiratory or gastrointestinal infection in the community, symptomatic individuals should be excluded from the nursery. Given these measures, there is no evidence that visiting by parents increases the incidence of infection among prematures.

Retrolental fibroplasia

Retrolental fibroplasia was first recognized in a premature infant in 1940. Determining that indiscriminate use of oxygen was the cause of this disorder required more than a decade, culminating in the report of a collaborative study in 1954[12]. In 1957 the Committee on The Fetus and Newborn of The American Academy of Pediatrics changed its statement regarding use of oxygen in premature infants to include a warning about the dangers of high concentrations.

Since 1957 little new information has been gained about retrolental fibroplasia. With restricted oxygen usage the disease has declined in frequency but has not disappeared. A later cooperative study in five university centers in the USA, reported in 1977, failed to define a relationship between arterial oxygen tension and occurrence of retrolental fibroplasia, using intermittent blood sampling techniques[11]. Current knowledge of the minute-to-minute fluctuations in arterial oxygen tension, revealed by transcutaneous oxygen monitoring, supports the belief that high arterial oxygen tension is indeed a causative factor, though not the only one. Duration of exposure to supplemental oxygen and the degree of immaturity of the retina are likely important etiologic factors.

Prevention of retrolental fibroplasia epitomizes the exacting technological requirements of *primum non nocere* in caring for preterm infants. The fine line between providing enough oxygen to prevent death or neurologic impairment and too much oxygen for the developing retina may be impossible to achieve in some very immature infants.

Psychosocial problems in the family of the premature infant

The birth, illness and prolonged hospitalization of a preterm infant may have profound emotional and sociologic effects on the family. The various components of stress are readily apparent. Parents experience intense disappointment and often guilt about having produced an 'imperfect' child. There is always anxiety over the uncertainty about whether the infant will live. After survival seems assured there is uncertainty about whether the child will develop normally. Almost always there are realistic concerns about the financial cost of medical care.

Preterm birth is more frequent among families who were previously experiencing serious problems – the very young, the poorly educated, the economically deprived. It is not surprising that ill preterm infants are more likely than full-term healthy infants to suffer abuse and neglect during the first years of life, nor that their parents are more likely to become divorced or separated.

Klaus and Kennel[13] have called attention to the importance of the early neonatal period in establishing a bond between mother and infant. This process, often thwarted by hospital routines following normal birth, is more difficult if birth has been premature. Major advances have been made, however, in 'opening' (both literally and figuratively) special care nurseries to parents. A wide range of counselling and supporting services, as well as nurses and physicians may be enlisted to help the family through this difficult time. After the infant leaves the hospital these efforts must be redirected but not discontinued.

Perinatal services

Regionalization of perinatal care

The medical and technological advances which characterize modern medical care of the preterm infant are costly. It is clear that not every hospital with obstetrical facilities can afford the personnel, equipment and space required to provide such care. In 1976 a committee on Perinatal Health, representing The American Academy of Family Physicians, The American Academy of Pediatrics, the American College of Obstetricians and Gynecologists and the American Medical Association recommended regional development of perinatal services[5]. In the recommended ideal system a geographic region having 8000 to 12 000 deliveries per year would develop perinatal resources in a cooperative and efficient way. The committee recommended that each region support a regional (tertiary or level III) center where complex problems could receive appropriate care and where research, education and leadership would take place. District (secondary or level II) centers, each serving a smaller population base within the region, would care for patients with problems of intermediate complexity. A larger number of community (primary or level I) hospitals would provide routine care for uncomplicated pregnancies and normal newborns.

Most of the 50 United States and some European countries have taken steps to implement regional perinatal programs. Participation by hospitals and physicians has generally been voluntary, although there are increasing incentives to provide perinatal care within the framework of this system.

Certain problems have been common in states which have implemented regional programs. The financial costs of providing high quality perinatal services were generally underestimated and many programs are inadequately funded. Regional planning is sometimes at odds with medical vested interests; unnecessary duplication of facilities continues to exist in many regions.

The provision of tertiary care in a facility distant from the patient's home requires transportation and communication resources which may not be readily available. For the family requiring tertiary services, the replacement of familiar surroundings and a trusted physician by strange places and people creates a significant stress. This problem is not insurmountable and it has been amply shown that regioal centers can provide a warm and caring environment. Indeed, in many cases the regional centers have led the way in serving the emotional needs of the family.

The overall effect of regional perinatal programs has yet to be adequately measured. Infant mortality in the USA has been declining rather steadily since about 1960 and many factors are probably responsible; the role of regioal perinatal care is uncertain. Several well-designed studies are being conducted to measure the specific impact of the regional approach.

How much effort, for how long, for how small a baby?

Scientific and technological advances of recent years have made it possible to support life in infants who would have been considered hopelessly immature only a few years ago. Survival of infants of 26–27 weeks gestation, weighing less than 750 g, is no longer rare. However, the cost of such survival is high and must be measured in human as well as financial terms.

With the simpler medical care of earlier times the crisis of prematurity was usually passed quickly, as death intervened. The crisis may now be prolonged, often for months, before survival is assured or death occurs. Decisions about whether to provide life support are inevitably influenced by such foreboding. The lower the birth weight, the higher the risk of death and the greater the possibility that survival may be associated with severe handicap.

The increasing substitution of technological systems for immature organs carries increasing risk of technical accidents and human error. Some of these are inconsequential, others are catastrophic. While these risks can be reduced by adequate staffing of nurseries with well-trained and conscientious physicians and nurses and by adequate supporting technical personnel, it is unlikely that they can be completely eliminated. Such risk must also be weighed in making decisions about life support in very immature infants.

Few guidelines have been established to assist the medical team and the family in determining how much medical support is appropriate, for how long, when the outlook seems nearly hopeless. The issues are ethical ones; several sets of values, each individually tenable, may seem to be in conflict. The physician's desire to sustain the baby's life may be modified by his desire to reduce the suffering of the family or society. It seems likely that in the future, scarcity of medical and economic resources will influence such decisions, even in developed countries, as is now the case in underdeveloped nations.

There is a tendency for a regional perinatal center staff to define a degree of immaturity below which ordinary care, namely warmth, fluids, nutrition and oxygen, but not extraordinary care in the form of mechanical ventilation is given. The degree of immaturity which separates these two levels of care will vary, depending on the experience and resources of the center. In the individual situation the condition of the infant at birth is also considered. Such an approach is tentative at best and will be subject to change with time and circumstances.

An understanding of the parents' values, attitudes and inner resources is essential, yet the burden of decision cannot be shifted solely onto the parents. Frequent and extended conversations are helpful, both to develop a plan as well as to provide a base of mutual trust which will be needed later. Conflicting values may need to be assigned relative priorities. In this way a plan of action (or inaction) may be developed jointly by the medical staff and the family.

The current intensive care approach to prematurity has been characterized as analogous to the treatment of poliomyelitis prior to the availability of an effective vaccine. The 'iron lung' represented a heroic, yet desperate attempt to defy a disease which had already exacted its toll. The solution was not a better machine but rather, prevention. Surely no 'vaccine' will emerge to prevent prematurity. Yet the ultimate reduction of infant mortality and childhood handicap requires a better understanding of the factors involved in preterm labor and how they may be modified to permit full-term gestation.

References

1 ALLEN, F. H., JR and DIAMOND, L. K. *Erythroblastosis Fetalis*. 38. Boston, Little, Brown and Co. (1957)

2 ATKINSON, S. A., BRYAN, M. H. and ANDERSON, G. H. Difference in nitrogen concentration in milk from mothers of term and premature infants. *Journal of Pediatrics*, **83,** 67–69 (1978)

3 BELL, E. F., WARBURTON, D., STONESTREET, B. S. and OH, W. Effect of fluid administration on the development of symptomatic patent ductus arteriosus and congestive heart failure in premature infants. *New England Journal of Medicine*, **302,** 598–604 (1980)

4 BOOK, L. S., OVERALL, J. C., HERBST, J. J., BRITT, M. R., EPSTEIN, B. and JUNG, A. L. Clustering of necrotizing enterocolitis: interruption by infection–control measures. *New England Journal of Medicine*, **297,** 984–986 (1977)

5 COMMITTEE ON PERINATAL HEALTH. *Toward improving the outcome of pregnancy*. White Plains, NY, The National Foundation-March of Dimes (1976)

6 DAHM, L. S. and JAMES, L. S. Newborn temperature and calculated heat loss in the delivery room. *Pediatrics*, **49,** 504–513 (1972)

7 ELMER, E. and GREGG, G. S. Developmental characteristics of abused children. *Pediatrics*, **40,** 596–602 (1967)

8 FITZHARDINGE, P. M., POPE, K., ARSTIKAITIS, M., BOYLE, M., ASHBY, S., ROWLEY, A., NETLEY, C. and SWYER, P. R. Mechanical ventilation of infants of less than 1501 g birth weight: Health, growth, and neurologic sequellae. *Journal of Pediatrics*, **88,** 531–541 (1976)

9 FORBES, G. B. Is human milk the best food for low birth weight babies? *Pediatric Research*, **12,** 434 (1978)

10 HUNTER, R. S., KILSTROM, N., KRAYBILL, E. N. and LODA, F. Antecedents of child abuse and neglect in premature infants: a prospective study in a newborn intensve care unit. *Pediatrics*, **61,** 629–635 (1978)

11 KINSEY, V. E., ARNOLD, H. J., KALINA, R. E., STERN, L., STAHLMAN, M., ODELL, G., DRISCOLL, J. M., ELLICOTT, J. H., PAYNE, J. and PATZ, A. PaO_2 levels and retrolental fibroplasia: a report of the cooperative study. *Pediatrics*, **60,** 655–668 (1977)

12 KINSEY, V. E. Retrolental fibroplasia: cooperative study of retrolental fibroplasia and the use of oxygen. *Archives of Ophthalmology*, **56,** 481–543 (1956)

13 KLAUS, M. H., and KENNELL, J. H. *Maternal–infant bonding*. St. Louis, C. V. Mosby (1976)

14 KLEIN, M. and STERN, L. Low birth weight and the battered child syndrome. *American Journal of Diseases of Children*, **122,** 15–18 (1971)

15 LAZZARA, A., AHMANN, P., DYKES, F., BRANN, A. W. and SCHWARTZ, J. Clinical predictability of intraventricular hemorrhage in preterm infants. *Pediatrics*, **65,** 30–34 (1980)

16 LOU, H. C., SKOV, H. and PEDERSEN, H. Low cerebral blood flow: a risk factor in the neonate. *Pediatrics*, **95,** 606–609 (1979)

17 NAEYE, R. L. and PETERS, E. C. Amniotic fluid infections with intact membranes leading to perinatal deaths: a prospective study. *Pediatrics*, **61,** 171–177 (1978)

18 NORTHWAY, W. H., JR., ROSAN, R. C. and PORTER, D. Y. Pulmonary disease following respirator therapy of hyaline membrane disease: bronchopulmonary dysplasia. *New England Journal of Medicine*, **276,** 357–368 (1967)

19 OH, W., WALLGREN, G., HANSON, J. S. and LIND, J. The effects of placental transfusion on respiratory mechanics of normal term newborn infants. *Pediatrics*, **40,** 6–12 (1967)

20 PAPILE, L. A., BURSTEIN, J., BURSTEIN, R. and KOFFLER, H. Incidence and evolution of subependymal and intraventricular hemorrhage: a study of infants with birth weights less than 1500 g. *Journal of Pediatrics*, **92,** 529–534 (1978)

21 POMERANCE, J. J., UKRANINSKI, C. T., URKA, T., HENDERSON, D. H., NASH, A. H. and MEREDITH, J. L. Cost of living for infants weighing 1000 grams or less at birth. *Pediatrics*, **61,** 908–910 (1978)

22 RIGATTO, H. Ventilatory response to hypercapnea. *Seminars in Perinatology*, **1,** 363–367 (1977)

23 SILVERMAN, W. A., FERTIG, J. W. and BERGER, A. P. The influence of the thermal environment upon survival of newly born premature infants. *Pediatrics*, **22,** 876–886 (1958)

24 WILMORE, D. W. and DUDRICK, S. J. Growth and development of an infant receiving all nutrients exclusively by vein. *Journal of the American Medical Association*, **203,** 860–864 (1968)

25 WINICK, M. and NOBLE, A. Cellular response in rats during malnutrition at various ages. *Journal of Nutrition*, **89,** 300–306 (1966)

16
Neurological assessment of the newborn infant – a new approach

Lilly M. S. Dubowitz and Victor Dubowitz

Introduction

Over the past decade there has been a marked proliferation of new anaesthetic and analgesic agents during labour, of new approaches to induction of labour, and of efforts to prevent or stall preterm labour. At the same time there still seems to be a universal sense of satisfaction and security amongst obstetricians and anaesthetists that as long as the Apgar score of the newborn infant is satisfactory at one or five minutes after birth, the drug used or procedure undertaken is innocuous. This misconception needs to be dispelled and evaluation of drugs and other agents in labour has to take account of the more subtle effects on the vulnerable developing nervous system of the preterm or full-term infant in addition to the more gross effects on respiratory or cardiac function[5]. Even if the apparent effects seem transient, they may still have long-term influences on the developing nervous system or on the child/mother interrelation in the newborn period and beyond. Moreover, whilst some of these factors may have less importance in optimal circumstances, they may well become potentially hazardous under other circumstances when compounded by additional stresses such as hypoxia, prematurity and poor social circumstances[9].

Over the years a number of attempts have been made to assess the neurological status of the newborn infant under the impetus particularly of Saint-Anne Dargassies and her co-workers in Paris[1,2,10,11,12] and Prechtl and his colleagues in Groningen[7,8], and more recently Brazelton[3]. The approaches of Prechtl and Brazelton have identified influences of perinatal drugs and other events on the newborn infant but have concentrated particularly on the full-term infant and have not been suitable for early assessment of the preterm infant. Moreover, the methodology has been complex and measurement (especially with the Brazelton technique) difficult, and so is not suitable for routine and repeated examination of large numbers of newborn infants. The examination of Dargassies has been geared to preterm infants but is also complex and needs considerable experience for its interpretation, and the tests used, which are mainly based on tone and primitive reflexes, are not particularly sensitive to drug and other minor insults.

We thus felt the increasing need for a neurological examination which would meet the following basic requirements.

(1) It should be suitable for use by staff with no particular expertise in neonatal neurology and therefore should have a recording system which is simple and objective.
(2) It should be applicable to preterm as well as full-term infants and reliable as soon after birth as possible in order to show the pattern of changes due to drugs, anoxia, difficult delivery and other environmental influences in the perinatal period.
(3) The same examination should be reliable for sequential examination of preterm infants after birth in order to compare their neurological behaviour with that of newborn infants of corresponding postconceptional age and also to assess the resolution or development of abnormalities.
(4) The full examination and its recording should not take longer than 10–15 min at most.

Method

Choice of items

To achieve the above aims the items selected had to meet the following requirements.

(1) Applicable to full-term infants within the first 3 days of life.
(2) Applicable to preterm infants in an incubator in the first few days of life and also suitable for sequential assessment of the preterm infant.
(3) Should be easy to define and show good inter-observer correlation.
(4) Should include some items covering aspects of higher neurological function.

Table 16.1 Items selected for assessment

Habituation	*Movement and tone*	*Reflexes*	*Neurobehavioural items*
Light (torch)	Posture	Tendon	Eye appearance
Auditory (rattle)	Arm and leg recoil	Palmar grasp	Visual and auditory orientation
	Arm and leg traction	Rooting	Alertness
	Ventral suspension	Sucking	Peak of excitement
	Head control	Walking	Irritability
	Head raising in prone		Consolability
	Arm release in prone		Cry
	Body movement during examination		
	Facial movement		
	Tremor and startles		

After personally testing all available neurological and neurobehavioural criteria from the studies of the earlier authors in a series of some 300 infants, we eventually selected a combination of neurological and neurobehavioural items for further assessment (*Table 16.1*).

Method of recording

We produced for our use a comprehensive manual of instructions for all the items in our protocol but found it was too time-consuming and impractical to use an approach of this type.

From our experience with the recording of the assessment of gestation we had found this was vastly improved in both accuracy and speed by using a flat sheet with the charts printed for each infant and recording the appropriate items by circling the item directly on the sheet. In this way the gestational assessment could be done and recorded within two or three minutes and this also provided a permanent objective record for each infant. We accordingly adopted a similar approach in the development of the neurological assessment.

We decided to record the items on a five-point scale as we found from experience that it provided a reasonable number of gradations to objectively categorise most neurological parameters. Because we found the nine-point scale of the Brazelton technique somewhat cumbersome and difficult to apply, we modified the Brazelton neurobehavioural criteria to fit our five-point scale. Clear instructions for the elicitation of each item were entered on the actual recording sheet, followed by descriptions of the five grades and, wherever possible, illustrative diagrams (*Figure 16.1*).

This scheme proved to be immensely practical and easy to handle in spite of the large number of items used. Over the past two years of use it has undergone a number of modifications and amendments. Some items have been deleted whereas others initially omitted have been subsequently included.

Timing and sequence of recording

Because many of the neurological items are influenced by the state of the baby, it is important to elicit the individual items with the infant in an optimal state for that item and also to record the state at the time. We accordingly decided to do the examination about two-thirds of the way between one feed and the next (irrespective of the frequency of feeding) in order to try to standardize the state of the infant as much as possible. Preterm infants on continuous feeding (intravenous or alimentary) were examined at any time.

The sequence of examinations was intentionally selected so that those assessments requiring the baby to be in a relatively quiet or sleep state (State 1 or 2) were done first, followed by those not particularly influenced by the state, and subsequently completing the examination with the Brazelton criteria for which the baby needed to be fully awake. We decided to use the six gradings of state as defined by Brazelton.

Assessment of gestation

During their first examination all infants had an assessment of gestation done in the course of their neurological examination.

Scoring of items

We intentionally decided not to summate the scores of individual items in order to arrive at a single total score as we felt this might mask variations in individual items and significant changes in opposite

NAME. | D.O.B./TIME | WEIGHT | E.D.D. L.N.M.P. | E.D.D. U/snd.

HOSP. | NO. | DATE OF EXAM | HEIGHT | GESTATIONAL ASSESSMENT | SCORE | WEEKS

RACE | SEX | AGE | HEAD CIRC.

STATES
1. Deep sleep, no movement, regular breathing.
2. Light sleep, eyes shut, some movement.
3. Dozing, eyes opening and closing.
4. Awake, eyes open, minimal movement.
5. Wide awake, vigorous movement.
6. Crying.

						State	Comment	Asymmetry
HABITUATION (⩽state 3)								
Light Repetitive flashlight stimuli (10) with 5 sec. gap. Shutdown = 2 consecutive negative responses	No response	A. Blink response to first stimulus. B. Tonic blink response. C. Variable response.	A. Shutdown of movement but blink persists 2-5 stimuli. B. Complete shutdown 2-5 stimuli.	A. Shutdown of movement but blink persists 6-10 stimuli. B. Complete shutdown 6-10 stimuli.	A. Equal response to 10 stimuli. B. Infant comes to fully alert state. C. Startles + major responses throughout.			
Rattle Repetitive stimuli (10) with 5 sec gap.	No response	A. Slight movement to first stimulus. B. Variable response.	Startle or movement 2-5 stimuli, then shutdown	Startle or movement 6-10 stimuli, then shutdown	A. B. C. – Grading as above			
MOVEMENT & TONE	Undress infant							
Posture (At rest - predominant) *			(hips abducted)	(hips adducted)	Abnormal postures: A. Opisthotonus. B. Unusual leg extension. C. Asymm.tonic neck reflex			
Arm Recoil Infant supine. Take both hands, extend parallel to the body; hold approx. 2 secs. and release.	No flexion within 5 sec. R L	Partial flexion at elbow >100° within 4-5 sec. R L	Arms flex at elbow to <100° within 2-3 sec. R L	Sudden jerky flexion at elbow immediately after release to <60° R L	Difficult to extend; arm snaps back forcefully			
Arm Traction Infant supine; head midline; grasp wrist, slowly pull arm to vertical. Angle of arm scored and resistance noted at moment infant is initially lifted off and watched until shoulder off mattress. Do other arm.	Arm remains fully extended R L	Weak flexion maintained only momentarily R L	Arm flexed at elbow to 140° and maintained 5 sec. R L	Arm flexed at approx. 100° and maintained R L	Strong flexion of arm <100° and maintained R L			
Leg Recoil First flex hips for 5 secs, then extend both legs of infant by traction on ankles; hold down on the bed for 2 secs and release.	No flexion within 5 sec. R L	Incomplete flexion of hips within 5 sec. R L	Complete flexion within 5 sec. R L	Instantaneous complete flexion R L	Legs cannot be extended; snap back forcefully R L			
Leg Traction Infant supine. Grasp leg near ankle and slowly pull toward vertical until buttocks 1-2" off. **Note resistance at knee** and score angle. Do other leg.	No flexion R L	Partial flexion, rapidly lost R L	Knee flexion 140-160° and maintained R L	Knee flexion 100-140° and maintained R L	Strong resistance; flexion <100° R L			

Popliteal angle Infant supine. Approximate knee and thigh to abdomen; extend leg by gentle pressure with index finger behind ankle.	180-160° R L	150-140° R L	130-120° R L	110-90° R L	< 90° R L			
Head lag * Pull infant toward sitting posture by traction on both wrists. Also note arm flexion.								
Head control (post.neck muscles) Grasp infant by shoulders and raise to sitting position; allow head to fall forward; wait 30 sec.	No attempt to raise head	Unsuccessful attempt to raise head upright	Head raised smoothly to upright in 30 sec. but not maintained.	Head raised smoothly to upright in 30 sec. and maintained	Head cannot be flexed forward			
Head control (ant.neck muscles) Allow head to fall backward as you hold shoulders; wait 30 sec.	Grading as above	Grading as above	Grading as above	Grading as above				
Ventral suspension * Hold infant in ventral suspension; observe curvature of back, flexion of limbs and relation of head to trunk.								
Head raising in prone position Infant in prone position with head in midline.	No response	Rolls head to one side	Weak effort to raise head and turns raised head to one side	Infant lifts head, nose and chin off	Strong prolonged head lifting			
Arm release in prone position Head in midline. Infant in prone position; arms extended alongside body with palms up.	No effort	Some effort and wriggling	Flexion effort but neither wrist brought to nipple level	One or both wrists brought at least to nipple level without excessive body movement	Strong body movement with both wrists brought to face or 'press-ups'			
Spontaneous body movement during examination (supine) If no spont.movement try to elicit by cutaneous stim.	None or minimal	A.Sluggish. B.Random, incoordinated. C.Mainly stretching.	Smooth movements alternating with random, stretching, athetoid or jerky	Smooth alternating movements of arms and legs with medium speed and intensity	Mainly: A.Jerky movement. B.Athetoid movement. C.Other abnormal movement.		1 2	
Tremors Mark: Fast (>6/sec) or Slow (<6/sec)	No tremor	Tremors only in state 5-6	Tremors only in sleep or after Moro and startles	Some tremors in state 4	Tremulousness in all states			
Startles	No startles	Startles to sudden noise, Moro, bang on table only	Occasional spontaneous startle	2-5 spontaneous startles	6+ spontaneous startles			
Abnormal movement or posture	No abnormal movement	A. Hands clenched but open intermittently. B. Hands do not open with Moro.	A. Some mouthing movement. B. Intermittent adducted thumb	Continuous mouthing movement	A. Continuously adducted thumb. B. Hands clenched all the time.			

Figure 16.1 Part of protocol for neurological examination of newborn infants

directions might merely cancel each other out. We accordingly preferred to document individual items on our proforma sheet so that patterns of responses could be readily seen. This approach allows one to use part of the proforma when the infant may be too ill to complete all the responses. It also allows flexibility and the possibility for modifications and adjustments within the overall protocol to meet particular circumstances or specific studies. The advantage of this approach is that individual items are objectively documented on the basis of the observed response, without any attempt to relate it to a preconceived normal response. The documentation can thus be used for preterm as well as full-term infants under both normal and abnormal circumstances.

The format of part of our final proforma is shown in *Figure 16.1*. We found that the examination could be readily recorded on a single flat sheet. Since the instructions are included on the sheet itself, and the recording is direct on the sheets, it can be done quickly and accurately (*Figure 16.2*). We have found that the average time for examination and recording done by one examiner is under 15 min; if a second person is available for recording it can be completed on a premature infant within 5–10 min. The whole procedure was well tolerated by preterm infants down to 28 weeks gestation and within 24 hours of birth[4].

Members of our junior medical staff with no prior expertise in neonatal neurology could readily be trained and showed good inter-observer recording on the same infant. This was observed by either one examiner doing the examination while the other was watching and both recording the data independently, or by two examiners doing the same examination independently of each other on the same day and in the same time relationship to the last feed of the infant.

Observations to date

Normal infants

Full-term infants born after normal pregnancy with minimal medication during delivery and no complications showed a fairly consistent pattern on the proforma. There was also a consistent difference in the pattern when examined on the fifth day of life compared with the first[4].

Item						Score		
Leg Recoil First flex hips for 5 secs, then extend both legs of infant by traction on ankles; hold down on the bed for 2 secs and release.	No flexion within 5 sec. R L	Incomplete flexion of hips within 5 sec. R L	Complete flexion within 5 sec. R L	Instantaneous complete flexion R L	Legs cannot be extended; snap back forcefully R L	3		
Leg Traction Infant supine. Grasp leg near ankle and slowly pull toward vertical until buttocks 1-2" off. Note resistance at knee and score angle. Do other leg.	No flexion R L	Partial flexion, rapidly lost R L	Knee flexion 140-160° and maintained R L	Knee flexion 100-140° and maintained R L	Strong resistance; flexion <100° R L	3		
Popliteal angle Infant supine. Approximate knee and thigh to abdomen; extend leg by gentle pressure with index finger behind ankle.	180-160° R L	150-140° R L	130-120° R L	110-90° R L	<90° R L	4		
Head lag * Pull infant toward sitting posture by traction on both wrists. Also note arm flexion.						4		
Head control (post.neck muscles) Grasp infant by shoulders and raise to sitting position; allow head to fall forward; wait 30 sec.	No attempt to raise head	Unsuccessful attempt to raise head upright	Head raised smoothly to upright in 30 sec. but not maintained.	Head raised smoothly to upright in 30 sec. and maintained	Head cannot be flexed forward	4		
Head control (ant.neck muscles) Allow head to fall backward as you hold shoulders; wait 30 sec.	Grading as above	Grading as above	Grading as above	Grading as above		4		
Ventral suspension * Hold infant in ventral suspension; observe curvature of back, flexion of limbs and relation of head to trunk.						4		
Head raising in prone position Infant in prone position with head in midline.	No response	Rolls head to one side	Weak effort to raise head and turns raised head to one side	Infant lifts head, nose and chin off	Strong prolonged head lifting	4		
Arm release in prone position Head in midline. Infant in prone position; arms extended alongside body with palms up.	No effort	Some effort and wriggling	Flexion effort but neither wrist brought to nipple level	One or both wrists brought at least to nipple level without excessive body movement	Strong body movement with both wrists brought to face or 'press-ups'	4		

Figure 16.2 Enlargement of part of protocol to show method of scoring/documentation

Abnormal infants

Full-term infants who were growth-retarded but had no other complications showed a consistently different picture from the appropriate size ones. There was increased flexor tone in the limbs, increased tremors and startles, deviant Moro response and significantly increased visual and auditory orientation. Infants delivered by forceps frequently showed during the first few days hyper-irritability, poor habituation, tremulousness, exaggerated adduction with the Moro response, and increased extensor tone in the neck muscles. These infants also showed marked lability of state.

Preterm and full-term infants recovering from hypoxia following either respiratory distress syndrome or birth asphyxia showed a similar pattern to the infants following forceps delivery, except for the absence of increased extensor tone in the neck.

Preterm infants

Some of our most interesting observations to date have been on the process of maturation in preterm infants. The method has enabled us to study the development of some of the functions not previously studied in newborn preterm infants, such as auditory and visual responses. It has also enabled us to follow longitudinally the evolution of some of the neurological signs previously only compared in preterm infants at term with full-term newborn infants. The results showed that visual fixation and orientation can be consistently documented in preterm infants from 30 weeks gestation onwards and that by the time they reach a maturity of 36 weeks, irrespective of their gestational age at birth, the pattern is fully mature and comparable to that of full-term newborn infants. Longitudinal studies in preterm infants born at 28–34 weeks gestation have shown a very different pattern of change in a number of neurological parameters as they approached term in comparison with full-term newborn infants. This is well illustrated by supine posture (*Figure 16.3*), arm traction, posture in ventral suspension (*Figure 16.4*) and the Moro response.

Other perinatal factors

We have been studying the effects of drugs and other influences during the perinatal period on the neurological status of the newborn preterm and full-term infant but the data are still insufficient to allow any firm general conclusions to be drawn. However, it has been strikingly

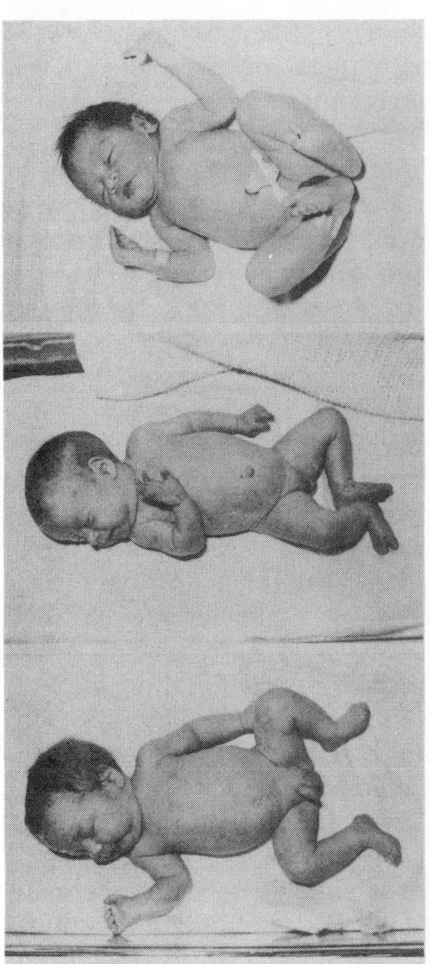

Figure 16.3 Comparison of posture in full-term newborn infant (top) and preterm infants (gestation 28 and 29 weeks) reaching term postconceptional age (centre and lower picture)

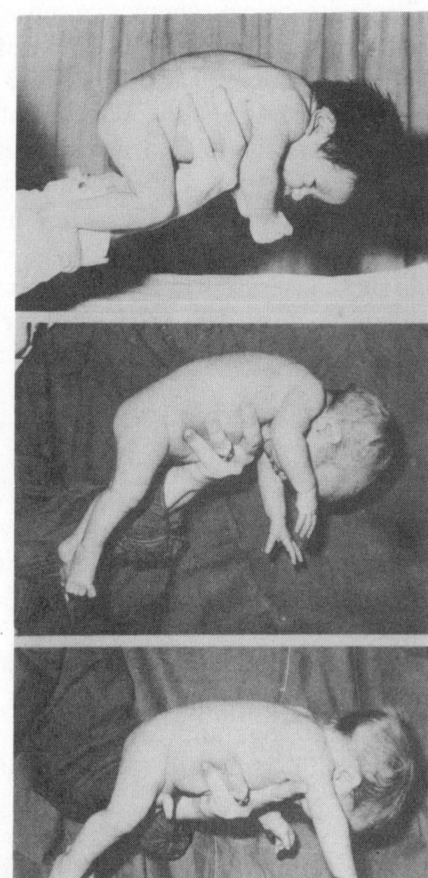

Figure 16.4 Ventral suspension showing posture of back, head and limbs in full-term newborn infant (top) and in two preterm infants (28 and 29 weeks gestation) reaching term (centre and lower picture). Note extended position of arms and legs in preterm infants

apparent that certain drugs, such as diazepam, seem to produce a very consistent and readily recognisable pattern of neurological and neurobehavioural response and various other influences during the perinatal period may also produce consistent changes. In a comparative study in progress on the early detection of intracranial haemorrhage in the newborn infant by the neurological assessment scheme and by ultrasonography done at frequent regular intervals, there are indications that early neurological signs of intracranial bleeding can be identified in preterm infants.

Conclusions

The neurological scheme we have evolved has proved to be practical and effective for the assessment of preterm and full-term infants and for the sequential study of the same infant. A combination of neurobehavioural and neurological criteria has proved feasible and the whole examination can be completed in most infants if the particular sequence of the examination is followed.

From our experience to date this scheme has the following to offer.

(1) It can be used to record objectively the neurological status of the preterm as well as the full-term infant within 24 hours of birth.
(2) It can provide a means to study the preterm infant under normal and abnormal circumstances.
(3) It can help to identify and document the effects of perinatal insults, such as drugs in the perinatal period, on the newborn infant.
(4) It provides a means of following sequentially the resolution of abnormal neurological signs and also for detecting the appearance of new abnormalities.

We have intentionally not tried to quantitate the items collectively and to give a single total score, as we thought this would mask individual deviations within the comprehensive assessment. The charts will readily show up a consistent pattern for the normal infant at varying gestational age, and any deviations in individual parameters readily become apparent. It is also likely that the 'normal' pattern may vary from one neonatal unit to another under the influence of aspects of management such as the use of drugs or even the posture in which the baby is nursed. Since the examination can be frequently repeated on the same infant, the evolution of various deviant features can be objectively recorded and followed.

The system has also enabled us to document and evaluate the progression of certain neurological parameters longitudinally in the preterm infant during its postnatal maturation outside the uterus and to directly compare these with the newborn infant of corresponding postconceptional age.

This has enabled us to put a new interpretation on some of the observations documented by earlier authors in preterm infants reaching term. Thus we believe that some of the neurological signs looked upon by Howard and Parmelee[6] as 'immature' are probably normal for the developing preterm infants because firstly they never develop the mature response shown by the full-term newborn infant (possibly due to the posture in which they are nursed and also the absence of the intrauterine restraint producing the flexed posture in the full-term infant), and secondly because of the frequency with which these 'immature' responses occur in preterm infants who subsequently have normal or even advanced motor development at follow-up. These results suggest that one probably ought to draw up a completely separate series of norms for the preterm infant and not to utilize the same criteria on which the full-term infant is assessed at follow-up.

Authors in the past have tried to predict the future neurological status of the infant some years later, with limited success. Our objective has been mainly to identify and document neurological abnormality in the newborn period. In view of the plasticity of the developing nervous system the long-term prognosis is likely to be influenced by many factors, including the management of the infant, apart from the initial abnormalities themselves.

While the actual interpretation of data will always depend to an extent on experience, the present scheme does provide a means whereby the inexperienced observer can objectively and accurately record meaningful criteria of neurological function in a standardised way. We hope that this will provide a useful baseline for future studies of deviation from the norm in relation to obstetrical and other perinatal factors that may influence it.

References

1 AMIEL-TISON C. Neurological evaluation of the maturity of newborn infants. *Archives of Disease in Childhood*, **43,** 89–93 (1968)

2 ANDRE-THOMAS C. Y. and SAINT-ANNE DARGASSIES. S. The neurological examination of the infant. *Clinics in Developmental Medicine* No. **1**, London, SIMP/Heinemann (1960)

3 BRAZELTON, T. B. Neonatal behavioral assessment scale. *Clinics in Developmental Medicine*, No. **50,** London, SIMP/Heinemann (1973)

4 DUBOWITZ, L. M. S. and DUBOWITZ, V. Neurological assessment of the newborn infant. *Clinics in Developmental Medicine*. London SIMP/Heinemann (in press)

5 DUBOWITZ, V. Neurological fragility in the newborn. *British Journal of Anaesthesia*, **47,** 1005 (1975)

6 HOWARD, J., PARMELEE, A. H. JR., KOPP, G. B., and LITTMAN, B. A neurologic comparison of pre-term and full-term infants at term conceptional age. *Journal of Pediatrics*, **88,** 995–1002 (1976)

7 PRECHTL H. The neurological examination of the full-term newborn infant, *Clinics in Developmental Medicine*, No. **63,** London, SIMP/Heinemann, (1977)

8 PRECHTL, H. and BEINTEMA, D. The neurological examination of the full term newborn infant. *Clinics in Developmental Medicine*, No. **12,** London, SIMP/Heinemann (1964)

9 ROSENBLATT, D. B., REDSHAW, M. E. and NOTARIANNI, L. J. Pain relief in childbirth and its consequences for the infant. *Trends in Pharmacological Science* (in press)

10 SAINT-ANNE DARGASSIES, S. La maturation neurologique du prématuré. *Revue Neurologique*, **93,** 331 (1955)

11 SAINT-ANNE DARGASSIES, S. Neurodevelopmental symptoms during the first year of life. *Developmental Medicine and Child Neurology*, **14,** 235–246 (1972)

12 SAINT-ANNE DARGASSIES, S. *Neurological Development in Full Term and Premature Neonate*. Amsterdam, Elsevier (1977)

17
The outcome for preterm infants

Rosamond A. K. Jones and Pamela A. Davies

Attempts to audit the later progress of preterm and low birth weight infants have been made for nearly three quarters of a century. Many such studies have followed the children in the first years of life only, to determine the extent of any neurological and sensory handicap; others have surveyed older children and assessed intelligence and school performance. Very few investigators have continued their enquiries into later life, and this omission must be cause for regret, for in the end what matters is whether such children will be able to take their place as adults in a competitive world to their own, their families' and society's satisfaction.

In recent years the approach to perinatal care has been increasingly complex and technological, and the coincident increase in survival of the most immature has led to renewed interest in their future potential. Has handicap increased with this fall in perinatal mortality, has it decreased or remained unchanged? Are the new techniques used in perinatal care safe in the short and long term? To a large extent these questions are still unanswerable, but in this chapter we shall try to review the evidence available from follow-up surveys and discuss its strengths and limitations.

Terminology

We shall use 'low birth weight' to mean one of 2500 g or below, and 'very low birth weight' one of 1500 g or less. A 'preterm' infant is one born before 37 completed weeks of gestation. A 'small for gestational age' infant, who may of course also be preterm, is one whose birth weight lies below the 10th centile for gestation. Follow-up surveys reported in the first half of this century did not distinguish between these two, and although our brief is to discuss outcome for preterm infants, the terms 'premature' or 'prematurity' when used will signify that the distinction was not made between the two in older studies, and in general referred to infants weighing 2500 g and below at birth, regardless of their gestation.

Follow-up surveys: general considerations

Later outcome for the preterm infant has to be viewed against the shifting background of a steadily falling mortality rate, subtly and constantly changing methods of perinatal management, and perhaps most important of all, the characteristics of the population from which the infants are drawn. Brief mention will be made of these, the question of controls, and other factors in design. It will be obvious that results of the childhood surveys which are most helpful – those that follow the children to the early school years and can include an assessment of learning difficulties – are always, when published, about 8–10 years out of date with current practices in perinatal care. This is unfortunately one of their major limitations.

Falling mortality

The gradual decrease in neonatal mortality reported from many parts of the world is exemplified in the figures for England and Wales shown in *Table 17.1* for infants weighing 2500 g or less and is self-evident[2]. It

Table 17.1 Twenty-eight day mortality for low birth weight infants, England and Wales*

	Mortality (%)				
Birth weight (g)	⩽2500	⩽1000	⩽1500	1501–2000	2001–2500
1953	15.4	No data	68.7	20.1	5.1
1958	14.2	No data	66.9	18.3	4.9
1963	12.8	85.1	62.6	16.2	4.0
1968	11.3	81.2	58.4	14.0	3.3
1973	10.1	80.8	54.3	12.8	3.1
1978	8.0	75.3	43.7	8.7	2.0

*Figures from Alberman[2] and personal communication

leads to ambiguities in reporting of results however; for the handicapped – when expressed as a percentage of ever increasing survivors – will almost certainly appear to be diminishing, when in fact this may not be so. For this reason, we believe it is most helpful when reporting follow-up results to give neonatal and post-neonatal deaths, handicapped, apparently normal and untraced survivors as percentages of total infants under review[58].

Perinatal care

Changes in the obstetric conduct of preterm labours are referred to elsewhere in this volume. Neonatal treatment of preterm infants has evolved gradually: from the scrupulous attention paid in the first quarter of the century by pioneers such as Pierre Budin of France and Julius Hess of America to keeping infants warm and nourished, to today's highly technological intensive care. Some of the major additions to treatment, and their implications for follow-up are shown in *Table 17.2*.

Characteristics of population

The population from which the majority of preterm and low birth weight infants are drawn is, in general, one of socio-economic disadvantage. The low birth weight rate in underdeveloped parts of the world is likely to be at least five times as great as that of the most prosperous Western country, but the data reviewed by Birch and Gussow[13] emphasize that socio-economic rather than ethnic considerations are the cause. It is the mothers' poor childhood and presumably nutritional status that correlates more closely with low birth weight than the fathers' social class[7]. The mothers are also more likely to be above average age or very young, to smoke more, to be unmarried and to have less antenatal care than those of normal weight infants[7, 31, 101]. There is a history of previous reproductive failure, involving infertility, recurrent abortions, stillbirths or previous small infants, and about half of the pregnancies are complicated[31].

The infants themselves may fit three aetiological categories each with a differing prognosis[34]. The first and probably smallest, includes those with the highest risk of handicap because of adverse factors in early gestation. The second may have been adversely affected in later pregnancy and show an increase in mild degrees of mental retardation and minor neurological abnormalities. The later status of the third group, potentially normal at their preterm birth, depends on neonatal care, though we believe that to add care in labour and/or in the birth process is essential.

Controls

This is a question of extraordinary difficulty. Douglas[29] for example, followed a National Cohort of low birth weight infants born in 1946 with controls who were considered well matched at the time for sex, ordinal position in the family, degree of crowding in the home as well as maternal age and social group. They concluded that where intelligence was concerned the lower scores of the low birth weight group compared with the controls were explained by poorer living conditions, less parental interest in educational progress and a lower standard of maternal care. The use of siblings as controls obviates these differences to a large extent, but they cannot be completely eliminated. The variable separation of the preterm infant from his parents after birth, the abnormal background of the neonatal intensive care unit, and his much greater risk of illness both after birth and during the first year or so, tend to set him apart. We have found the difficulties of controls for the most part insuperable, and like many others are usually forced to make comparisons within the study group itself. However as serious neonatal illness occurs more frequently in the least mature, this leads to a comparison of infants of unlike gestational age.

Other factors in design

In the past, follow-up surveys have been of two main types. Firstly they have followed groups of infants chosen by weight or gestation, or because of some specific illness associated with preterm birth such as respiratory distress syndrome, jaundice or recurrent apnoea; or secondly they have sought to assess the results of specific forms of treatment such as some of those outlined in *Table 17.2*. It is unfortunate that the majority in recent years have come from individual referral centres whose clientele at best must be considered unrepresentative of any well-defined community. The numbers they report are often small, making precise correlation with perinatal events difficult or impossible,

Table 17.2 Some possible long-term effects of neonatal treatments

Neonatal treatment	*Harmful effect*	*Possible implications for follow-up*
Oxygen	Hyperoxaemia	Varying degrees of retrolental fibroplasia – late retinal detachments ? Pulmonary damage
Incubator	Noise	? Hearing deficit
Umbilical vessel catheterization	Thrombi, emboli and infection	? Hypertension if renal vessels involved
Alkali	Osmolality changes if rapidly injected	? Increased incidence of GLH/IVH[80]
Intravenous fluids	High intake (and oral) leading to necrotizing enterocolitis[8]	Intestinal stricture formation and obstruction
	Tissue infiltration with skin necrosis	Scarring
Glucose	Hyperglycaemia in very low birth weight[37]	? Central nervous system abnormality
Mechanical ventilation	Bronchopulmonary dysplasia	Increased susceptibility to respiratory infection and obstructive airways disease
with endotracheal tube	Tracheal damage Alveolar ridge damage	Subglottic stenosis Defective primary dentition[75]
with nasotracheal tube	Damage to nostril	Stenosis of anterior nares
with face mask	Cerebellar infarcts[80]	Central nervous system abnormality
CPAP	Pneumothorax	Drainage scars, possible interference with breast development in female
Total parenteral nutrition	Hyperaminoacidaemia	? Central nervous system abnormality
with Intralipid	Obstructive jaundice	? Permanent liver damage
Repeated blood transfusions	Possible cytomegalovirus infection[11]	? Central nervous system damage

GLH = Germinal layer haemorrhage; IVH = Intraventricular haemorrhage; CPAP = Continuous positive airway pressure.

particularly as numbers of untraced survivors may vary from a very small percentage of the total to up to one half of the children under review. True population surveys have been few and far between, and there is an urgent need for studies based on geographically defined areas to determine the real impact of present care of the preterm on their outcome. The issue of whether or not those involved in neonatal care should also be involved in follow-up is a contentious one. Our personal view is that some dual involvement can be of benefit, for a first-hand knowledge of perinatal events often makes the search for physical as well as developmental abnormality more thorough and comprehensive. It must also be acknowledged that the relationship formed between doctors and other workers anxious to keep a cohort together, and the means they adopt to achieve this, may subtly influence results.

Routine care: older survey results

Although we are concerned here with present rather than past outcome, some review of previous work must be given for a true perspective. This will be divided into two time periods, although overlap is inevitable.

1900–1940

Results from the early years of the century, reviewed extensively by Benton[12], are conflicting. Standards of care were very variable, and assessments often based on clinical impressions which did not always take note of social circumstances. The incidence of mental retardation reported varied widely: one paediatrician found only one retarded child among 73 legitimate, premature children of 'high socio-economic status'; in another study 29 per cent of 70 children below 2000 g, of 'poor socio-economic background' (30 per cent of whom were illegitimate) were thought by their parents to be subnormal. The work of many of the authors reviewed by Benton reported a high incidence of 'nervous disorders'. Hess had opened his Premature Infant Station in Chicago in 1922, and despite high neonatal and infant mortality survivors appeared to do remarkably well[54]. A detailed survey of 250 of them born between 1922 and 1933 was carried out, using standardized intelligence tests. The conclusions drawn were that if age was corrected for prematurity, there was no difference in intelligence quotient (IQ) between premature survivors and their sibling controls. However, the few survivors whose birth weight or subsequent weight was below 1000 g had a high risk of handicap (three out of nine); as did infants in whom intracranial haemorrhage had been suspected at birth (29 out of 69). Infants whose birth weight was 1500 g or less remained lighter and shorter than their siblings, whereas larger premature babies caught up fully. Behaviour problems, as well as ear and respiratory infections were increased in the premature infants compared with sibling controls.

Alm[4], one of the few to have recorded the fate of the premature infant in adult life, pursued the fortunes of 999 premature boys born in wedlock in Stockholm between the years 1902–1921 inclusive. He excluded the 'lowest social stratum', and only 25 of the 999 were of very low birthweight. The only significant differences in adult life between them and 1002 male controls of normal birth weight were that they required institutional care more often, and their mean height and weight were lower. As members of the Swedish Armed Forces or in dealings with the Criminal Courts, those born prematurely were no more of a burden on the community than controls. Howard and Worrell[55] have reported on 22 'unselected' infants as children and adults, born between 1930 and 1942, who weighed between 1000 and 1820 g. They were unable to show any relation between intelligence using standardized tests, and birth weight. However, over half were considered to have made unsatisfactory personality adjustments, for which parental over-protectiveness, poor physical endowment and degree of prematurity were held to be the main contributory factors. The economic status of six was given as 'welfare', but the remainder were in gainful employment, including one with an IQ of 56. No correlation of their abilities with social class was made however.

It was towards the end of this period, in 1931, that Hess introduced the use of oxygen and reported a sudden increase in survival, especially amongst infants 1500 g or less. Before long, unlimited oxygen was widely used, but it was a further 20 years before the hazards of this treatment were fully recognised[6].

1941–1960

The period of the late 1930s, 1940s and early 1950s saw the first obvious appearance of iatrogenic disease as many nurseries were set up; oxygen-induced blindness from retrolental fibroplasia was probably the first such condition to occur on any scale (*see Table 17.2*). Although mortality continued to fall steadily, between one and two-thirds of the survivors appeared handicapped (*see Table 17.3*), and in addition to the retinopathy, cerebral palsy, moderate and severe mental retardation and neurosensory deafness were all common, particularly among the very low birth weight babies[25,33,70,73].

Table 17.3 Mortality and handicap from specialist centres in very low birth weight infants born between 1940 and 1960

Reference	*Date of birth*	*Birth weight (g)*	*Neonatal mortality (%)*	*Number of survivors traced (% total)*	*Handicapped* (% traced survivors)*
25	1940–52	≤1000†	No data	94 (84)	60
70	1947–50	≤1500	47	73 (78)	70
33	1948–60	≤1360	No data	99 (95)	53
73	1951–53	≤1360	No data	206 (98)	33
104	1952–56	750–1500	56	65 (93)	46

*Handicap includes cerebral palsy, visual and hearing loss, IQ below 90 and epilepsy
†Birth or subsequent weight

Many of the children had multiple handicaps, and those blind and severely deaf from birth were often of low intelligence; though had they been without such gross sensory deprivation it seems reasonable to assume that many of them might have achieved a more normal IQ score. Several workers showed that intellectual outcome depended not only on birth weight, but was strongly influenced by social class[32, 39, 85, 100], and by the standard of maternal care[32]. The Baltimore study needs further amplification because of its large numbers, which included controls, and its longitudinal nature. Low birth weight infants born there in 1952 and full term controls were followed[51, 66, 98, 99, 100]. Of the originally selected sample of 1170, 992 (85 per cent) comprising 500 prematures and 492 controls, were examined 40 weeks after birth, and then recalled at varying ages through childhood to adolescence. By the time of their final assessment at 12–13 years[98], 848 (85 per cent) of the group of 992 or 72 per cent of the original, could be traced. A significant correlation was found at 8–10 years[100] between birth weight and the Verbal, Performance and Full Scale IQ scores (Wechsler tests) and the Bender Gestalt score, increasing impairment occurring with decreasing birth weight. The authors pointed out that the depressed average performance in the lower weight groups was largely due to an excess of children with greater neurological disability while the majority of low birth weight children had normal intelligence. However, at 12–13 years[98] relative impairment in tests of reading and arithmetic, more pronounced for arithmetic, and independent of race or socio-economic status, was found among the low birth weight. Using covariance and multiple regression analyses birth weight *per se* was shown to be highly significantly correlated with academic achievement, though its effect was small compared with socio-economic factors.

Physically, survivors were often smaller than children born at term, with as many as 48 per cent remaining below the 10th centile for height at age 10 years[70]. The often low calorie intake allowed during the first weeks of life at that time may have some relation to this poor growth, and possibly to some of the handicap[32], though there is no certain proof. It may have placed those well grown *in utero* at the same nutritional disadvantage as those already undernourished at birth[26]. Infants small for gestational age tended to have less retrolental fibroplasia and cerebral palsy, but lower intelligence with an overall rate of handicap similar to those who were appropriately grown at birth[33,73].

Most of these unfavourable results came from specialist centres with mortality rates below national figures. Conversely, the survey which studied all singletons weighing 2000 g or less who were legitimately born in one week in England, Wales and Scotland in 1946[30], a time when special care was not generally available in these countries, showed a high mortality but no handicap at 18 years among 14 survivors of birth weight of 1500 g or less; and the whole group showed no significant excess of severe physical, mental or behavioural handicap compared with controls weighing more than 2500 g at birth, matched as already described[29].

Intensive care: present results

The last two decades have seen a burgeoning of technological skills applied to the preterm newborn. The ability of doctors and, when encouraged, nurses to intubate the larynx and cannulate or puncture the veins and arteries of even the tiniest infants is now taken almost as a matter of course; it has been paralleled by an increase in equipment of all sorts, both simple and sophisticated. These developments have led to increasingly effective treatment of birth asphyxia and later hypoxia, more precise use of oxygen with blood gas monitoring, and the supplementation of 'inadequate' oral feeding by intravenous fluid, or even the total provision of calories for growth by the intravenous route. Mechanical ventilation for severe respiratory distress syndrome and respiratory failure, first applied in the 1950s, with isolated survivors[10], has been used more and more, with refinements in technique leading to improved results[84]. However, controlled trials of newly introduced methods of treatment have been noticeably few. Kitchen *et al.*[62] undertook the basic one of intensive versus routine care in Melbourne, Australia, between 1966 and 1970. Two hundred and thirty eight infants weighing between 1000 and 1500 g at birth were allocated on an alternate basis to one or other types of care. Intensive care, its intensity a pale shadow of that practised today, significantly improved the survival rate of infants with respiratory distress syndrome during the latter part of the study.

Is handicap decreasing, increasing or static?

Some definition is first necessary. Mitchell[74] has defined a handicapped child as one who has a disability of body, intellect or personality proving to be a disadvantage in his environment. Authors use varying definitions in their reports. Stewart and Reynolds[91] described handicap as an abnormality sufficiently severe to interfere with present or future normal function in society. We have included as major handicap cerebral palsy, IQ of less than 70, and visual or hearing defect sufficient to require special schooling[58]. A more detailed breakdown has been given by Kitchen *et al.*[63] who divide handicap into profound, severe, significant and minimal.

The survivors of the Melbourne trial[61] were examined at eight years, and it was apparent that there were significantly more severely/profoundly handicapped children among the intensively treated; the handicaps were more likely to be serious deafness and impaired vision than cerebral palsy. The beginning of the 1970's however, saw a number of publications from centres practising the technological approach to the care of the very low birth weight, all giving enthusiastic reports of falling mortality and/or falling morbidity[3, 22, 28, 45, 69, 83, 91, 92].

Those from University College Hospital, London were foremost in suggesting a striking improvement in outcome[83, 91, 92]. One hundred and ninety seven infants born in, or cared for there, between 1966–1970 inclusive, who weighed between 500 and 1500 g at birth, were shown to have a 28 day survival rate of 55 per cent; a further 11 infants died subsequently between 29 days and 25 months. Of the 98 long-term survivors, 95 were followed up with repeated physical examinations and developmental assessments. Stewart and Reynolds[91] found that 90.5 per cent of the children had no detectable handicap at a mean age of 5 years 2 months (range 2 years 10 months–7 years 10 months). A further report from that hospital[92] gave the results over a 10 year period, 1966–1975, for inborn and outborn infants weighing 1000 g or less at birth. Neonatal and post-neonatal mortality combined was 74 per cent;

major handicap was present in as few as seven per cent of the 27 oldest survivors.

Calame and Prod'hom[22] reported from Lausanne, Switzerland that 75 per cent of their long-term survivors born between 1966 and 1968 weighing 1500 g or less at birth were developing normally between 15 months and 4.5 years; in a further 14 per cent development was doubtful but in only 10.5 per cent was it frankly abnormal. Among 165 survivors of the same birth weight cared for at Hammersmith Hospital, London between 1961 and 1970, Davies and Tizard[28] found no cases of cerebral palsy in the last six years of the study among 107 children, compared with seven of 58 (12 per cent) in the first four years. Six of these children had spastic diplegia. The mean full scale IQ measured in 105 of 120 of the same consecutive long-term survivors born between 1961 and 1968 was 97.0 using the Wechsler tests; the 15 children who were not tested mainly for geographical reasons were not thought to differ from the whole sample[46]. Small for gestational age children had a significantly lower mean IQ (92.0) than children who had been appropriately grown at birth in whom the IQ was 99.0. Social class seemed the most important determinant of IQ, and there was no direct correlation with birth weight.

These and other results all seemed to suggest a greatly decreased incidence of handicap among survivors at a time of decreasing mortality, especially when compared with those in the larger studies carried out among infants born between 1940 and 1960, reported in *Table 17.3*. This gave grounds for increasing optimism. Retrolental fibroplasia in particular, though not completely abolished, was extremely rarely seen as a cause of total blindness and the incidence of deafness in recent surveys seemed lower[27], perhaps because of more carefully controlled dosage of ototoxic drugs. These two factors inevitably led to a reduction in the numbers of severely handicapped children.

Caution should be exercised before these reports are taken at face value and it is assumed that there has been a continuing and marked reduction in handicap. The ever-decreasing mortality rates, in very low birth weight infants particularly, introduce an artefact when the handicapped are calculated as a proportion of survivors. This is illustrated by the two hypothetical samples shown in *Figure 17.1* in which major and minor handicap in sample A occurs in 50 per cent of survivors, (the situation perhaps for the very low birthweight in the 1940s) and in sample B in 17 per cent (the situation at present?). Ten per cent of the whole group are handicapped in both samples, so that the

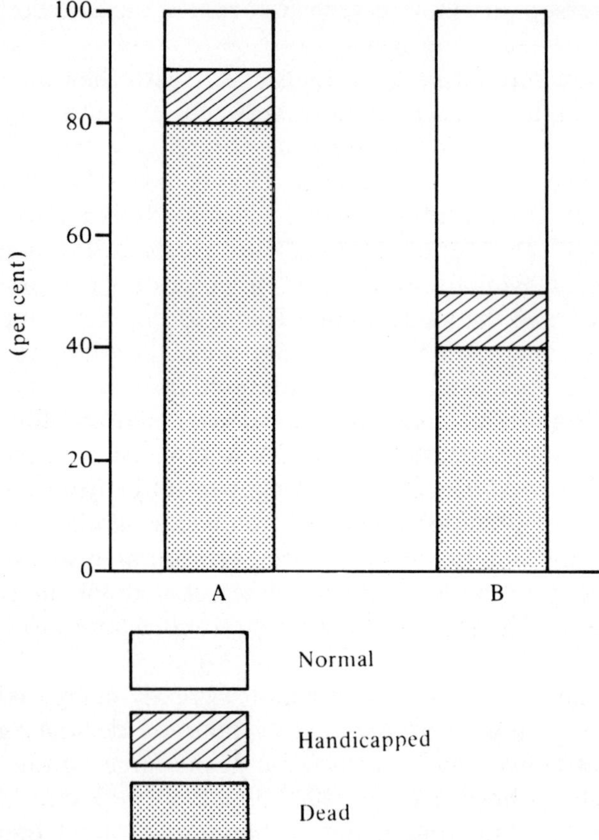

Figure 17.1 Handicap in samples of differing mortality. A = Handicap in 50 per cent of survivors (10 per cent of total sample). B = Handicap in 17 per cent of survivors (10 per cent of total sample)

burden to the community, and to individual families, is unchanged. Jones, Cummins and Davies[58] could show no decrease in major handicap calculated as a percentage of total births from an intensive care unit over a 15 year period, during which time care had become increasingly complex. The figures and those from University College Hospital, calculated in this way are shown in *Table 17.4*. Assuming Drillien's hypothesis regarding the aetiology of handicap to be correct, results could be significantly influenced by subtle variations in social

Table 17.4 Major handicap expressed as percentage of total births 501–1500 g

	1961–65	*1966–70*	*1971–75*
Hammersmith Hospital	5.6	3.9	6.7
University College Hospital*		4.0	4.8

*500–1500 g (Figures by courtesy of Prof. E.O.R. Reynolds and Dr A. L. Stewart)

class affecting fetal growth rates. She too has noted a disappointing lack of improvement in major impairment in Edinburgh infants born between 1953 and 1955, and those born between 1966 and 1970, once the earlier born who had suffered the 'iatrogenic disaster of imposed starvation' were omitted[35]. Survivors born in the latter period with birth weights of 2000 g or less have been followed to school age and 31 of 299 (10 per cent) have moderate or severe handicap. In only seven of these children could the handicap be attributed to perinatal complications; in 17 it was either familial or associated with congenital abnormalities, and six were healthy small for gestational age infants.

Thus although there is national[82] and regional data[89, 95] to confirm that intensive care saves lives, the evidence that it improves the quality of survival is more difficult to come by. Some causes of handicap such as hypoglycaemia, hyperbilirubinaemia and hyperoxaemia are now largely preventable. However, damaged children, from whatever cause, who would previously have died may now live, so that the nature of handicap changes. Some have claimed that conservative management applied with equal supervision and enthusiasm produces equally low mortality and morbidity as does intensive care[56, 90]. Steiner *et al.*[90] have recently reported the long term outcome in 236 infants of very low birth weight born in King's Mill Hospital, Mansfield, between 1963 and 1971 inclusive. Throughout this period the standard of nursing and medical supervision was good and uniform. However, energetic resuscitative measures, and X-ray and laboratory facilities were not used to any extent and 'active medical intervention', much of which is described in *Table 17.2*, was deliberately eschewed. Careful follow-up with intelligence testing showed that the incidence of major handicap was no greater among inborn infants than that reported from two units practising highly technological care[58, 91, 93].

The lack of population surveys which would allow a more objective measure of handicap than that obtainable from individual small units is regrettable, though optimism is expressed by the Swedish cerebral palsy study[49, 50]. This showed a continuing decline in the total incidence of all forms of cerebral palsy between 1954 and 1970 within one geographically defined area. The reduction of nearly 50 per cent was largely due to a significant drop in the number of cases of spastic/ataxic diplegia among low birth weight children. However a further report from 1971 to 1974 showed a slight increase in cases of mild diplegia mostly among infants of normal intelligence and weighing between 1000 and 1500 g at birth[48]. A survey from Western Australia[24] suggested that low birth weight and small for gestational age infants with neonatal illness treated in neonatal intensive care units had added significantly to the number of cerebral palsy cases between 1968 and 1975.

Factors associated with handicap

General aspects

Many past and present surveys have tried to define the perinatal factors which are most likely to be associated with handicap among low birth weight infants. Apart from knowing of the harmful effects associated with hyperbilirubinaemia, hypoglycaemia, excessive oxygen and possibly extremes of starvation, it occasionally appears we are little further forward than 30 years ago. However Stewart *et al.*[93] studied very low birthweight infants and tried to identify factors affecting their long-term prognosis. Significant correlations were found between developmental quotient and both later IQ and handicapping abnormality. A multiple regression analysis using developmental quotient as the dependent variable found illness associated with convulsions and low arterial pH within two hours of birth to be the most significant contributions. Among children who had weighed 2000 g or less at birth, Drillien, Thomson and Burgoyne[35] found that problems at school were related to social class, evidence of intrauterine insult, male sex, postnatal complications and neurological and developmental status during the first year of life. Kitchen *et al.*[63] reported that unsatisfactory outcome, defined as profound, serious or significant handicap, among very low birth weight children was significantly correlated with a gestational age of less than 30 weeks, birth weight of less than 1200 g, severe apnoeic episodes, a lowest postnatal weight at 6 or more days of age, birth weight regained later than 21 days, a peak serum bilirubin of more than 255 μmol/l (15 mg/100 ml) and low socio-economic status.

It is presumably the integrity of the cerebral circulation that is so vital for intact neurological survival yet the measurement of intracranial pressure and cerebral blood flow in the newborn is still in its infancy. Until we know much more about the factors compromising it, there will be difficulty in defining the gestational age below which a normal brain cannot be supported outside the uterus[80]. Since 1975 increasing numbers of infants below 1000 g have been surviving, some of whom have required intensive care, in particular mechanical ventilation, for weeks rather than days after birth. Respiratory aspects of such cases are discussed below, but our own unpublished data and the preliminary observations of others[9, 36, 38, 77, 86] lead us to believe that neurological outcome can be disappointing. It will be another few years before full details of these children will be available. Very low birth weight infants transferred long distances after birth, and who arrive at referral units both hypothermic and acidotic are known to have a high mortality, as well as high incidence of major handicap among survivors[44]. This can be reduced by anticipation of premature delivery, and the transfer of the mother to an intensive care unit with the baby still *in utero*.

Specific aspects

Intraventricular haemorrhage. New radiological techniques such as computerized axial tomography (CAT scan), and more recently ultrasonography, allow a more confident diagnosis of certain intracranial abnormalities. Intraventricular haemorrhage of varying degrees has been shown by CAT scan to be present in 44 per cent of 100 consecutively delivered very low birth weight infants[21]. A preliminary report on the 65 survivors[81] suggested that at one year infants who had subependymal haemorrhage, listed as Grade I, and blood rupturing into the lateral ventricles without distension, listed as Grade II, during the neonatal period had no major developmental handicap; whereas those with blood distending the lateral ventricles, listed as Grade III, or additional rupture into cerebral substance, listed as Grade IV, were likely to have major neuromotor and developmental handicap. Krishnamoorthy *et al.*[67] reported the same findings in a series of 15 infants surviving intraventricular haemorrhage similarly diagnosed during the early neonatal period. Recurrent apnoea may be among the presenting features of intraventricular haemorrhage, and reports of neurological outcome in infants mechanically ventilated for recurrent apnoea are often less favourable than for those ventilated for respiratory distress syndrome[16, 44], though this is not invariably so[71].

Differences in the population and gestational age of the babies may account for discrepancies between the samples. Also, ventilation for apnoea was often carried out by face mask held in place by an inch-thick rubber band round the occiput – the latter causing localised skull distortions – which is now known to be associated with cerebellar infarcts[79,80], and a high risk of handicap in surviving infants. When face masks are held in place by elastic netting covering the entire head, skull distortion is less. No major deleterious effect of this practice was found by Tuck and Ment[96] who compared treated infants with controls of like birthweight and gestational age. However, some treated infants who died were found to have similar though less marked cerebellar pathology to that found by the Toronto group[79].

Presumed hyaline membrane disease and other respiratory disorders
Most previous follow-up studies of infants who had respiratory distress syndrome have suggested that major neurological handicap is no more frequent than in those of similar gestation who did not have it[5,41,52,57,59,84,88]. Handicap has been variably recorded in 6–20 per cent of survivors, with motor development being disproportionately delayed in the early years. Residual lung damage – termed bronchopulmonary dysplasia[78] still lacks precise definition, having a variable incidence and somewhat controversial aetiology[103]. It can cause considerable morbidity during the first year of life when respiratory infections are common and is accompanied by abnormal lung function[20,94]. Both these groups of workers showed greater damage to infants who survived mechanical ventilation than in the unventilated survivors of respiratory distress, though presumably the latter infants had less severe disease. The ill-effects of ventilation used for other neonatal disorders, such as apnoea, aspiration syndromes and persistent hypersecretion are similar[102]. Persistent airway obstruction has been demonstrated in these other groups through the latter half of the first year of life and may rarely require tracheostomy. At particular risk of respiratory handicap are these recent very immature survivors who have been ventilated for several weeks. A reduction in dynamic compliance, that is, stiff lungs, commonly found as an aftermath of neonatal mechanical ventilation, has been particularly severe following interstitial emphysema. The long-term significance of these findings to individual children is of course not yet known. It has however also been shown[23] that expiratory flow rates are low in preterm children who have had *no* neonatal lung disease, and the suggestion made that this finding

could be secondary to pulmonary growth retardation. Diffuse radiographic changes are also occasionally seen in the lungs of very immature infants who have had neither presumed hyaline membrane disease nor ventilator treatment. Susceptibility to respiratory infections in the first year or two of life was a feature of low birth weight infants long before mechanical ventilation was a contributory factor; overcrowding and poor home conditions may be at least in part responsible.

One potentially harmful aspect of repeated upper respiratory tract infections is that of otitis media. Abramovich *et al.*[1] recently reported on the hearing of 111 infants of less than 1500 g born in or cared for at University College Hospital between 1966–1972. Ten children (nine per cent) had sensorineural loss, one (one per cent) had a congenital conductive loss, but 21 (19 per cent) had exudative otitis media with a mean loss of 25 dB.

Intrauterine growth retardation. Some authors[16, 63, 97] have recorded little difference in outcome between small for gestational age and other very low birth weight children; and intrauterine growth was not closely related to school problems in Drillien's Edinburgh cohort of children weighing less than 2000 g at birth[35]. However this is not a universal finding[43, 46, 87]. A population survey was made on a random sample of Newcastle children born between 1960 and 1962[76]. This study observed that children whose birth weight had fallen below the 10th centile (mean birth weight 2537 g), performed significantly worse than preterm children (mean birth weight 2415 g), who in turn performed less well than appropriately grown full term infants (mean birth weight 3508 g), over a wide range of psychometric, neurological and behavioural tests at age five to seven years. The differences shown persisted even when correction had been made for a variety of social factors, and suggested that the deleterious effects of intrauterine growth retardation were more marked than those of preterm birth. These authors also emphasised the particular vulnerability of a subgroup of very light for dates infants to the effects of adverse social factors. The timing of the start of intrauterine growth constraint and its duration – now known more accurately through ultrasonic cephalometry during pregnancy – may well be important to the outcome[40, 53], and may account for the variability of results. Head circumference less than the 10th centile at birth, together with an abnormal neurological examination in the neonatal period, were important predictors of a later poor outcome in 118 infants weighing between 750 and 2000 g at birth[47].

Physical growth. Unless their immediate postnatal growth is severely curtailed by illness in the first weeks of life most infants appropriately grown at birth now reach normal size in later childhood[14,17,26,60]. Although some have also reported normal growth and head circumference centiles for small for gestational age, very low birth weight infants[60] this has not always been the experience of others[14,17,26,27,42]. However these children are a heterogeneous population, their immediate postnatal growth is also important with regard to final size, and longitudinal assessments on very large samples will be needed before some of these differences can be settled. Certainly as Kitchen, McDougall and Naylor[60] have emphasised, longitudinal assessments at given ages are an important counsel of perfection where study of growth of the preterm is concerned.

Psychological aspects of preterm birth. Much recent interest has centred on the damaging effects of early separation on the mother–child relationship[18,64]. Child abuse is more common amongst low birth weight infants, particularly if parental visiting in the neonatal unit is delayed or infrequent[65]. The increase in behaviour problems noted[15,32,76] may be in part related to disturbance in family relationships. Rigid visiting policies and transfer of babies without their mothers from distant hospitals increase the amount of separation. A greater awareness of this problem should lead in future to more liberal visiting policies with positive efforts being made to involve parents directly from an early stage in the care and progress of their preterm infant. So called intervention programmes both in the nursery and after discharge, which have stimulation of the infant and maximum interaction between him and his parents as their aim, are at present being assessed in some centres[19,68,72].

Conclusions

Previous follow-up surveys of low birth weight children which used full term controls of like social class, all born before the advent of neonatal intensive care, showed that – spared certain well defined handicaps – they were often indistinguishable from their full term peers except for a tendency to be shorter and lighter. The handicaps of cerebral palsy, most frequently spastic diplegia, low intelligence, learning and behavioural difficulties, as well as visual and hearing impairment, were certainly more common than in the controls, and tended to occur most frequently at the lowest gestations and birth weights, which had a high mortality.

The present situation is that intensive care has reduced mortality, and larger numbers of very low birth weight children in particular now survive. Most of the recently published follow-up studies which concern them usually dispense with controls, and have relatively small numbers. They also come from individual units practising intensive care, and population surveys, which are greatly needed, have been few and far between. The results suggest that the great majority of the new survivors will go to normal school where they will not stand out conspicuously from their contemporaries of a similar socio-economic background unless very searching and detailed tests of intelligence are made. Although the evidence is difficult to extract from the previously published reports, there is a suggestion that the numbers of handicapped children, expressed as a proportion of total very low weight births, may not have changed greatly. On the other hand the nature of their handicap may have changed, with retrolental fibroplasia diminishing since the 1950s, and complex forms of cerebral palsy becoming more common. The long term safety of many of the new methods of treatment has yet to be established. The survival of larger numbers of extremely immature infants (below 28 weeks gestation) who have been mechanically ventilated sometimes for several weeks after birth is very recent. This means that details about them must be far from complete. Preliminary observations suggest however that the neurological, intellectual and respiratory function as well as physical growth of those that were smallest and sickest at birth may be compromised, sometimes seriously.

Further refinements in and widespread application of neonatal intensive care are probably unlikely to reduce the level of handicap and may even increase it. Thus prevention of preterm birth and of fetal growth retardation have greater potential. However this may require profound social rather than obstetric changes.

References

1 ABRAMOVICH, S. J., GREGORY, S., SLEMICK, M. and STEWART, A. Hearing loss in very low birthweight infants treated with neonatal intensive care. *Archives of Disease in Childhood*, **54,** 421–426 (1979)

2 ALBERMAN, E. Stillbirths and neonatal mortality in England and Wales by birthweight, 1953–71. *Health Trends*, **6,** 14–17 (1974)

3 ALDEN, E. R., MANDELKORN, T., WOODRUM, D. E., WENNBERG, R. P., PARKS, C. R. and HODSON, A. Morbidity and mortality of infants weighing less than 1000 grams in an intensive care nursery. *Pediatrics*, **50,** 40–49 (1972)

4 ALM, I. The long-term prognosis for prematurely born children: a follow-up study of 999 premature boys born in wedlock and of 1002 controls. *Acta Paediatrica Scandinavica*, **42,** supplement 94, 9–116 (1953)

5 AMBRUS, C. M., WEINTRAUB, D. M., NISWANDER, K. R., FISCHER, L., FLEISHMAN, J., BROSS, I. D. J. and AMBRUS, J. L. Evaluation of survivors of respiratory distress syndrome at 4 years of age. *American Journal of Diseases of Children*, **120,** 296–302 (1970)

6 ASHTON, N., WARD, B. and SERPELL, G. Role of oxygen in the genesis of retrolental fibroplasia; a preliminary report. *British Journal of Ophthalmology*, **37,** 513–520 (1953)

7 BAIRD, D. The epidemiology of prematurity. *Journal of Pediatrics*, **65,** 909–924 (1964)

8 BELL, E. F., WARBURTON, D., STONESTREET, B. S. and OH, W. Effect of fluid administration on the development of symptomatic patent ductus arteriosus and congestive heart failure in premature infants. *New England Journal of Medicine*, **302,** 598–604 (1980)

9 BENNETT-BRITTON, S., FITZHARDINGE, P. M. Is intensive care justified for infants weighing less than 801 g at birth? *Pediatric Research*, **14,** 590, (1980) (Abstract)

10 BENSON, F., CELANDER, O., HAGLUND, G., NILSSON, L., PAULSEN, L. and RENCK, L. Positive-pressure respiratory treatment of severe pulmonary insufficiency in the newborn infant. A clinical report. *Acta Anaesthesiologica Scandinavica*, **2,** 37–43 (1958)

11 BENSON, J. W. T., BODDEN, S. J. and TOBIN, J. O'H. Cytomegalovirus and blood transfusion in neonates. *Archives of Disease in Childhood*, **54,** 538–541 (1979)

12 BENTON, A. Mental development of prematurely born children. *American Journal of Orthopsychiatry*, **10,** 719–746 (1940)

13 BIRCH, H. G. and GUSSOW, J. D. *Disadvantaged Children, Health, Nutrition and School Failure*. 46–80. New York, Grune and Stratton (1970)

14 BJERRE, I. Physical growth of 5-year-old children with a low birth weight. Stature, weight, circumference of head and osseous development. *Acta Paediatrica Scandinavica*, **64,** 33–43 (1975)

15 BJERRE, I. and HANSEN, E. Psychomotor development and school-adjustment of 7-year-old children with low birthweight. *Acta Paediatrica Scandinavica*, **65,** 88–96 (1976)

16 BLAKE, A., STEWART, A. L. and TURCAN, D. M. Perinatal intensive care. *Journal of Psychosomatic Research*, **21,** 261–272 (1977)

17 BRANDT, I. Growth dynamics of low birth weight infants with emphasis on the perinatal period. In *Human Growth*, Vol. 2, edited by F. Falkner, J. M. Tanner, 557–617. London, Baillière Tindall (1978)

18 BRIMBLECOMBE, F. S. W., RICHARDS, M. P. M. and ROBERTON, N. R. C. Separation and special-care baby units. *Clinics in Developmental Medicine*, No. **68,** London, Heinemann (1978)

19 BROMWICH, R. M. and PARMELEE, A. H. An intervention program for pre-term infants. In *Infants Born at Risk*, edited by T. M. Field, 389–411. New York, S P Medical and Scientific Books (1979)

20 BRYAN, M. H., HARDIE, M. J., REILLY, B. J. and SWYER, P. R. Pulmonary function studies during the first year of life in infants recovering from the respiratory distress syndrome. *Pediatrics*, **52,** 169–178 (1973)

21 BURSTEIN, J., PAPILE, L.-A., and BURSTEIN, R. Intraventricular hemorrhage and hydrocephalus in premature newborns: a prospective study with CT. *American Journal of Research*, **132,** 631–635 (1979)

22 CALAME, A. and PROD'HOM, L. S. Pronostic vital et qualité de survie des prématures pesant 1500 g et moins á la naissance, soignés en 1966–1968. *Schweizerische Medizinische Wochenschrift*, **102,** 65–70 (1972)

23 COATES, A. L., BERGSTEINSSON, H., DESMOND, K., OUTERBRIDGE, E. W. and BEAUDRY, P. H. Long-term pulmonary sequelae of premature birth with and without idiopathic respiratory distress syndrome. *Journal of Pediatrics*, **90,** 611–616 (1977)

24 DALE, A. and STANLEY, F. J. An epidemiological study of cerebral palsy in Western Australia, 1956–1975. II: Spastic cerebral palsy and perinatal factors. *Developmental Medicine and Child Neurology*, **22,** 13–25 (1980)

25 DANN, M. LEVINE, S. Z. and NEW, E. V. The development of prematurely born children with birth weights or minimal postnatal weights of 1,000 grams or less. *Pediatrics*, **22,** 1037–1053 (1958)

26 DAVIES, P. A. Perinatal nuitrition of infants of very low birthweight and their later progress. *Modern Problems in Paediatrics*, edited by F. Falkner, N. Kretchmer, E. Rossi, **14,** 119–133. Basle, Karger (1975)

27 DAVIES, P. A. and STEWART, A. L. Low-birth-weight infants: neurological sequelae and later intelligence. *British Medical Bulletin*, **31,** 85–91 (1975)

28 DAVIES, P. A. and TIZARD, J. P. M. Very low birthweight and subsequent neurological defect (with special reference to spastic diplegia), *Developmental Medicine and Child Neurology*, **17,** 3–17 (1975)

29 DOUGLAS, J. W. B. 'Premature' children at primary schools. *British Medical Journal*, **1,** 1008–1013 (1960)

30 DOUGLAS, J. W. B. and GEAR, R. Children of low birthweight in the 1946 national cohort: behaviour and educational achievement in adolescence. *Archives of Disease in Childhood*, **51,** 820–827 (1976)

31 DRILLIEN, C. M. The social and economic factors affecting the incidence of premature birth. Part 1. *Journal of Obstetrics and Gynaecology of the British Empire*, **64,** 161–184 (1957)

32 DRILLIEN, C. M. *The growth and development of the prematurely born infant*. Edinburgh, Livingstone (1964)

33 DRILLIEN, C. M. The incidence of mental and physical handicaps in school age children of very low birth weight. II. *Pediatrics*, **39,** 238–247 (1967)

34 DRILLIEN, C. M. Aetiology and outcome in low-birthweight infants. *Developmental Medicine and Child Neurology*, **14,** 563–574 (1972)

35 DRILLIEN, C. M., THOMSON, A. J. M. and BURGOYNE, K. Low-birthweight children at early school-age: a longitudinal study. *Developmental Medicine and Child Neurology*, **22,** 26–47 (1980)

36 DRISCOLL, J. M. JR., DRISCOLL, Y. T., STARK, R. I., DANGMAN, B. C. and KRITZ, P. Mortality and morbidity in infants less than 1000 g birth weight. *Pediatric Research*, **14,** 596 (1980) (Abstract)

37 DWECK, H. S. and CASSADY, G. Glucose intolerance in infants of very low birth weight. I *Pediatrics*, **53,** 189–195 (1974)

38 EGAN, E. A., BUCKWALD, S., TOPPER, W. H., ZORN, W. A. and JOHNSON, C. B. Extreme prematurity (600–799 g): survival and early follow-up. *Pediatric Research*, **14,** 433 (1980) (Abstract)

39 ETO, K. Studies on the physical and mental development of prematurely born children from the viewpoint of social medicine. *Psychiatria et Neurologia Japonica*, **68,** 609–628 (1966)

40 FANCOURT, R., CAMPBELL, S., HARVEY, D. and NORMAN, A. P. Follow-up study of small-for-dates babies. *British Medical Journal*, **1,** 1435–1437 (1976)

41 FIELD, T. M., DEMPSEY, J. R. and SHUMAN, H. H. Developmental assessments of infants surviving the respiratory distress syndrome.

In *Infants Born at Risk*, edited by T. M. Field, 261–280. New York, S P Medical and Scientific Books (1979)

42 FITZHARDINGE, P. M. Follow-up studies on the low birth weight infant. *Clinics in Perinatology*, **3,** 503–516 (1976)

43 FITZHARDINGE, P. M., KALMAN, E., ASHBY, S. and PAPE, K. E. Present status of the infant of very low birth weight treated in a referral neonatal intensive care unit in 1974. In *Major Mental Handicap: Methods and Costs of Prevention*, edited by K. Elliott, M. O'Conner, Ciba Foundation Symposium No. **59,** 139–144. Amsterdam, Elsevier (1978)

44 FITZHARDINGE, P. M., PAPE, K. ARSTIKAITIS, M., BOYLE, M., ASHBY, S., ROWLEY, A., NETLEY, C., and SWYER, P. R. Mechanical ventilation of infants of less than 1,501 gm birth weight: health, growth and neurologic sequelae. *Journal of Pediatrics*, **88,** 531–541 (1976)

45 FITZHARDINGE, P. M. and RAMSAY, M. The improving outlook for the small prematurely born infant. *Developmental Medicine and Child Neurology*, **15,** 447–459 (1973)

46 FRANCIS-WILLIAMS, J. and DAVIES, P. A. Very low birthweight and later intelligence. *Developmental Medicine and Child Neurology*, **16,** 709–728 (1974)

47 GROSS, S. J., KOSMETATOS, N., GRIMES, C. T. and WILLIAMS, M. L. Newborn head size and neurological status. Predictors of growth and development of low birth weight infants. *American Journal of Diseases of Children*, **132,** 753–756 (1978)

48 HAGBERG, B. Epidemiological and preventive aspects of cerebral palsy and severe mental retardation in Sweden. *European Journal of Pediatrics*, **130,** 71–78 (1979)

49 HAGBERG, B., HAGBERG, G. and OLOW, I. The changing panorama of cerebral palsy in Sweden, 1954–1970. I. Analysis of the general changes. *Acta Paediatrica Scandinavica*, **64,** 187–192 (1975)

50 HAGBERG, B., HAGBERG, G. and OLOW, I. The changing panorama of cerebral palsy in Sweden, 1954–1970. II. Analysis of the various syndromes. *Acta Paediatrica Scandinavica*, **64,** 193–200 (1975)

51 HARPER, P. A., FISCHER, L. K., RIDER, R. V. Neurological and intellectual status of prematures at three to five years of age. *Journal of Pediatrics*, **55,** 679–690 (1959)

52 HARROD, J. R., L'HEUREUX, P., WANGENSTEEN, O. D., and HUNT, C. E. Long-term follow-up of severe respiratory distress syndrome treated with IPPB. *Journal of Pediatrics*, **84,** 277–286 (1977)

53 HARVEY, D. R., PRINCE, J., BUNTON, W. J. and CAMPBELL, S. Abilities of children who were small for dates at birth and whose growth in utero

was measured by ultrasonic cephalometry. *Pediatric Research*, **10,** 891 (1976) (Abstract)

54 HESS, J. H., MOHR, G. J. and BARTELME, P. F. *The Physical and Mental Health of Prematurely Born Children*. Illinois, University of Chicago (1934)

55 HOWARD, P. J. and WORRELL, C. H. Premature infants in later life. Study of intelligence and personality of 22 premature infants at ages 8 to 19 years. *Pediatrics*, **9,** 577–584 (1952)

56 HUGHES-DAVIES, T. H. Conservative care of the newborn baby. *Archives of Disease in Childhood*, **54,** 59–61 (1979)

57 JOHNSON, J. D., MALACHOWSKI, N. C., GROBSTEIN, R., WELSH, D., DAILY, W. J. R. and SUNSHINE, P. Prognosis of children surviving with the aid of mechanical ventilation in the newborn period. *Journal of Pediatrics*, **84,** 272–276 (1974)

58 JONES, R. A. K., CUMMINS, M. and DAVIES, P. A. Infants of very low birthweight: a 15-year analysis. *Lancet*, **1,** 1332–1335 (1979)

59 KAMPER, J. Long term prognosis of infants with severe idiopathic respiratory distress syndrome: II. Cardio-pulmonary outcome. *Acta Paediatrica Scandinavica,* **67,** 71–76 (1978)

60 KITCHEN, W. H., McDOUGALL, A. B., and NAYLOR, F. D. A longitudinal study of very low-birthweight infants. III: Distance growth at eight years of age. *Developmental Medicine and Child Neurology*, **22,** 163–171 (1980)

61 KITCHEN, W. H., RICKARDS, A., RYAN, M. M., McDOUGALL, A. B., BILLSON, F. A., KEIR, E. H., and NAYLOR, F. D. A longitudinal study of very low-birthweight infants. II: results of controlled trial of intensive care and incidence fof handicaps. *Developmental Medicine and Child Neurology*, **21,** 582–589 (1979)

62 KITCHEN, W. H., RYAN, M. M., RICKARDS, A., GAUDRY, E., BRENTON, A. M., BILLSON, F. A., FORTUNE, D. W., KEIR, E. H. and LUNDAHL-HEGEDUS, E. E. A longitudinal study of very low-birthweight infants. I: study design and mortality rates. *Developmental Medicine and Child Neurology*, **20,** 605–618 (1978)

63 KITCHEN, W. H., RYAN, M. M., RICKARDS, A., McDOUGALL, A. B., BILLSON, F. A., KEIR, E. H. and NAYLOR, F. D. A longitudinal study of very low birthweight infants. IV: an overview of performance at eight years of age. *Developmental Medicine and Child Neurology*, **22,** 172–188 (1980)

64 KLAUS, M. and KENNELL, J. H. *Maternal-Infant Bonding*. St. Louis, Mosby (1976)

65 KLEIN, M. and STERN, L. Low birthweight and the battered child syndrome. *American Journal of Diseases of Children*, **122,** 15–18 (1971)

66 KNOBLOCH, H., RIDER, R., HARPER, P. and PASAMANICK, B. Neuropsychiatric sequelae of prematurity. A longitudinal study. *Journal of the American Medical Association*, **161,** 581–585 (1956)

67 KRISHNAMOORTHY, K. S., SHANNON, D. C., DeLONG, G. R., TODRES, I. D. and DAVIS, K. R. Neurologic sequelae in the survivors of neonatal intraventricular hemorrhage. *Pediatrics*, **64,** 233–237 (1979)

68 LIPSITT, L. P. Learning assessments and interventions for the infant born at risk. In *Infants Born at Risk*, edited by T. M. Field, 145–169, New York, S P Medical and Scientific Books (1979)

69 LUBCHENCO, L. O., BARD, H., GOLDMAN, A. L., COYER, W. E., McINTYRE, C. and SMITH, D. M. Newborn intensive care and long-term prognosis. *Developmental Medicine and Child Neurology*, **16,** 421–431 (1974)

70 LUBCHENCO, L. O., HORNER, F. A., REED, L. H., HIX, I. E., METCALF, D., COHIG, R., ELLIOTT, H. C. and BOURG, M. Sequelae of premature birth. Evaluation of premature infants of low birth weights at ten years of age. *American Journal of Diseases of Childhood*, **106,** 101–115 (1963)

71 MARRIAGE, K. J. and DAVIES, P. A. Neurological sequelae in children surviving mechanical ventilation in the neonatal period. *Archives of Disease in Childhood*, **52,** 176–182 (1977)

72 MASI, W. Supplemental stimulation of the premature infant. In *Infants Born at Risk*, edited by T. M. Field, 367–387. New York, S P Medical and Scientific Books (1979)

73 McDONALD, A. D. *Children of Very Low Birth Weight*. London, Heinemann (1967)

74 MITCHELL, R. G. The nature and causes of disability in childhood. In *Neurodevelopmental Problems in Early Childhood. Assessment and Management*, edited by C. M. Drillien, M. B. Drummond, 1. Oxford, Blackwell (1977)

75 MOYLAN, F. M. B., SELDIN, E. B., SHANNON, D. C. and TODRES, I. D. Defective primary dentition in survivors of neonatal mechanical ventilation. *Journal of Pediatrics*, **96,** 106–108 (1980)

76 NELIGAN, G. A., KOLVIN, I., SCOTT, D. M. and GARSIDE, R. F. Born too soon or born too small. *Clinics in Developmental Medicine* No. **61,** London, Heinemann (1976)

77 NELSON, R., RESNICK, M., NELSON, L., ROSSLEY, K., DICKMAN, H. and EITZMAN, D. Differential outcomes: Mortality and morbidity for extremely premature infants. *Pediatric Research*, **14,** 437 (1980) (Abstract)

78 NORTHWAY, W. H., JR. ROSAN, R. C. and PORTER, D. Y. Pulmonary disease following respirator therapy of hyaline-membrane disease: broncho-

pulmonary dysplasia. *New England Journal of Medicine*, **276,** 357–368 (1967)

79 PAPE, K. E., ARMSTRONG, D. L. and FITZHARDINGE, P. M. Central nervous system pathology associated with mask ventilation in the very low birthweight infant: a new etiology for intracerebellar hemorrhages. *Pediatrics*, **58,** 473–483 (1976)

80 PAPE, K. E. and WIGGLESWORTH, J. S. Haemorrhage, ischaemia and the perinatal brain. *Clinics in Developmental Medicine* No. **69/70,** London, Spastics International Medical Publications (1979)

81 PAPILE, L. A., MUNSICK, G., WEAVER, N. and PECHA, S. Cerebral intraventricular hemorrhage (CVH) in infants < 1500 grams: developmental follow-up at one year. *Pediatric Research*, **13,** 528 (1979) (Abstract)

82 PHAROAH, P. O. D. and ALBERMAN, E. D. Mortality of low birthweight infants in England and Wales, 1953–1977. *Archives of Disease in Childhood* (1980) (in press)

83 RAWLINGS, G., REYNOLDS, E. O. R., STEWART, A. and STRANG, L. B. Changing prognosis for infants of very low birth weight. *Lancet,* **1,** 516–519 (1971)

84 REYNOLDS, E. O. R. and TAGHIZADEH, A. Improved prognosis of infants mechanically ventilated for hyaline membrane disease. *Archives of Disease in Childhood*, **49,** 505–515 (1974)

85 ROBINSON, N. M. and ROBINSON, H. B. A follow-up study of children of low birth weight and control children at school age. *Pediatrics*, **35,** 425–433 (1965)

86 ROTHBERG, A. D., MAISELS, M. J., and BAGNATO, S. Outcome for infants weighing 1250 grams or less at birth. *Pediatric Research*, **14,** 636 (1980) (Abstract)

87 SABEL, K-G, OLEGÅRD, R. and VICTORIN, L., Remaining sequelae with modern perinatal care. *Pediatrics*, **57,** 652–658 (1976)

88 STAHLMAN, M. L., HEDVALE, G., DOLANSKI, I., FAXELIUS, G., BURKO, H. and KIRK, V. A six-year follow-up of clinical hyaline membrane disease. *Pediatric Clinics of North America*, **20,** 433–446 (1973)

89 STANLEY, F. J. and ALBERMAN, E. D. Infants of very low birthweight. I: Perinatal factors affecting survival. *Developmental Medicine and Child Neurology*, **20,** 300–312 (1978)

90 STEINER, E., SANDERS, E. M., PHILLIPS, E. C. K. and MADDOCK, C. R. Very low birth weight children at school age: comparison of neonatal management methods. *British Medical Journal*, **281,** 1237–1240 (1980)

91 STEWART, A. L. and REYNOLDS, E. O. R. Improved prognosis for infants of very low birthweight. *Pediatrics*, **54,** 724–735 (1974)

92 STEWART, A. L., TURCAN, D. M., RAWLINGS, G. and REYNOLDS, E. O. R. Prognosis for infants weighing 1000 g or less at birth. *Archives of Disease in Childhood*, **52,** 97–104 (1977)

93 STEWART, A., TURCAN, D., RAWLINGS, G., HART, S. and GREGORY, S. Outcome for infants at high risk of major handicap. In *Major Mental Handicap: Methods and Costs of Prevention*, edited by K. Elliott, M. O'Connor. Ciba Foundation Symposium No. **59,** 151–164. Amsterdam, Elsevier (1978)

94 STOCKS, J., GODFREY, S. and REYNOLDS, E. O. R. Airway resistance in infants after various treatments for hyaline membrane disease: special emphasis on prolonged high levels of inspired oxygen. *Pediatrics*, **61,** 178–183 (1978)

95 THOMPSON, T. and REYNOLDS, J. The results of intensive care therapy for neonates. I. Overall neonatal mortality rates. II. Neonatal mortality rates and long-term prognosis for low birthweight neonates. *Journal of Perinatal Medicine*, **5,** 59–75 (1977)

96 TUCK, S. and MENT, L. R. A follow-up study of very low birthweight infants receiving ventilatory support by face mask. *Developmental Medicine and Child Neurology,* **22,** 633–641 (1980)

97 VOHR, B. R., OH, W., ROSENFIELD, A. G., COWETT, R. M. and BERSTEIN, J. The preterm small-for-gestational age infant: a two-year follow-up study. *American Journal of Obstetrics and Gynecology*, **133,** 425–431 (1979)

98 WIENER, G. Scholastic achievement at age 12–13 of prematurely born children. *Journal of Special Education*, **2,** 237–250 (1968)

99 WIENER, G., RIDER, R. V., OPPEL, W. C., FISCHER, L. K. and HARPER, P. A. Correlates of low birthweight: psychological status at 6–7 years of age. *Pediatrics*, **35,** 434–444 (1965)

100 WIENER, G., RIDER, R. V., OPPEL, W. C. and HARPER, P. A. Correlates of low birthweight: psychological status at eight to ten years of age. *Pediatric Research*, **2,** 110–118 (1968)

101 WILSON, M. G., PARMELEE, A. H., JR. and HUGGINS, M. H. Prenatal history of infants with birth weights of 1,500 grams or less. *Journal of Pediatrics,* **63,** 1140–1150 (1963)

102 WONG, C., BEARDSMORE, C., STOCKS, J. and SILVERMAN, M. (personal communication)

103 Workshop on bronchopulmonary dysplasia. *Journal of Pediatrics*, **95,** 815–920 (1979)

104 WRIGHT, F. H., BLOUGH, R. R., CHAMBERLIN, A., ERNEST, T., HALSTEAD, W. C., MEIER, P., MOORE, R. Y., NAUNTON, R. F. and NEWELL, F. W. A controlled follow-up study of small prematures born from 1952 through 1956. *American Journal of Diseases of Childhood*, **124,** 506–521 (1972)

18

Directions for future work and expectations

M. G. Elder

Before considering future developments it is important to consider the present situation. When preterm labour is diagnosed, and the difficulty of making this diagnosis in some cases must be stressed, one of a number of tocolytic drugs may be administered either orally or parenterally, while corticosteroids and antibiotics may or may not be administered in addition. The justification for trying to prevent preterm labour is to allow time for surfactant production to increase either naturally or as a result of enzyme induction by corticosteroids given to the mother, thereby diminishing the incidence of respiratory distress syndrome. The effect of other factors such as antenatal and intrapartum hypoxia on the incidence of RDS has not been adequately considered.

Effective prevention or treatment of any condition depends on an understanding of its aetiology. Until the complex interaction of events that precede and cause labour are known many questions will remain unanswered. For example, what is the role of the incompetent cervix in the aetiology of preterm labour and consequently what are the benefits of cervical cerclage? A large, multicentre, prospective case control study is necessary before conclusions can be drawn. However, the strongly-held views of individual physicians based on personal clinical experience and the fact that doctors feel happier doing something rather than nothing, make the study difficult to carry out. However, the setting-up of such a study despite these problems is a priority.

A second unanswered question is 'what is the best tocolytic drug to use?, or indeed, are they of more value than bed rest alone?' The current division of medical opinion is fully discussed in Chapters 7, 8 and 9.

Studies of one tocolytic drug versus another are easier to carry out and a number have contributed in limited fashion to our present knowledge. Nevertheless, there is a need for case-controlled studies of β-mimetic treatment versus no treatment both for the therapeutic and prophylactic use of these drugs.

The third uncertainty concerns the use of corticosteroids to reduce the incidence of RDS. The pros and cons of this therapy have been argued in Chapters 10 and 11. It appears that their use is only of significant benefit at a certain period of gestation and that their effects last for a limited time. At present they are being used in some centres in a haphazard way, thereby apparently providing reduced benefits whilst incurring the possible risks of an increased incidence of intrauterine infection in cases with ruptured membranes as well as any other possible drug effects. Further studies of the physiology of surfactant production and the factors influencing it, as well as a more precise definition of the possible benefits and risks are needed. The difficulties inherent in setting up such clinical and laboratory studies are obvious but despite these they should be carried out to clarify the current confused clinical situation.

The incidence and effects of intrauterine infection in cases of preterm labour have not been adequately investigated. Questions arise such as:

(1) does chorioamnionitis precede rupture of the membranes or does it follow rupture?
(2) What is the role of infection in causing myometrial contractions?
(3) Is there increased prostaglandin production and release from the infected membranes?
(4) Do bacterial endotoxins have any effect on myometrial activity?
(5) What are the bactericidal agents in liquor amnii, and what factors influence these?
(6) Does the use of corticosteroids increase the risk of intrauterine infection?

While it is known that infection of the fetus is often rapidly lethal, the effect of small amounts of bacterial endotoxins is unknown.

Long-term follow-up of preterm infants, particularly those of very low birth weight is necessary so that the effects of drug therapy, as well as those of prematurity and its treatment, can be properly assessed.

Conditions such as retrolental fibroplasia, bronchopulmonary dysplasia, and necrotizing enterocolitis are undoubtedly serious and are due in whole or in part to the treatment necessary for the survival of the low birth weight baby.

The assessment of motor and mental deficiencies resulting from preterm birth, particularly among very low birth weight infants, together with the possible effects of drugs administered to these babies while *in utero* is more difficult. The widespread use of the neurological assessment of the newborn described in Chapter 16 could provide valuable information at an early stage of the child's life. This would complement the need for the careful long-term follow-up studies described in Chapter 17.

If the energetic treatment of the very low birth weight infant is to become standard practice then we must be sure that we are not doing more harm than good and that we minimize the risks of iatrogenic handicap.

The best method of delivery of the preterm infant has still not been determined. There is some agreement that the very low birth weight infant presenting by the breech should be delivered by caesarean section. This has been discussed in Chapter 12 and 14 as has the role of caesarean section in the delivery of the low birth weight infant presenting cephalically. Large, adequately controlled, prospective studies of the mode of delivery are needed; again the strongly-held views of individual obstetricians, particularly on such an emotive subject as mode of delivery, as well as all the other variables involved, make this a very difficult task, but nevertheless one that should be attempted. Whatever the mode of delivery the obstetrician must manage the pregnancy and delivery so that the low birth weight baby is exposed to little, if any, antenatal or intrapartum hypoxia or trauma. It is our impression that delivery of the infant weighing over 1000 g by lower segment caesarean section, before hypoxia compromises it to any degree, reduces the likelihood of RDS whether or not corticosteroids or β-mimetics have been administered.

Finally there is still some controversy about the best place to manage these patients. Can they and their babies be adequately cared for in district hospitals?, or does the mother need to go to a regional centre where the necessary neonatal and obstetrical expertise is available? The advantages of the former and the disadvantages of the latter, such as ease of visiting and maternal bonding to the preterm infant while in the intensive care unit, are relatively short-term. The long-term threats of physical and mental handicap are surely much greater and if these can be reduced then the development of regional centres are justified.

The optimum treatment of preterm labour is not clear and in the present relatively confused situation the interests of the mother and her baby will be served best by a joint obstetric and neonatal paediatric approach. This joint approach will only flourish if both parties are interested, skilled, and committed to improving the care of the preterm baby. The necessary senior medical expertise, back-up staff and complex monitoring and laboratory equipment will only be available in regional centres. Any attempt to spread these throughout the country will dilute the resources below the level where the best care can be given and will inhibit the development of new therapeutic approaches.

Index